Neural Rainbow

The Center, the Perimeter, and the Brain –

A new view of human nature

⌇

In Three Volumes

⌇

VOLUME ONE
THE ORIGINS OF THE RAINBOW

⌇

Judith Lauter

Library of Congress Control Number: 2022921860
ISBN: Hardcover   978-1-6698-5722-8
            Softcover   978-1-6698-5720-4
            eBook   978-1-6698-5721-1

Credits & permissions: All graphics and cover wraparound photo are by the author; author photo on back cover by Ken Lauter, used with permission.

Print information available on the last page.

Rev. date: 11/29/2022

To order additional copies of this book, contact:
Xlibris
844-714-8691
www.Xlibris.com
Orders@Xlibris.com
841826

Neural Rainbow
is dedicated to:

Charles Darwin, Alfred Russel Wallace,
Ashley Montagu, and Lynn Margulis for
their astounding work that over many years
has helped guide me

Michael McKaig, an eclectic thinker,
devoted to the study of nature, and willing
to spend long hours asking questions and
listening to my answers about the mysteries
of Neural Rainbow Theory

and most of all, to my dear life companion
Ken Lauter for undertaking the exhausting
editorial hours that made this book possible,
and for his lifetime of unstinting love and
support for me and my work – including
Neural Rainbow Theory, for which he has
been my principal advocate, as well as my
iconic model of the loving Center Male

Neural Rainbow

SUMMARY TABLE OF CONTENTS
FOR ALL THREE VOLUMES
(Chapters 1-16, titles only)

[bolded = current volume]
*[an expanded contents for Volume One begins p. 20;
see Appendix for expanded contents of all three volumes]*

Preface (2022)

Neural Rainbow (first draft written between 2000 and 2005) is a very personal book for me. It has grown out of my thirty years as a behavioral neuroscientist, but its conclusions are the product of my entire life – personal experiences from cradle to old age; undergraduate and graduate work in the humanities, primarily literature; my later multidisciplinary education in basic and applied sciences related to brain and behavior; university teaching of subjects ranging from embryology and general anatomy and physiology, to the physics of sound, psycho-physiological linguistics, and developmental learning disorders; research on human brain and behavior using noninvasive brain imaging (PET, MRI, qEEG, evoked potentials, etc.) and other methods; and life-long reading in the biology and behavior of animals including humans.

   This is a thoughtful but not a 'scholarly' book. The format is unconventional, with no footnotes or endnotes, and the chapter bibliographies are more like 'related readings' than an accounting of works cited (I don't agree with all of them, some are included only for completeness). They are based for the most part on the personal library I gathered by the time I wrote the 2005 draft. My process and the ideas expressed depart from the 'state of the art' scientific mainstream in many ways, primarily because I also have a very different Point-of-View (POV) on these issues compared with most of the experts, a perspective not derived from any single discipline. Though other writers are referenced, my goal is not a general overview and critique of previous theories – instead, I will tell the story strictly as I see it – from the POV of a longtime student of literature, a poet, a behavioral neuroscientist, and a woman. As a result, this is a book that few scholars in the fields included will agree with or approve of. But that didn't deter me twenty years ago, and it won't deter me now.

* * *

In science, powerful and precious as it is as a tool for thought, there is 'many a slip twixt cup and lip' – i.e., between what the world actually is, and the almost metaphorical way it is represented in the data and conclusions of scientific descriptions. Science is supposed to render the reality of things, free of the subjective limitations of individuals from specific cultures and times. My own early introduction to science was presented as that myth: a shining, objective, truth-oriented activity, free of personal bias and shortcomings. However, after decades as a scientist, I have lost my early naiveté, and realized that science, like all human endeavors, is influenced by personal agendas, preferences, and assumptions, almost all of them unacknowledged, unexamined, and often beyond the awareness of the individual practitioner.

Science can be as subjective as art – and a scientist may find it much more difficult than an artist would to separate the influence of culture and personal experience from her or his way of doing their work. This is especially – and poignantly – true in the case of studies of animal behavior, human and otherwise. For some scientists, it can be almost impossible to take off their cultural and personal glasses in order to view the world of animal behavior in an unfiltered way.

Of course, I too have my own 'filters' – but I am as interested *in* them, and how they influence (I prefer to say guide) my observations, as I am in the other issues I discuss. In a way, it was the process of learning the crucial importance of Point-of-View in science – in this case, *how to see my own identity, who and what I am, in the bio-neuro-ethological sense I explore here* – which provided the final piece in the puzzle that *Neural Rainbow* attempts to solve, the real pot of gold at the end of the rainbow – 'a new view of human nature.'

* * *

The biosocial thesis described in this book is called Neural Rainbow Theory (NRT). It derives from three sources: 1) my brain-and-behavior research; 2) my years of general reading in science and the humanities, including ethology, history, and other social sciences; and 3) my personal experience of and intuitions about life, gender, and human possibilities.

NRT is rooted in the new set of multidisciplinary sciences known as psycho-immuno-neuro-endocrinology (the PINE sciences), but goes considerably beyond current conclusions, to apply them to recent findings from many other areas of study, including but not limited to: archeology, anthropology, pre- and postnatal brain development, the biology of sex hormones, ethology (the science of natural animal behavior including social organization), sociology, psychology, and medicine. Each of these scientific areas provides one small piece of a complex puzzle, that in isolation can address only one aspect of human life. The goal of NRT is to view these pieces from an expanded perspective, attempting to 'connect the dots' in a new way, letting us see how the pieces of the puzzle may fit together. The result is a picture we may not have seen before, but hopefully bears an uncanny resemblance to what some have always suspected was true.

NRT focuses on understanding the 'neuroethology' of humans, this term based on the dual assumption that ethology is ethology, no matter the species, and that the behavior of any animal is intimately related to the structure and function of its nervous system. Defined in this way, neuroethology offers a way of looking at human behavior that is quite different from the point of view of many recent studies of the links between biology and human society, including those about 'brain sex.' It is certainly at odds with the vision of the group of writers who insist on the 'nature red in tooth and claw' version of primate/human life, a modern version of Social Darwinism, to which NRT offers an alternative, a means of escaping many fatalistic, self-limiting 19th-century preconceptions about gender, evolution, and the biological nature of human beings that are still with us today.

The NRT point of view offers a novel approach to describing human behavior that also helps us consider the behavior of other animals in a new way, and thus leads us to the realization that the fundamental rules of species survival are the same for all animals, and we break them at our peril. As applied to humans, NRT can be summarized in terms of four major topics: 1) hormone-based brain types, 2) social roles, 3) social organization categories, and 4) stages of human history. Each of these, discussed in terms of their biological origins, will be examined in detail across the book's three volumes. The goal is to understand human nature in a way that shows how we as a species relate to all animals and all life, and gain a new comprehension of who we are on the planet, and what kind of future we might expect.

To do that, NRT encourages us to find out more about our long-term history, and understand more about our biology. We have been here much longer than the blindered history books tell, and for most of that time, humans have lived in peace under the guiding influence of women and the loving values of what we will call 'the Center.' As with many other things in this book, such a concept may be difficult to accept. Listening to my story may be painful because it requires a certain amount of 'cultural un-learning' – being willing to set aside much of what we have been taught, and consider the possibility that things might have happened differently than we've been told. If one is open to un-learning and then re-learning a new way of thinking, it can be liberating to find that our 'present' – the short human experience of the last 10,000 years – is not the standard, but a *neuro-ethological aberration*, and that its hallmark of violence is a testimonial to the radical *unnaturalness* (and mal-adaptiveness) of organizing human (or any mammalian) society according to values that are destructive rather than nurturing; NRT also describes the biological origins of both sets of values.

The Point of View that valorizes destructive values such as 'might makes right,' and 'the strong deserve to take from the weak' which dominate many current societies, and also color scientific interpretations of human nature, is not the only one possible. It has been *imposed* on the rest of us, not only with regard to how we live our everyday lives, but what we think of ourselves as human beings – and thus represents a crisis in POV that this book hopes to challenge. If we want to continue as a species, we must stop internalizing the poisonous idea that human nature is as dark as the destructive forces in our societies want us to believe.

Clearly, then, this is an ambitious book. It attempts to tell a story that combines many facts and observations about humans and other animals, with the goal not only to describe a new approach to understanding how all animals live (in terms that show how humans are bound by the same rules), but also to explain the consequences of certain *historical accidents* that have happened to humans fairly recently which have transformed us into *an invasive species*, both to ourselves and many other species on Earth.

With the help of NRT, the old curse 'biology is destiny' is transformed into a message of hope and wisdom far older than the cultures we live in today. Trusting in the power of biology (and seeking to comprehend even factors that shape each of us during prenatal growth) does not mean a loss of 'free will.' To the contrary, it offers a firm biological foundation for improving human life, a strategy for helping every human being to have the widest repertoire of capabilities possible.

This is the vital lesson to be taken from our long and successful past – that our brains are superbly built to prepare us for living in nurturing societies. By recognizing that fact, and acting on it, we can bestow on ourselves and the generations to come a life that is fulfilling as well as purposeful. We can once again live together in human communities that flourish because they are in harmony – not only with our brains within, but also with the greater community of our planet.

* * *

On the flyleaf of her edition of Charles Darwin's autobiography, his grand-daughter Nora Barlow quoted a letter he wrote to Joseph Hooker in 1869, a decade after *Origin of Species* was first published:

> If I lived twenty more years and was able to work, how I should have to modify the *Origin*, and how much the views on all points will have to be modified! Well it is a beginning, and that is something . . .
> – C. Darwin, quoted in Barlow (1958)

As I write now, in 2022, it is two decades since I completed the first (unpublished) draft of *Neural Rainbow*; but like Darwin (who was 60 when he made the above comment – I am currently 78), I also must be realistic about the time I have left to re-examine what I wrote about these issues back when this book was new to me.

Had Darwin been granted those additional 20 years, he would no doubt have spent them not only modifying his ideas, but also collecting new data. After my original draft was finished, the demands of my university job increased significantly, and I stopped working on the book itself, though I did prepare a synopsis of its basic concepts, published in 2008 as a popular-neuroscience book, *How is Your Brain Like a Zebra? A new human neurotypology* (see Preface bibliography). I used the 'Zebra book' in teaching, and presented summaries of it at a series of research conferences.

Since retiring from teaching in 2012, I have focused my creative energies on nature photography and writing and publishing poetry, favored pastimes from my younger years (a multi-volume autobiography describing that history is in progress – see the About the Author summary at the end of this volume). The last public presentation I gave on the ideas included in the first draft of *Rainbow*, and the 'Zebra book,' was in 2012, as a keynote address (also cited in the bibliography) presented to a regional conference of the American Association for the Advancement of Science (AAAS).

I am excited to bring together in this revised edition the ideas from the first *Rainbow,* the Zebra book, and my 2012 presentation, regarding the links between sex hormones, brain types, gender, social roles, and social organization. I believe my hypotheses on these themes have not been described before, and that collectively they represent an idea whose time has come.

Lynn Margulis, one of my scientific heroes, all her life championed the attitude that she called 'against orthodoxy.' She even chose that phrase as the title of an inspiring autobiographical chapter in *Symbiotic Planet* (1998), and I could wish for no better precedent. And with Darwin, I ask the indulgence of my readers to attend to my humble plea for this book – that I realize these ideas are embryonic, but feel I have to deliver them, premature as they may be. As Darwin put it:

". . . It is a beginning, and that is something . . ."

....

Barlow N (Ed) (1958) The autobiography of Charles Darwin, 1809-1882. NY: WW Norton & Co., Inc.

Lauter JL (2008) How is your brain like a zebra? A new human neurotypology. Bloomington IN: Xlibris.

Lauter JL (2012) SPINE: A new sociobiology for the 21st century based on socio-psycho immuno-neuro-endocrinology (SPINE). Plenary Lecture to 87th Research Conference of the SouthWest and Rocky Mountain (SWARM) division of the American Association for the Advancement of Science (AAAS), Tulsa OK. [excerpt in the Appendix]

Margulis L (1998) Symbiotic planet; A new look at evolution. NY: Basic Books.

– J. Lauter, October 2022

Preface (2005 draft)

As I sit down (in June 2000) to begin this book, it is a beautiful Oklahoma summer day. A slight breeze, cool for this time of year, is pushing big snowy cumulus clouds from the south (out of Texas) to the north (into Kansas) across a wide blue sky, and the grass and black-jack oaks around our house are very, very green. Geraniums stand tall in their damp clay pots on the front porch – they are gloriously red, bobbing from time to time in the breezy shade. A mockingbird chatters his circle around our yard to show that he owns it, and a robin stops for a moment outside my window holding a precious straw in her mouth.

Sitting at my computer, looking back at the robin, I am 56 years old. My husband is in the living room reading a book on Wallace Stevens. It's good to have him there, while I sit in my study with pictures of zebras and elk on the walls. His presence a room away, doing something he loves, makes me feel safe and cared for in a way I don't tell him about often enough.

* * *

I grew up in a family of three generations of women. I was the oldest of four girls, cared for by my maternal grandmother and my mother (both were their parents' only children) and my father, the youngest of four boys. My grandmother was a major influence on my life. She was a great gardener, and even when we lived in houses with small yards, she would line the porch and border the sidewalk with pots of flourishing plants and flowers. At the dinner table, she sat at one end opposite my schoolteacher father; she cooked our meals to save my mother work after her long days as a secretary. Grandma didn't drive, but she loved car rides. She would go just to go, and sit patiently in the car while we ran errands or shopped.

My family worked hard to take care of us, and even after leaving my nurturing home, I have been lucky enough to have a good living. I have never gone hungry or been without a comfortable, loving home. But although my life has not been hard, and I have never experienced or witnessed serious violence, I have learned terrible, unthinkable things about human beings – the awful things they do to other animals, and to each other. I know about animals imprisoned and helpless in slaughterhouses, laboratories, and backyards. I know about the amazing deliberateness with which humans inflict misery on each other – in the jails and prisons of every country in the world, and in houses where men secretly batter women, and attack children as though they mean to kill them and eat them whole.

Nothing of the kind has ever happened to me or anyone that I love, but just knowing about them has been a heavy psychological burden. I have to 'think away' from them in order to stay sane. I can't imagine them in detail –

I am too good at making mental pictures and feeling vicariously the fear and pain, "the horror, the horror," as Joseph Conrad's Kurtz says.

* * *

Recently, however, I have begun to see such things differently – not to accept them, but to understand *where they come from, why they exist.* I believe with all my heart and brain that to understand the origins of something is the first step toward peace – the peace that *is* understanding, that provides confidence and hope. Knowing the origins of something good encourages us to value, nourish, and keep it; and knowing the origins of something terrible gives us insight about how to stop it.

My new perspective is not the result of any kind of religious experience, though it has answered the need that religion once did for me. It is in fact a *scientific* experience, one that has risen like a living, growing thing out of my entire life, from my own research of more than 30 years, and from my reading in sciences outside my own discipline.

I am NOT, however, writing this book for the experts. In fact, I predict that most of them won't like this book. My experience has been that an incredible amount of their time and effort is spent attacking other experts. Some of Galileo's peers refused even to look through his telescope, for fear that what they saw there would force them to change their picture of the universe and their place within it. That story is not merely a historical curiosity, a fable about provincialism in a primitive time. I would say that as a group, scientists are *more* likely than most people *not* to look through any telescope besides the one they and their friends prefer. In many instances, they live by the motto, 'If it's true it's not new, if it's new it's not true, unless it was written by me.'

* * *

So I am not writing for the experts. Rather, I am writing for the girl in middle school who begins to notice that the boys around her seem to grow younger and more childish every day – even as she is getting the message from many quarters that girls aren't as smart as boys, and that her widening hips are a curse and not a gift to be celebrated. I am writing for the middle-school boy who starts wetting his bed or having erections night and day (which no one has properly prepared him for) – and who may even be experiencing violent feelings toward the girls who arouse him, or toward the tall, athletic boys whom the girls seem to like instead of him.

I'm writing for the nurse who is ordered by doctors to shove plastic tubes down the raw, narrow throats of premature babies, forcing them to breathe when all signs are clear that what they need above all is to *stop* breathing, the nurses who are told to constantly push babies away from the sheltering corner of the "isolettes," back into the exposed middle where there is nothing reassuring to press against, much less the beat of a mother's heart.

I'm writing for the older boy who returns from a war, traumatized for life, who signed up out of a passion for defending women and children, but who encounters nothing but incompetence and confusion, and senseless violence to his body and soul and those of his dear comrades in arms. And I'm also writing for all those who have made the unforgivable "mistake" of loving someone of the same sex; and for the millions of children who find it hard to learn to read no matter how hard they try.

In short, I am writing for all those who are attacked by the human world's violence either actually, or vicariously, those who can't comprehend how or why people can be so *inhuman,* why so much in our society is unloving, cruel, and – like the wars that color our history with their toxic glow – "unhealthy for children and other living things."

* * *

One of the main messages of this book is that for any conclusion about human behavior that comes from European so-called "civilization," it is probably safe to assume that *exactly the opposite is true* – 180 degrees out of phase. If they say that pesticides and lawn chemicals won't hurt the oceans, the opposite is true. If they say that nicotine is not addictive, the opposite is true. If they say women are hysterical and men aren't, the opposite is true. If they say white people are better than people of color, and men are better than women ... well, you get the picture.

In other words, this book is about how to figure out if you're being lied to, about how to know for yourself who YOU are, why you think and feel and sleep like you do, how and why you are both like and unlike other people, and why humans can be so beastly that they sometimes behave worse than any beast, as Shakespeare's Richard III bragged of himself – "No beast so fierce but knows some touch of pity. But I know none, and therefore am no beast."

This book *will* consider humans as animals, with all the glory – and the potential for being cursed – which that entails; but I will describe human animals in ways that I think are new, that provide a new basis for hope that we can in fact change things about ourselves which we don't like. I'm not talking about eugenics or gene transplantation, which is all the rage today as a 'quick fix' for our problems. I'm talking about learning more about our biology – and especially about ourselves as *mammals*, not just primates – and how this knowledge suggests that we are better and more loving animals than we thought, more prone to nurturance than most history books allow, and more capable of framing a future in which every child is a wanted child, a future where *every* human being – not just the property-owning adult white males

14

specified in the Declaration of Independence – is assured the birthright of "life, liberty, and the pursuit of happiness."

* * *

I write this book as a woman, a scientist, and (although I'll have some rather harsh things to say about males as we know them in our current patriarchal world) as the life-companion of a loving man who is an example of what I will define below as a "Center male." The result may read at times like a political manifesto – but my real interest is not 'movements,' political slogans (feminist or otherwise), or adding more laws to already overstuffed statute books. It is in capturing a new sense of the past, the present, and the future – in seeing how the nature of the human/mammalian brain has been reflected in our history for tens of thousands of years into the past, and also how it directly impacts the most intimate and crucial aspects of our lives now on a day-to-day, minute-by-minute basis.

The picture I paint is sometimes somber, sometimes funny, sometimes horrifying, sometimes reassuring. If I am right about the Neural Rainbow and its influence on individual lives and human history, then the general outlook may be good, though not without daunting challenges in the near term. My goal was always to find the face of hope– and I think I have.

* * *

When I was a little girl, one of my grandmother's favorite pastimes was to sit on a park bench and 'people-watch.' I sometimes joined her, and we spent many hours, fascinated by the variety of faces, bodies, and ways of walking that people exhibit. When I remember that now, I see us as anthropologists. Without thinking about it, we took in details that both differentiate and group people – how people held their bodies, balanced packages in one arm or carried a child, whether they walked fast without looking at anything, or strolled casually, enjoying the world around them, including other people.

Human diversity still fascinates me. As a student of literature, and then as a behavioral neuroscientist, I've studied it for more than sixty years. You'd think that by now science would have come up with a good theory of human variety – but that isn't the case. Instead, education still arranges children in rows and columns, like little machines, and insists that they all learn in the same way. There is a discipline called "differential psychology," but it deals with things like IQ tests, and so individual differences in everyday skills (such as the ability to do several things at once, or to hear shades of emotion in a voice) still remain a mystery. Medicine isn't much better. It's practiced more like car repair than a science. It treats "patients" not people, as though they are made of interchangeable parts. Everyone gets the same dose of a medicine, or is dosed by trial and error.

Scientists have, however, long been fascinated by individual differences. The Greeks theorized that people contained different mixes of the four physical elements – earth, air, fire, and water. Others were more biological, and attributed individual differences to the proportions of body fluids or "humours" – blood, digestive juices, lymph. Nineteenth century phrenologists thought it all depended on how different parts of the brain grew. If your "math area" was well developed, you would not only be good at arithmetic, but also have a "math bump" over that part of the skull.

By the 20th century, some researchers concluded that individual differences could be understood in terms of a small set of human types, which brought together details such as body proportions, academic skills, sex life, handedness, eating habits, general health, and personality. They didn't know where the types came from or why they were important, but they predicted that if there ever came a day when we could study individual differences in the brain directly, these questions might be answered.

I believe that time has finally come. The brain-imaging tools of modern neuroscience offer powers far beyond what early researchers dreamed – making it possible to take brain 'fingerprints' in such detail that we can even detect clues to how each brain grew before birth. Recent developments in neuroscience may provide new insights into some of the oldest, most profound mysteries about human beings. For example, where do individual differences come from? Are they organized into categories linking health, special abilities, and personality? Are these categories related to gender and social organization? Are there secrets buried in the human brain that can help us understand concepts like good and evil? In the course of this book, we will look closely into these matters and many more.

* * *

It's twilight now, and my husband has been mowing the yard for the last couple of hours. The delicious scent of cut grass and the sounds of crickets and twilight are rising around the house. The mockingbird is quiet, and the robin has gone back to her nest. The breeze has fallen, and the sky is gathering filmy clouds as though for sleep. I shut down the computer and go out on the porch to look at the moon. I remember from last night that she is waxing, a graceful crescent of light, like a woman just starting to show. By 9:00, she'll be straight overhead, and looking a little milky in the haze.

– J. Lauter, June 2000

ᕦ

How this book is different from most Evolutionary-Psychology/ Eco-Apocalypse/New-Humanist Treatises

Today there are many books attempting to explain human history, which often share a certain structure. They typically begin with a description of 'human nature' defined in terms of our biological and evolutionary beginnings, then go on to review the events of both 'prehistory' and recorded history up to the present day.

At this point such books often peer with horror into our truncated future, the cliff of species extinction (our own and many others) and the environmental breakdown toward which we seem to be rushing. I suspect that it is precisely the growing realization of the reality of that cliff which has inspired authors from such a wide range of backgrounds to try to understand how this crisis came about.

My book follows a similar curve, but differs crucially in its details. Some of these have to do with mechanisms, which I will discuss later. However, there are also several major assumptions that seem to lurk behind virtually all other books on these topics – assumptions which I *reject* at the outset. These (often unstated) assumptions are:

1) The best if not exclusive source of information regarding the biological basis of individual human psychology and group behavior is found in our "closest relatives" the great apes – in particular, chimpanzees, including bonobos.

2) The most natural social organization for humans is living in female/male pair-bonds, within relatively large groups – like migrating Canada geese. The implication is that we have *always* lived as pair bonds, an arrangement supposedly as much a part of our species definition as the shape of our pharyngeal cavities or our upright posture. Some authors even suggest that it was the adoption of this type of social organization which accelerated the evolutionary expansion of human intelligence – "Monogamy is Mental."

3) Humans have *always* killed and eaten other animals for food. Carnivorism too is supposedly part of our species definition, and some, hailing our status as an 'apex predator,' suggest that, like monogamy, the practice of eating other animals may have nurtured brain enlargement – "Meat is Mental."

4) Humans have *never* lived for any significant amount of time, or in appreciable numbers, in a sustainable way characterized by peaceful relations with neighbors and the surrounding world. Any contentions to the contrary are scoffed at as instances of the "Golden Age fantasy" or the "Rousseauian

myth." The complexity of thought required for personal and organized violence is often suggested as a factor leading to the equally complex human brain – "Murder & Mayhem are Mental."

5) Over the past 10,000 years, in spite of the nagging persistence of war, violence, and genocide, things in general have been getting better for humans as a species – we have been "rising from animals," "rising from chimps," "rising to civilization."

6) *All* humans are capable of *evil* – 'we are all genociders,' says one author.

7) Finally, the assumption that may be the basis for all the others – that *maleness* is the measure of all things. Explanations of human nature, including its connections to other animals, typically begin with and focus on adult-male psychology and behavior. Females and children are considered only as satellites to males and male motivations. The intelligence of the adult male of a species is implicitly assumed to be superior to that of either children or females, and human societies dominated by men are judged as more 'advanced' than those managed by women – thus, "Maleness is Mental."

I reject all these assumptions – not via wishful thinking, fantasy, or religious faith, but for purely scientific reasons, which derive in part from facts that were not available to most of the other authors, and in part from a new interpretation of other facts which have been known for some time.

For compositional reasons, this book is not organized according to these rejected assumptions; but as it proceeds, I will discuss my alternatives to them in detail. In doing so, I hope to draw the outlines of a deeper, more accurate and nuanced understanding of the biological nature of human nature, our unusual history, and our most uncertain future.

Neural Rainbow

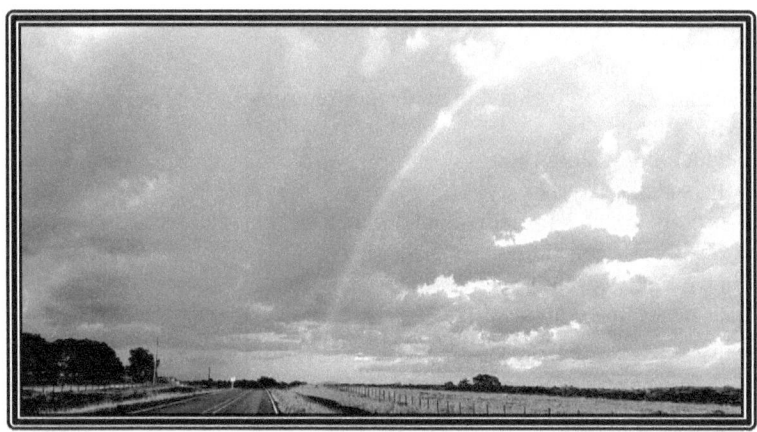

❧

Volume One

The Origins of the Rainbow

❧

The Origins of the Rainbow
CONTENTS

Sex hormones and the developing brain
    Brain connectivity and asymmetries
    'Gendering the brain'
    Making three brain types, shaping six genders
        1. 'Hormone-free' prenatal development (XX only): Gender One
        2. Testosterone exposure in other XX individuals: moderate & high:
           Genders Two and Three
        3. Testosterone exposure in Xy individuals: low, moderate, high:
           Genders Four, Five, Six
    Summary of the origins of the three brain types/six genders complex
Trimodal Model catalog of individual features by brain type
    Brain hallmarks: Polytropic, Middle, Focal
    Handedness
    Birth order
    Body type
    Age of puberty
    Height
    Coloration
    Autonomic emphasis
    Handshaking relations
    Skills
        1. Phonemic Awareness (PA)
        2. Eye-movement coordination
        3. Fine-motor control
        4. Mental imagery
        5. Cortical visual acuity
        6. Emotional intelligence
        7. Social skills
        8. Athletic intelligence
        9. Artistic ability
    Health
        1. Immune function
        2. Cardiac function
        3. Eating habits
        4. Sleep habits
        5. Emotional health
    Group membership
        1. Preferred structure
        2. Choice of professions
        3. Natural societies
    Developmental and learning disorders (DLDs)
        1. DLDs and polytropics
        2. DLDs and middle-brains
        3. DLDs and focal-brains
    Other conditions
        1. Psychiatric conditions
        2. Substance abuse
        3. Violence
Chapter Three Summary: Taking stock

THE HISTORY OF TYPOLOGIES: PATTERNS OF INDIVIDUAL VARIATION

One of the most striking features of human beings is their individuality. As we all know from everyday experience, there are general differences between people, such as height and weight and hair color, but in addition, every person seems to be a set of rules unto her or himself. These involve personality, abilities, the tendency to be healthy or sickly, social preferences, etc. There are even different degrees of susceptibility to specific types of problems – heart disorders vs. allergies, anxiety attacks vs. difficulty with reading, etc.

At the same time, we know that people also seem to fall into categories – again, not just the usually-named ones such as gender and ethnicity, but other things that are more intriguing, stereotypes such as the Natural Athlete, the Geeky Scientist, the Good Parent, which science hasn't really helped us understand. We still don't know whether such stereotypes are only cultural biases (and therefore, as we are warned these days, Politically Incorrect), or whether they might actually have a basis in biological fact – and if so, where do they come from, and what is their significance? Even modern genetics doesn't offer very good answers to such questions.

Yet there is every reason to suspect that people have always been this way – and even that other animals show the same combination of highly recognizable individuality plus categories of types. For example, of two Siamese cats, one may be friendly, while the other is irascible; or of two Arabian horses, both of whom are gentle and loving, one might be able to learn almost any trick, while the other is always slow to catch on. Recently, students of non-human animal behavior have begun trying to categorize such differences, attempting to link behavior to clusters of anatomical and physiological features, in order to characterize what are called different 'behavioral phenotypes,' 'styles of aggression,' 'coping styles,' or 'animal personalities.' The terms can change from species to species, perhaps indicating this new scientific approach is in its early stages. In contrast, the study of human categories, generally referred to as 'typologies,' has a much longer history.

An introduction to human typologies

Before continuing, we need to acknowledge that the science of human 'types' has a bad reputation. Charles Darwin and his contemporaries acknowledged the existence of 'individual variation' – the evolutionists recognized it as the crucial component common to all organisms which allowed natural selection to work – but other than conventional group distinctions such as gender and race (their biological nature poorly understood at the time), the idea of '*systematic* variation' was not a central topic of mainstream 19th century evolutionary thought. Because 'systematic variation' is at the heart of Neural Rainbow Theory, it will be a focus for the first few chapters of this book, beginning with a brief review of some of the most famous 'typologies' of the past.

The fascination with the idea of human 'types' is very old – suggesting there is something there that needs study – but sadly, attempts to do so have been plagued with non-scientific factors such as cultural biases and personal prejudices. As a result, modern research on human behavior tends to prefer 'averaging over subjects' (even when raw data clearly show that something much more interesting is going on), and most conventional statistical techniques treat variation from person to person only as experimental 'noise,' that is, random, instead of a potential source of information. This is true even in research that employs the new brain-imaging techniques, in spite of the fact that they all reveal individual characteristics in dramatic, 'fingerprint' levels of detail (cf. Lauter 2001, 2008).

It is true that there are scattered pockets of professional interest in individual characteristics, and occasionally one runs across a scientist or even a whole laboratory working according to the belief that in order to understand humans in general we need to study each individual in particular – but I have found these are few and far between. Personality psychologists (e.g., research on 'temperament' or 'personality types'), and students of sexual behavior have developed a variety of scales for describing individuals. However, to my knowledge, these are for the most part 'one-topic' scales, limited to a single application, and considered as an end in themselves.

In contrast, in this chapter, and in the *Neural Rainbow* book overall, we will be more interested in approaches that seek to *characterize each individual as a whole* in a *multivariate* way, combining several biological, psychological, and social features – all assumed to represent *continua* – in order to create individual profiles that can then be used as a basis not only for framing categories of individual types, but also for assessing how any given individual fits into the category-types described.

Such an approach offers a scientifically-sensible means of exploring whether and how the 'variation' across individuals, which can sometimes seem chaotic and random ('noisy') can be shown to be also 'systematic,' roughly divisible into identifiable-if-fuzzy-edged categories, much as a rainbow is both (physically) a *continuum* of wavelengths of light and, when viewed through the human eye (i.e., psycho-physiologically), six main bands – '*categories*' – of color. The physical fact that the rainbow is a continuum does not erase the perceptual fact of the categories, and vice versa, and knowing about the co-occurrence of both types of facts enriches our understanding of the interface between the nervous system and the outside world.

It is true that some of the scientists who study individual differences in humans remain reluctant to talk about *categories*, beyond obvious things such as gender or different types of handedness (though these topics themselves cause great confusion – perhaps unnecessarily, as we will see). Such reluctance may grow out of a distrust in the way that 'category' has been used in the past for describing humans, as something that is rigid, unchanging, and unchangeable. Recognizing that the categories we will be talking about represent continua should help to allay these fears. In our discussions, we will focus on measurement approaches assumed to represent continua under the same assumption expressed by Albert Kinsey and colleagues: "The living world is a continuum in each and every one of its aspects" (1948); and "Many persons do not want to believe that there are gradations in these matters from one to the other extreme" (1953) – both from KinseyInstitute.org/research/publications/kinsey-scale, viewed on 10/1/22.

In general, however, the bad reputation of attempts to frame rules for human categories, or 'types,' has come about for cultural/sociological reasons rather than scientific ones. The 'sociology of types' has suffered from abuses related to racism and discrimination. We will see later where such impulses come from, and how they are in opposition to the broad-minded scientific quest to understand more about human beings.

The scientific failings of approaches to human typology are due in part to the incompleteness of individual and category descriptions (that is, only a few features may be targeted, while many others are left out, naturally leading to mismatches and inconsistencies). In fact, if science had done a better job of describing and explaining individual differences and similarities – the *systematic patterns* of what Darwin called individual 'variation' – in a biological way, simplistic categories used to support racial and gender prejudices might have been shown for what they are – anti-scientific manifestations of self-interest and fear.

Typologies have also fallen into scientific disrepute because in many cases, as a system is applied over time by its founder and his (usually *his*) disciples, the categories are allowed to degenerate into rigid labels that are more restricting than explanatory. There is also the concern that admitting scientifically what we already know perfectly well – that people are different, but they also fall into categories – will lead to abuse. The argument is that 'different' has to imply 'greater vs. lesser.' We surely need to get beyond that – after all, Darwin's finches were 'different' from each other, and for him that turned out to be the difference that made all the difference, as he recognized that the categories of beak types were *adaptive,* with each one matched to an environmental feature, like a key in a lock. If he had not accepted the testimony of his eyes, and instead gave up trying to understand the *significance in such individual variation*, we might still be stuck thinking that speciation (differences between species) is just another form of biological 'noise.'

Finally, people are sometimes nervous that categorizing individuals, particularly in terms of their biology, will somehow restrict a person's ability to make choices, to exercise 'free will.' We can't 'choose' to fly, or depend on nitrogen instead of oxygen, or be a member of a different species – yet these and many other biological facts about humans are not seen as restrictions on free will. I've even heard one person say he would like to be able to choose his gender, his body type, or his blood type on a day-to-day basis – I'm not sure what planet he's living on, but I know it's not the one where I was born.

If those who are suspicious of typologies could be convinced that humans are as fully biological as any other organism, they might see that accurate information about the rules that govern our brains and bodies is liberating, not restricting. Willfully choosing to remain blind to the rules of our existence – when those rules have the potential for helping us help ourselves – is surely the greatest mental prison of all.

Typologies before the 19th century

Many systems for distinguishing-and-grouping individual humans begin by identifying some set of basic properties, which are then combined and recombined in different ways to make differences in people.

The Four Elements

For example, one Greek theory said that, like everything else in nature, each individual human was a combination of 'the four elements:' earth, air, fire, and water (note this is a good description of the basic ingredients for photosynthesis, upon which all life on earth ultimately depends: 'earth' = minerals like phosphorus and magnesium, 'air' = carbon dioxide/oxygen/ nitrogen, etc., 'fire' = sunlight, 'water' = water). (A similar Chinese five-element system substituted 'wood' and 'metal' for air.)

With reference to humans, the theory had three tenets: 1) every person is made up of the same basic elements; 2) individual *differences* are due to different proportions of each; and 3) *categories* of individuals result when a set of individuals had pretty much the same proportions. This was a truly scientific approach, in that it attempted to abstract from the highly-specific 'fingerprint' features of any individual human, to explain how each person could not only differ from all others, but at another level, be a member of a category – sharing similarities with some, and differences with others.

The Four Elements approach was rather like saying that all humans are versions of the same type of pastry, where all have basically the same ingredients, only in different proportions – a cup of flour vs. a cup and a half, a fourth cup of sugar or only a third, etc. The suggestion was that the different proportions made all the difference – a person with a higher proportion of fire might be quick to anger – we would say they have a 'fiery temper' – while another who had somewhat more of the earth element would be very solid and reliable – we might say such a person is 'well grounded' or 'very down to earth.' A person's four-element 'recipe' was associated with many features of the individual – biological, psychological, social, medical (propensity for different diseases, etc.). As these catchphrases show, whether we've ever heard of the Four Elements theory or not, our day-to-day descriptions of other people indicate that we still recognize the aptness of these categories, whatever their origin.

The Humours

A very similar concept, that is, the same components mixed in different proportions, was expounded by other thinkers who took a more biological approach and described individual differences and categories in terms of four types of body fluids – blood, phlegm, yellow bile, and black bile. This was known as the Humours theory, and again, attributed individual differences to differences in the predominance of one or another component – in this case, fluids involved in body functions. Thus a person in whom the blood was predominant would have a healthy, highly-oxygenated view of life – he would be 'sanguine' (the word's meaning is 'optimistic,' but its root is the word for 'blood') – while another whose gall bladder manufactured too much yellow bile would be sour and grumpy, with a 'bilious' nature. Again, when we read descriptions of these types of categories, we can recognize forms of them in the people we know.

So we can see that these old attempts to account for the combination of individual differences and human categories, were not all that inaccurate from a descriptive standpoint – but at the same time, we might suspect that they were quite limited in an explanatory way. (Later we'll see that the Humours approach might have had a grain of explanatory truth, and its problem was in attributing *causal* power to something that was itself the effect of a more primal cause, a cause-of-the-cause – we'll return to this logical difficulty in another chapter.)

The Astrologies

At the time the Four-Elements and Humours theories were being put forth and discussed in Europe, many cultures around the globe had already developed systems, some of them very old, for understanding individual differences based on facts about the time when a person was born. 'Time' in this case included: time of year, time of month, and even time of day. We know now these systems were actually ways of talking about the influence of *natural biological cycles*, well-established 'biorhythms,' changes in the body and brain that occur in a rhythmic way. Some cycles occur around the course of a day ('circadian'), others over the course of a month, and still other cycles are played out from month to month in the year. There are even supra-year cycles, such as those associated with sunspots; supra-year cycles are also referred to in many astrologies.

The changes in the body associated with some of these cycles are so basic that it is entirely possible some of them could have dramatic effects on a baby conceived at a certain time and carried within the mother's body during certain months of the year. Medical research today recognizes such influences to at least some extent, in the growing literature on 'season-of-birth,' which has found associations between birth month and different types of psychiatric and learning disorders.

It is not surprising that these systems, some of them of great antiquity, have usually been referred to as different types of 'astrology,' since the markers for their 'clocks' were all celestial – position of the sun in the sky marked time of day, phase of the moon divided the month, and changes in the appearance of stars in the night sky provided a handy external map of the yearly cycle of seasons as the earth travels its long ellipse around the sun.

When we recognize that the astrologies are really based on biological rhythms, we see that we might re-interpret distinctions between two people, such as a Taurus vs. a Sagittarius, as due not to some magical influence exerted by constellations 'presiding' at their birth, but rather the direct *neurobiological effect of the hormonal state prevailing in a mother's uterus at conception and during gestation.* It may be crucial for many aspects of a child's nature, whether she is conceived when hormones for mating are high in the fall and then carried in the mother's warm body during the winter (the case for a Taurus), or conceived in spring when hormones for birthing are high and then carried through the hot summer and dry fall (for a Sagittarius). We will see that there may be every reason to believe that, as the writer of Ecclesiastes remembered, there really is a preferable 'time to be born' – directly related to the cycle of the seasons.

(Interestingly, many of these older systems also made reference to a harmonious norm, with disease seen as an imbalance, a disharmony – examples are the balance of yin and yang in the East, or between opposites such as hot vs. cold or sweet vs. sour in Greece. Modern formulations referred to as 'alternative medicine' or 'behavioral medicine' retain these older ideas of harmony and disharmony, which many older cultures saw as extending even beyond the individual's body to involve the social, biological, and even meteorological environment of the individual.)

Of course, astrologies of different forms are generally looked down on by scientists, though they have not lost their attraction for the general population. Many countries still rely on astrologers to provide advice about personal and political decisions, and many citizens of industrial states turn to the astrology column in the daily newspaper or on their morning internet search, for hints as to how they should approach the day. This continuing fascination suggests that there is at least a half-truth in astrology (certainly if it embodies some very old knowledge about biorhythms), and that it is only the overelaboration and exaggerated claims made for such schemes that have called them into question.

19th-century psychology and individual differences

Body types

It was not until the 19th century that psychology, as the scientific study of behavior, was born in Europe, and almost immediately took up the question of individual variation. One of the first groups to address this concentrated on the idea of *body types*. They recalled an old suggestion by Hippocrates that the people he saw in his clinical practice tended to have one of two body types, susceptible to very different types of disorders: the long, thin body, that he reported was particularly vulnerable to tuberculosis, and the short, thick body, prone to heart problems.

Workers in 19th-century France, Germany and Italy agreed that individual differences did seem to fall into categories based on physical appearance, and they also hypothesized that body type might be an outward reflection of a wide range of individual features, not only including disease susceptibility but also behavioral characteristics such as personality.

Several versions of this approach, based on a set of three types, were developed, with details that were very reminiscent of the old Humours theory (a sign that even over a space of 2000 years, researchers were after all looking at the same kind of creatures). That is, the "new" three types were described as characterized by the predominance of different organ systems. In one, the viscera seemed most important (round, fleshy body type), another was remarkable for its muscular development (a solid, athletic type), and the third was very thin, considered to be highly cerebral but also prone to difficulties such as immune problems (similar to Hippocrates' thin type vulnerable to tuberculosis).

Some of these investigators even did dissections on the bodies of individuals representing different types, and measured internal organs including the intestines. On the basis of such measures, one group suggested that the visceral body type might be called 'herbivorous' since it typically had long, massive intestines, clearly capable of handling large amounts of fiber. In contrast, they designated the thin body type as 'carnivorous,' having shorter and less bulky intestines (the difference was marked even when corrected for weight and height) – more in the direction of the very short intestines found in true carnivores. (Humans are not 'true' carnivores – many features of our digestive systems identify us as frugivores. In carnivores, the digestive system, from oral saliva to large intestine, is designed to process ingested flesh as rapidly as possible before it becomes actively toxic.)

Phrenology

Other scientists began focusing on the *brain* as the source of individual differences, advancing the set of ideas known as *phrenology*. This approach was based on a very reasonable suggestion, that different parts of the brain supported different types of abilities, and that individual differences in the degree of development in one neural area or another could result in individual differences in levels of skill. The phrenologists agreed that there were three body types, and extended the body-type formulations by suggesting that one feature of these categories might involve brain function. However, over time, their work fell into disrepute, as their original idea became complicated to absurd extents – much as has happened for astrology and many other type-based schemas for understanding human behavior.

Personality psychology

The various schools of psychoanalysis which emerged in the 19th century represented another angle on describing human characteristics, but these systems proved over time to be more interested in the distinction between normal vs. abnormal (a 'medical model' – we'll talk more about this later), than in understanding individual differences in general. This was definitely true for Jung, who sought to describe human psychological universals, with little or no concern for their biological origins or for individual differences other those than needed for designing treatment.

Freud originally expressed interest in a biological approach to human behavior. He read the writings of the great neurologist John Hughlings Jackson, in which Jackson reviewed clinical evidence that more recently-evolved levels of the nervous system were important for maintaining executive control over motor responses (use of body muscles) of hyper-reactive older levels. Freud thought this might be a helpful metaphor for human psychology, and used it to create his model of the psyche, positing that the psychological function of more advanced neural levels have evolved to control certain emotions and reactions originating in more primitive ones.

Although this was a very suggestive application of Jackson's basic idea, and may actually be a good approximation to the way the nervous system supports different levels of our behavior (we will talk later about the 'Triune Brain' model), Freud himself never sought to explore the implications of reinterpreting his psychological model in a true biological context.

These psychological ideas of the 19th century gave birth to several ways of classifying humans, generally referred to as 'personality psychology.' However, few of these systems sought to connect personality-type descriptions to wider issues related to behavior in general, special skills, or health. Our review will next focus on only those attempts that took this latter type of 'whole-organism' approach, out of the conviction that the best way to learn about the nature of humans is to understand more about them as *biological entities*.

20th-century systems for individual differences

It was not until the 20th century that two schemes were suggested which did focus on the individual as a whole, attempting to see psychology in a biological context, and considering many aspects of each individual, such as body shape, personality, immune function, eating habits, and special abilities.

Sheldon's "constitutional psychology"

W.H. Sheldon first described his approach in the early 1940s. Sheldon, who had both a PhD in psychology and an M.D., was the godson of William James; Sheldon's father was a naturalist and animal breeder, and his mother was a midwife. During a two-year fellowship in Germany after receiving his medical degree, Sheldon studied with Carl Jung and also visited Freud and Ernst Kretschmer (a German psychiatrist who had been writing about his own scheme of body types for several years).

Sheldon began by reviewing the previous work on body types described above (including Kretschmer's), and proposed to address the question of individual differences and similarities by body type in a highly quantitative way, employing methods developed by physical anthropologists for their own explorations of human variation. To these 'physical anthropometry' techniques, which were focused on external body morphology, Sheldon brought his belief that the biological nature of an individual, expressed in one way in body dimensions, must be intimately related to everything about that person, whether mental or physical.

He used state-of-the-art photography to generate a large database of pictures of individuals, and from these photographs made painstaking measurements of physical dimensions of different details of external body morphology. (We should note that Sheldon began by studying Caucasian males, but intended to extend the methods to women, to children of both genders, and to other ethnic groups. Details describing his approach are included in both of his books referred to below, one of which offers a preliminary survey of Caucasian women.)

Based on these observations, he then designed a classification system of 'somatotypes,' based on three characteristics – endomorphic (fleshy), mesomorphic (muscular), and ectomorphic (thin), reminiscent of the three general body types discussed by earlier researchers. But Sheldon went beyond this, stressing the importance of recognizing a *continuum* of individual differences.

He suggested that this continuum could be systematically described if each individual were considered as a mix of the three characteristics, with different proportions from person to person (shades of the Four Elements and Humours!). This was done by ranking the morphological features of a given person against a 7-point scale for each of the categories, and then citing this 'recipe' in the order endomorphy-mesomorphy-ectomorphy. Thus one individual might be designated as 6-2-2, that is, with endomorphy predominating, while another might be 3-6-1, with mesomorphy accentuated, and a third 1-1-7, high in ectomorphy.

Sheldon then conducted in-depth interviews of selected individuals representing points along the *somatotype continuum*. The interviews addressed many aspects of personal history, abilities, and preferences. The results of all this work are reported in two major publications (see bibliography for references), which include not only a description of Sheldon's measurement methods, but also verbal 'sketches' of the characteristics of representatives of a variety of somatotypes. The descriptions are uncanny in their vivid reality – it is possible to recognize similarities to people you know in his type-summaries, which include specifics of hair color, body size, skin tone, personality, and lifestyles.

For example, sketches for the three individuals whose somatotypes were given above went as follows: the 6-2-2, high in endomorphy, was described as "the traditionally jolly fat boy, fond of good company but with low sexuality, likes to eat and drink to excess;" the 3-6-1, with mesomorphy accentuated, was "a big man physically, a supreme football athlete, popular, wherever he goes the world pays attention;" and the 1-1-7, predominating in the ectomorphic component, was "thin, physically weak, sickly, but highly sexual."

Sheldon acknowledged that his approach was necessarily uneven, combining state-of-the-art quantitative methods for measuring and categorizing physical dimensions, with relatively crude and non-quantitative means of characterizing all other features. He looked forward to the time when more quantitative means would be available for assessing psychological features as well as more analytical aspects of basic biology – in particular, means of describing individual differences related to the brain and biochemistry.

Nyborg's "hormotyping"

Fifty years later, the techniques that Sheldon wished for in the 1940s had finally arrived. Methods in molecular biology made it possible to study details of body and brain biochemistry that were previously unavailable. Also, a variety of new 'noninvasive' devices gave researchers a revolutionary set of windows on the inner workings of the body, including the brain – that could be used on living, healthy people. How Sheldon would have loved to get his hands on a Magnetic Resonance Imaging (MRI) scanner, to examine the *anatomy* of the digestive and cardiac systems and the brain of each of his subjects, or a technique for studying body and brain *physiology and function*, such as Positron Emission Tomography (PET) or quantitative Electro-encephalography (qEEG), to observe ongoing activity inside those 6-2-2 or 1-1-7 or 3-6-1 individuals while they rested or did some type of task!

During the 1980s and 1990s, a new area of multidisciplinary research, which came to be known under various names – we will use *psycho-immuno-neuro-endocrinology* (PINE) – began to generate information regarding the *organizational effects of sex hormones on the brain*. The name used here, if 'read' in reverse, provides a handy summary of the general conclusions of this research: namely, that a number of hormones, including sex hormones, which are produced within the body (*endocrinology*) have direct effects on the nervous system (*neuro-*), and as a result impact many aspects of health and function, including immune response (*immuno-*) along with a spectrum of behaviors (*psycho-*), impacting personality, special skills, and social preferences.

With two publications in 1994, H. Nyborg, a Danish developmental psychologist, summarized his attempts to gather many details from this new research together to create a new scientific model, and apply it to the very topic we've been discussing – understanding individual differences and categories in humans. In these books, Nyborg recounted his impatience with the long history of psychology, which professed interest in individual differences, but continued the practice of averaging over subjects without first establishing the homogeneity of the groups being described. He was particularly distressed at the lack of insight regarding a *continuum of gender,* which he took for granted based on his own experiences, and which he believed contributed to the lack of gender effects in many studies.

For example, he discussed how sorting participants into "women" vs. "men" on the basis of general anatomical gender was fraught with difficulties, since individual differences *within* each group were so great. This went far beyond mixing apples and oranges – Nyborg suggested that the multitude of gender types along the continuum resulted in overlaps and offlaps that hopelessly confused the issue. His solution was not to abandon gender as a grouping variable, but do the opposite – examine it in more detail, and accept that "gender" might be more or less a continuous variable instead of one with only two states – female vs. male. Nyborg predicted that if studied properly, gender differences would provide important clues to the biological bases of individual characteristics. He recalls how he set about looking for a research methodology for more accurately classifying individuals. He found that the sciences included in PINE provided the techniques and conclusions he needed.

The result was a formulation he termed "physicology," a science of the biological bases of behavior emphasizing specific details of individual differences and similarities which were created by the dramatic influences of *sex hormones* throughout the brain and body, acting at all stages of life, from conception till death. Nyborg's conclusions were based on a variety of data from many sources, including results of his own work using many research approaches, ranging from experimental studies of behavioral changes in women with Turner's syndrome being treated with hormones, to detailed retrospective analyses of the medical histories of large numbers of men enrolled in the Danish military.

As detailed in his 1994 publications, Nyborg's physicology predicted that: 1) there is a *continuum of gender* based on exposure to prenatal hormones; 2) prenatal hormones interact with genes to 'prime' the nervous system so that each individual's biology responds in its own way to environmental influences, both before and after birth; 3) this priming also affects future production and responses to hormones, including the timing and nature of puberty, and other cycles related to hormones, throughout life; and 4) an individual's place along this neurobiological continuum is expressed in details involving virtually all aspects of life, from gender behavior to special skills (which can themselves fluctuate over time in response to ongoing hormonal changes), from general health to choice of profession, and extending to lifestyle issues such as preferences regarding marriage and children. Nyborg's model was at once the most detailed with regard to mechanisms, and at the same time the most sweeping with regard to implications, of any that had been proposed up to that time.

[Nyborg later became controversial when, instead of using his model to reveal new insights into human behavior, he began re-interpreting the results along *conventional* sexist and racist lines, a fate that has haunted the history of typologies. The problem for typology is, there *are* differences between humans – the difficulty is how best to specify and interpret them, in order to get closer to the truth of where they come from, and what they mean. The situation is exactly analogous to what Darwin and his colleagues struggled with more than a century ago: there *are* differences between biological forms ('species,' 'varieties,' etc.) – the question is, how best to specify and interpret those differences in order to advance our understanding of their origins, their 'meaning,' the insights they provide into universal principles of biology.

Nyborg's case, and the 19th century controversy over the origin of species, both provide excellent demonstrations of the ever-present challenge in science of *the gap* between data and interpretation. If you are a scientist, no matter the area of work, you must constantly be on guard not to allow unexamined assumptions (which are frequently culturally-biased, especially when the topic involves humans) interpret the data for you. The scientist's job is to be as objective as possible, to *let the data speak for themselves* without any 'ventriloquism' on your part, and then to follow where they lead. Only then can you reasonably hope each experiment will be a step forward, a move closer to the truth, an opening of new horizons.]

Nyborg may have failed the challenge of 'the gap' by ending up putting his new wine in old bottles, but that doesn't affect our interest in his methodology for quantifying individual differences in humans. Our discussion will focus on his *early* predictions about the spectrum of individual differences, and how to quantify them. He suggested that individual differences in exposure to prenatal sex hormones will create a spectrum of brain sex types which is permanent. These differences, put in place prenatally, provide a basis on which subsequent environmental influences can work, including postnatal hormonal events, but that by birth, the essential foundation has been laid. The result is a spectrum of individual types which he proposes can be identified by "hormotyping" at any age, accomplished by measuring levels of sex hormones in the blood. For women, this is based on measuring estrogens, which he called "estrotyping," and for men, androgens are measured to do "androtyping." He cautioned that one must be careful to control time of day, month, and year in comparing across different individuals, to account for biorhythms in hormones that follow those cycles.

With these controls in place, Nyborg claimed that a continuum of hormonal levels is observed, which he suggested can be usefully divided into five different categories by level, separately for each gender. Women range from type E1 (very low estrogens) through E3 (moderate levels) to E5 (very high levels), while men range from type A1 (very low androgens) through A3 (moderate levels) to A5 (very high levels). He pointed out that this approach can offer a useful means of helping us move away from considering gender as an either/or variable – 'the women vs. the men.' For example, in comparisons related to behavior, skills, and general health, A1 men may prove to be more similar to E1 women than to A5 men.

With this as a beginning, the research that Nyborg conducted himself, (while inviting additional contributors) focused on studying the correlations between these hormotypes and a wide range of individual characteristics such as height, weight, time of puberty, the nature of fluctuations in hormone levels seen for each type, skills, personality, health, sociability, etc. For instance, he reported that A5, or what we'll call 'high-T,' males show a high degree of masculinization measured in several ways, with few feminine traits, while the opposite is true for A1 males. Women can be shown to become somewhat more male-like (for example, in general behavior and on tests of special skills) during different parts of the monthly cycle, but the degree of change will differ depending on the individual's underlying estrotype.

What is exciting about Nyborg's use of PINE as the basis for his approach, is his suggestion that *the fundamental effects of sex hormones can be associated with such a wide range of individual differences, which are thus seen not as magically co-occurring, but as different facets of the same underlying set of fundamental biochemical mechanisms.* Thus he predicted that A5 males will be short, muscular, and early-maturing, while A1 males will be tall, fatty, and slow maturing – all governed by specific, known influences of prenatal testosterone. High-T males are also predicted to be extroverts, physically active, somewhat inhibited verbally, and prone to a variety of conditions such as coronary failure and prostate cancer.

We recall that Sheldon's approach for his research on individual differences and categories was to collect subjects, measure their physical dimensions, then interview individuals representing different types to study correlations between physically-measured body type vs. other features. Nyborg proceeded in much the same way; for example, in his studies on sets of military records containing measures of plasma androgens, he first sorted individuals on the basis of measured levels of testosterone, then statistically tested the distribution by androtype group of other features such as height, weight, age at time of test, verbal and performance IQ, scores for psychoticism/ extraversion/neuroticism, incidence of allergies, use of medicines, use of alcohol and nicotine, highest grade level of school completed, etc.

He concluded that the results supported his model, though with qualifications, since many other variables were involved. He emphasized that he considered his findings in this and other studies to be preliminary, and called for much more research to test out the predictions of his model. But he also expressed hope that this type of neurobiological approach to understanding human behavior and individual differences could provide a new and more scientific means of exploring human characteristics, with implications ranging from strategies for education, to identification of risk factors for a variety of disorders.

Genetics and individuality

We have not paid much attention to Charles Darwin and the concept of natural selection in this discussion so far, primarily because Darwin was interested in describing universal forces that act similarly on every individual of every species. Of course it is true that the individual organism is at the heart of natural selection, since it is The Individual who is the vehicle of features which are either passed on to the next generation, or not.

Darwin did not have the mechanism of genes to help him describe how transmittable features were coded biologically, or how features of two parents are combined in their children, or how environmental factors such as nutrition can affect inheritance, but he recognized the surface phenomena that signaled the presence of some kind of units that not only: 1) give rise to individually-specific features, but 2) can also be combined between parents to create either copies or variations in their children.

Once the concept of the gene was advanced and the science of genetics as we know it began, an obvious application of genetics was to study individuals as well as the nature of categories, for humans and for other organisms. However, most research in genetics has focused on cross-species comparisons, essentially addressing 19th-century questions related to speciation rather than newer questions about individuation.

Genetic research on individual characteristics is primitive at best – having got not much further, and that quite recently, than the DNA fingerprinting used primarily in forensics. This of course is due to the incredible complexity, not only of the genetic material itself (only recently have complete genomes for some species been completed), but also the complexity of how the genetic makeup of an individual is expressed in the sorts of features we have been talking about.

It is interesting that in genome work, material from many different individuals from a species is pooled to do the research, clearly erasing the very individually-specific features that are the focus of Neural Rainbow Theory. Thus this research practice represents the latest version of 'averaging over subjects' criticized by Nyborg and others, though in this case it might be excused as a necessary evil required in the early stages of a new science. Once an 'average-species genome' has been established, it can provide a basis for studying within-species individual differences and categories in the form of variations around that crude 'species mean,' but such studies are clearly far in the future.

Of course, the relevance of an 'average-species' genome for understanding individual differences, remains to be seen. It is true that a very few features seen in individuals may be genetically encoded and transmitted in a fairly straightforward way – they are said to be determined by 'simple Mendelian inheritance' – but apparently the great majority are not. The biomedical sciences are understandably searching for genes associated with diseases and even complex behavioral conditions such as developmental disorders. For the most part, these have not been forthcoming, and some geneticists do not hold out much hope that the situation will be very different in the future, even with dramatic advances in genetic techniques.

There is one school which has already thrown up its hands with regard to the sufficiency of a genome description, even when established on an individual basis, for helping us understand more about the transmission of features. These researchers admit that the genome must be considered as a starting point, but they emphasize that it is only that. They point to the incredible complexity of inter-gene interactions which are known to exist but not at all understood, the similar complexity of interactions between the genomes of two parents, and the overwhelming influence that prenatal and postnatal environments must have on virtually all aspects of genetic expression; some of this very newest of genetic research falls under the heading of 'epigenetics,' an area of study very relevant to this book.

But even as epigenetics advances, some researchers still express doubt regarding the usefulness of using genes at all to understand individual differences. Some have suggested that even if a particular genome can be analyzed as having a limited number of forms (called norms of reaction, that is, 'one genotype can be expressed as a limited number of specific phenotypes'), there is still a multitude of influences that may never be knowable – which these researchers summarize in rather a hopeless way as 'developmental noise.'

It seems rather premature, given the state of genetics (including epigenetics) and our understanding of development, to conclude that between the 'norms of reaction' (dependent on the genome), and the final state of the new organism, there is nothing but an intimidating blank space called 'noise.' We might want to remember that to call something 'noise' is often a scientist's way of judging (dismissing?) a phenomenon as completely random.

However, if the history of science has taught us anything, it is that such a dismissal very often really means: 'it is something that I do not know how to analyze and thus do not understand.' Such a judgement can be a reflection of one scientist's point of view (perhaps encapsulated as 'one man's signal is another man's noise,' frequently the most accurate interpretation of the often-condescending response "that's another issue," so often heard in scientific exchanges) – or, more dangerously, it can reflect the state of an entire specialization.

The history of science offers many illustrations that one of the principle paths by which science advances is by discovering 'signal' (that is, something systematic) in what was previously thought to be noise – that is, where what on the surface can appear as a bewildering diversity is found to reveal *an underlying pattern*. We can find instances in physics, chemistry, astronomy, biology, medicine. A simple example is provided by recent developments in cardiology, where the variation from heartbeat to heartbeat, previously dismissed as random (i.e., 'noise') has been found to be highly systematic. In fact, this has come to be recognized as life-and-death information: the detail of *heartbeat variability* have been shown to reveal early warning signs of heart trouble at a stage when the 'snapshot' heartbeat waveform, or a waveform averaged over beats, may appear to be entirely normal.

Chapter One Summary: Taking stock

We have seen that a typological approach to understanding individual differences and similarities has a long history. While that history has been marked by ups and downs, many of the approaches seem to provide a rough fit to everyday experience, exhibiting what is called 'face validity.'

From the examples we have discussed, it is clear that these typologies have several things in common: 1) they take human diversity as a given, and value knowledge about the features of each individual; 2) they seek to frame categories based on close observation of multiple individuals, allow the individual details to group the subjects, and in the most ambitious cases, to formulate categories which 'account for' a large number of features – biological, medical, psychological, and social; and 3) their formulations are assumed to apply to each and every human.

In these characteristics, the typological approach stands in marked contrast to others which have unfortunately governed most of the history of psychology, medicine and even human sociology, where: 1) human diversity is considered as experimental noise, not a source of information; 2) any hint of individual distinctions or group differences (except according to the 'medical model' of whole vs. broken) has come to be distrusted as a possible basis for prejudice and exclusion; and 3) the overruling goal is the distinction named above between normal vs. abnormal, standard vs. outlier, healthy vs. unhealthy.

None of the typologies makes such a mistake – within each system, all *types* are considered to be equal in integrity, though of course they may differ in their susceptibility to problems. A Sagittarius is not considered to be a pathological form of a Taurus, Sheldon's mesomorph is not judged as a failed version of either an ectomorph or an endomorph, or vice versa. As Nyborg suggested, if psychological and medical research had put their resources into studying individual variation as a basis for *categories of individuals*, we might be much closer to understanding human behavior than we are now. Neural Rainbow Theory is based on that assumption.

✄

Chapter One Bibliography

Kinsey AC, WB Pomeroy, CE Martin, PH Gebhard (1948) Sexual behavior in the human male. Philadelphia PA: WB Saunders.
Kinsey AC, WB Pomeroy, CE Martin, PH Gebhard, J Bancroft (1953) Sexual

behavior in the human female. Philadelphia PA: WB Saunders.

Kinsey Institute webpage, article about *The Kinsey Scale*. (viewed 10/1/22)

Lauter JL (2001) Neuroimaging: How understanding individual differences can improve your clinical practice [3-hr educational video with manual]. Rockville MD: American Speech-Language-Hearing Association.

Lauter JL (2008) How is your brain like a zebra? A new human neurotypology. Bloomington IN: Xlibris.

Mead M (1949) Male and female; A study of the sexes in a changing world. NY: Dell Pub. Co.

Montagu A (1959) Human heredity. Cleveland: The World Pub. Co.

Nyborg H (1994a) Hormones, sex, and society; The science of physicology. Westport CT: Praeger.

Nyborg H (1994b) The neuropsychology of sex-related differences in brain and specific abilities. *In* PA Vernon (Ed) The neuropsychology of individual differences. San Diego: Academic Press, pp. 60-113.

Rolfe R (2002) The four temperaments; A rediscovery of the ancient way ['four humours'] of understanding health and character. NY: Marlowe & Co.

Sachs G (1998) The astrology file. NY: Plenum.

Sheldon WH (1940) The varieties of human physique; An introduction to constitutional psychology. NY: Harper & Brothers.

Sheldon WH (1942) The varieties of temperament; A psychology of constitutional differences. NY: Harper & Brothers.

Sheldon WH (1954) Atlas of men; A guide for somatotyping the adult male at all ages. NY: Harper & Brothers.

Smith DL (1999) Freud and Jackson: Dualism and anti-Localizationism, *In* DL Smith, Freud's philosophy of the unconscious (Ch. 7), pp. 71-80. Dordrecht: Springer Science + Business Media.

SEX HORMONES AND BRAIN CONNECTIVITY

The goal of this chapter is to lay the groundwork for understanding the neurological aspects of Neural Rainbow Theory. To do this, we need to review briefly some research about three basic topics: 1) how sex hormones can influence the brain and human development; 2) the different patterns of connections linking different parts of the brain, and the ways brain and behavior can undergo radical changes if these connections are altered; and 3) a new way of thinking about a specific category of brain connection, involving specializations of the right vs. the left sides of the brain.

Once these three topics have been reviewed separately, we will be able to go on in the next chapter to tell the story of how they are related to each other. That story will describe how sex hormones working before birth can dramatically transform brain connectivity, particularly with regard to how the two sides of the brain develop, to shape the 'fingerprint' characteristics of each and every individual.

Possibilities for prenatal sex-hormone exposure

As mentioned at the end of Chapter One, the new multidisciplinary sciences of psychoimmunoneuroendocrinology (PINE) have given us an entirely new way of looking at sex hormones. 'Sex hormones are not just for sex anymore' – at least, not just for controlling the limited functions we were taught in school. (In a larger sense, *everything* sex hormones do is about sex – that is, reproduction – but in the service of a more fundamental aspect of biology – but we'll get to that later.)

Actions of sex hormones: overview

Of course, it has been known for some time that sex hormones are incredibly powerful chemicals for controlling the body and behavior. They are involved in the onset of puberty, create radical changes in the shape and size of body parts from genitals to larynx, prepare a woman's body to conceive, carry, and nurse a baby, and can affect our emotions in radical ways during the 'hormonal storms' that men as well as women know all too well.

But these powers are puny compared to the new information coming out of the PINE sciences. The new findings reveal widespread actions of sex hormones throughout the body and brain which at first glance do not seem to be related to reproduction at all. These include: the ability of sex hormones to serve as neurotransmitters (chemicals that allow brain cells to talk to each other), their actions regulating other neurotransmitters, other effects on nerve cells such as enhancing growth and connectivity (the estrogens) or counteracting the 'nerve-growth factor' action of estrogen (the androgens). Receptors for both estrogens and androgens have been found in many parts of the brain and body; testosterone has been shown to retard growth of the thymus gland, an important part of the immune system, while prolactin (the nursing hormone) seems to boost immune response.

[Note that in my discussion of the role sex hormones play in shaping the brain and body, I will use names such as estrogen or testosterone as a kind of shorthand, with the caveat that all biochemical processes involve networks of chemical relationships, and temporal chains of causation, and it is seldom easy to identify the 'proximal' (that is, direct, immediate) *cause* of any one *outcome*.

I don't have the specifics of all those webs and chains at my fingertips (in many if not most cases, I suspect they have yet to be discovered), to use in my descriptions and predictions, just as Darwin did not have genetics to explain how the observable facts of inheritance, variation, and changes in species over time were achieved.

Yet he was confident that the observations and data he did have pointed to the importance of individual differences (he would have called it 'variation') and that *something* about such variation – whatever its source, however it was inherited – was central to the 'origin of species.' In the same way, I am confident that certain biochemical changes related to sex hormones (in particular, androgens such as testosterone) are biological agents used to accomplish a crucial feature in all animals, the *shaped (that is, systematic) variation* of individuals, with life-and-death consequences for the survival of individuals *and* species.]

Sex hormones may have such basic effects on the brain and body as a result of their relation to cholesterol, one of the oldest biological molecules, a crucial component of every animal cell. Sex hormones are ultimately made from cholesterol, the reason for their being called 'steroids,' and possibly also the basis for the fundamental differences in food processing and cholesterol metabolism that are often associated with gender.

Perhaps most importantly, it has been established that sex hormones are *epigenetic factors*: they have the capability of entering the nucleus of a cell, whether in the body or in the brain, and there regulate gene expression. Sex hormones have the power to turn genes on and off.

Earlier we said that some geneticists despair of unravelling the connections linking genome and actual individual, claiming that environmental factors influencing gene expression are so complicated that only 'developmental noise' can be invoked as bridging between genome and the individual, between genotype and phenotype. As we have already suggested, new information from the PINE sciences predicts that things might not be quite that bad, that prenatal exposure to sex hormones in particular might represent *a systematic influence on gene expression* that is not random at all.

The powers of sex hormones for regulating genes, other proteins, and the properties of nerve cells, may be too basic to be classed generically as 'environmental,' and we might want to say rather that sex hormones are a *third factor* that interacts with the genetic blueprint of an individual, and environmental influences such as nutrition and stress, both before and after birth, to create the body, brain, and personality of each individual. In later portions of this book, we will show how Neural Rainbow Theory describes *the larger, nonrandom way* in which this 'third factor' is designed to work, and how it may function in the same way in all humans (and presumably all animals) as a 'final filter' for determining many aspects of individual health, personality, and social identity.

Such an impact on individual behavior is not beyond the bounds of reality. The PINE sciences have shown, for example, that sex hormones alone can reverse the behavior expected for an individual based on its sex chromosomes. In newborn mice, the brain has not yet been shaped for gender-specific behaviors such as nest-building (for females) or aggression (for males). Researchers have found that if a newborn mouse carrying XX sex chromosomes is given testosterone, that individual will grow up to have behaviors that cannot be distinguished from Xy individuals – territorial exploration, courting receptive females, aggression against other males. The opposite is also true – a newborn Xy mouse given estrogen will grow up to show typical female behaviors, inviting males to mate, building a nest, and (although it may lack the internal plumbing for conception and gestation) skillfully caring for pups.

In humans, as in some other mammals, these changes in the brain are accomplished *before* birth, and thus it is possible that prenatal exposure to sex hormones gender-shapes the brain for future behaviors. (For a long time, farmers have known that if a cow or horse has twins, and one is a female, she may be sterile – apparently affected by the testosterone produced by her twin brother while in the womb. This happens frequently enough that this type of individual is called a 'freemartin.')

In order to understand how such things can happen, and what changes can be created in this way, we need to review just how the brain can be exposed to sex hormones before birth.

Prenatal sources of sex hormones

It may be surprising to hear about 'prenatal exposure to sex hormones.' We tend to think of sex hormones being produced only by the gonads starting at puberty – estrogens from a girl's ovaries, and androgens from a boy's testes. If this is the whole story, how can a developing fetus be exposed to testosterone? What could be the source, when only the mother and a fetus are involved?

There are two answers to this. First, every woman (and every man) has an organ in their bodies called the adrenal cortex, which makes androgens (such as testosterone) and estrogens. The adrenal cortex is a 'paired organ' – there is one sitting on top of each of the left- and right-side adrenal glands (which as the name 'ad-renal' tells us, themselves sit on top of the kidneys). The adrenal cortex actually begins making sex hormones at around eight or nine years of age, an event called "adrenarche," or 'onset of adrenal cortex function.' (Adrenarche also occurs in other mammals, of course. For example, adrenarche in a buck fawn will help grow the foundation 'pedicels' where antlers will eventually grow, well before the little buck is sexually mature.)

Adrenarche is an important detail all by itself – given the effects of sex hormones on the brain we've already reviewed, adrenarche may be related to many of the changes commonly observed in children of this age (eight/nine), which otherwise might have no obvious explanation. These include: transformations in personality, improvements or regression in certain academic skills, and clinical features such as onset (or offset) of epileptic seizures, clearing of 'developmental' stuttering, and changes in immune function (allergies may get better or worse, depending on the child; frequency of ear infections might decrease). Sex hormones produced at adrenarche might be responsible for more general changes associated with this age, such as the dramatic diminishment in some people of the brain's ability to acquire a new language, or to recover easily from damage.

Starting with adrenarche then, the adrenal cortex goes on producing sex hormones throughout life. Predictably there are individual differences in this process – from person to person, the adrenal cortex may make different levels of hormones in general, or different levels of each category – estrogens vs. androgens. Among other things, this could be one of the reasons for individual differences in menopause symptoms. For instance, women whose adrenal cortex tends to make relatively high levels of androgens (we will later refer to these as "high-T" women), should experience some degree of 'masculinizing' following menopause. This is because when their ovaries stop making estrogen, the relatively high levels of testosterone produced by the adrenal cortex are no longer masked, and are free to create changes such as the appearance of hair on the upper lip, and lowering of voice pitch.

In contrast, women whose adrenal cortex tends to make relatively little testosterone may have a much easier time with menopause. This type of woman may also be blessed with a moderate degree of body fat (not too much and not too little), which provides additional help with menopause symptoms, because fatty tissue has the ability to transform testosterone into estrogen. As a result, some women's bodies naturally provide them with post-menopausal 'estrogen treatments' – i.e., adrenal-cortex estrogen, plus adrenal-cortex testosterone-turned-into-estrogen by body fat. (Note that for fatty tissue in this case, 'more may *not* be better' – if a woman (or man) is very heavy, this may be a sign of a body that has basic difficulties with food metabolism in general, and problems with sex hormones (recall their connection to cholesterol) may be part of this larger picture.)

So we've seen that one answer to the question of 'where can prenatal testosterone come from?' is – from the mother's adrenal cortex. And recall that this can be graded, ranging from very little in some mothers, to very much in others, with overall levels changing from time to time. For instance, the adrenal cortex may tend to make more testosterone during certain kinds of stress. We will see later that all these differences in levels of adrenal-cortex T may be extremely important for the outcome of pregnancy.

There is a second answer to the question of sources of prenatal T that may seem even more surprising, but to understand it, we need to talk in somewhat more general terms about embryology. It is known that if a mammalian embryo is allowed to grow in a hormone-free environment, it will develop into a female – with a female body, psychology, health, and social behaviors. This will be the result no matter the sex chromosome make-up of that individual. This is why developmental biologists make a basic distinction between *sexual identity* (according to sex chromosomes) vs. *sexual differentiation* (according to what a person really becomes – anatomically, behaviorally, etc. – which depends on the nature of hormone exposure during prenatal development).

Note that a sex-hormone-free environment can occur for any embryo if the mother does not make much testosterone from her adrenal cortex. Estrogens are present throughout gestation, and can fluctuate dramatically in the fetal bloodstream. But the developing baby's brain is shielded from estrogen exposure by a chemical called alpha-fetoprotein (AFP), produced by the fetus and absorbed into the mother's bloodstream, and which 'binds' any estrogens in the fetal bloodstream and keeps them from crossing the baby's blood-brain barrier and affecting the brain. (In fact, the appearance of this protein in a mother's blood is used as one of the signals that she is pregnant – the presence of AFP means that her body is ready to protect a developing child from the changes in estrogens that occur during the stages of pregnancy, no matter the chromosomal identity of the fetus.)

[I have recently seen statements that although AFP *is* known to protect the developing brain of other mammals such as mice from estrogens, a similar role in humans remains controversial. I believe that protecting the developing brain from estrogens is critical for achieving the shaping-of-individuals that is the focus of NRT, and thus – whether AFP proves to be the active agent, or something else – the end result is the same.]

Given this background, we can re-cast the concept of individual differences in 'prenatal sex-hormone exposure' as 'individual differences in prenatal *testosterone* exposure.'

We've already described how both XX and Xy embryos and fetuses can be exposed to graded levels of testosterone, from the mother's adrenal cortex. Later we will describe what these levels of maternal T can mean for XX embryos, but for now we need to see how Xys can experience *additional* prenatal testosterone exposure, sometimes reaching extremely high levels.

Very early in development (for a human, around six to eight weeks post-conceptual age, or PCA), a gene known as SRy located on the short arm of the y chromosome begins a cascade of events that initiate and guide the development of testes. [I have previously read that the SRy gene itself is triggered to begin this process by the presence of adrenal-cortex testosterone in the fetal bloodstream, but as of 2022 I have been unable to find the original reference for this statement. Also, I use a lower-case *y* to refer to the y chromosome, reflecting the fact that it is much smaller than the X.]

Given these conditions – that is, a y chromosome with a functional SRy gene (plus, perhaps, sufficient T for triggering), the same structures that in an XX embryo would have eventually become ovaries, begin changing into testes. (Note that this delicate interaction between levels of blood-borne T and the y chromosome may be one of the contributors to 'ambiguous' development of sexual parts, which can cause tremendous difficulties in a culture which demands that every child's primary sex parts be unambiguously female or male. We will return to the abuses of 'sexual assignment' in a later section, to discuss how such practices are just another facet of certain societies' refusal to embrace the biological fact of individual differences.)

Once complete, fetal testes themselves begin making testosterone, and continue production throughout gestation, right up to birth. The levels of testosterone made by fetal testes can vary dramatically from time to time – in some unfortunate Xys, the developing brain will be exposed to levels of testosterone that are as high or higher than they will be at puberty. This 'roller-coaster' production of testosterone means that in many Xy fetuses, the developing brain is exposed to radically differing levels of testosterone during highly sensitive periods of growth, when different parts of the brain and body are being formed.

Thus we have seen that the overall pattern of prenatal T exposure varies from fetus to fetus, whether XX or Xy, ranging from overall very low to overall very high, from consistent levels throughout (usually very low) to a roller-coaster pattern of dramatic peaks and valleys. Across individuals, then, this can be described as *a 'biochemical rainbow' of prenatal T exposure, where each and every person ends up representing a particular point along the spectrum of exposure.*

Of course, there are other opportunities for the brain to be exposed to testosterone that occur *after* birth. Many Xys, predictably those with higher prenatal T, will continue to have high T in their bloodstream during the first year of life, some extending later than this. (This again gives the lie to the idea that girls and boys are "the same" until postnatal experience and cultural biases shape their brains – the nature of hormone exposure has done its job well before any caregiver gets hold of what is anything but a "blank slate.")

As with prenatal T, continuing production after birth in Xys can clearly affect the developing brain. At adrenarche (around eight or nine years of age) in both girls and boys, the adrenal cortex begins making both estrogens and androgens such as testosterone, providing another chance for brain shaping by T in both chromosomal genders; and at puberty, Xys dose themselves with a new 'testosterone storm' as the testes revisit their prenatal life and again begin producing testosterone in great quantities.

Of course, the graded nature of prenatal T will be reflected in all these postnatal events, as well – XXs with at least some prenatal T will predictably give themselves more at adrenarche than XXs who did not have such prenatal 'priming,' and they will have somewhat later puberty than XXs who enjoyed a hormone-free gestation. Xys with low to moderate prenatal T will give themselves less in childhood and at puberty (and should have somewhat delayed puberty), while Xys who experienced high levels of prenatal T will be fated to endure this again at adrenarche and at the (early) close of their childhood years.

The curve of T production for most Xys continues rising from puberty through adolescence, presumably continuing to change the brain during all those years, to peak in the mid-20s. The testosterone-mediated events occurring in Xys in the young-adult years are generally understood to be the origin of psychological and sociological expressions such as restlessness, aggression, and risk-taking behaviors seen among many males during the same years. In Chapter Five we will look again at these behaviors which can be so disruptive in our society, and explain *why* they are happening in a larger sense, why they are *natural* for Xys, and how they were completely *adaptive* in the past, when humans lived in a way that was a much better fit to our brains than the way we live now.

But it is the experience in the womb, the individual differences in prenatal hormone exposure, that are primarily responsible for setting the stage for individual differences in postnatal life. In the next chapter, we will describe in more detail how the 'biochemical rainbow' of prenatal T exposure gives rise to a 'neural rainbow' of individual differences in brain structure and function, which in turn supports many other 'rainbows' of features of individual differences, such as distinctions in immune function, gender behavior, personality, skills, and even physical characteristics, which we recognize in people around us every day.

Eventually we will use the rainbow metaphor to show how these individual differences are *grouped* into categories, and how (and why) the categories are distributed in the general population. The rainbow metaphor is useful because although a rainbow is actually a continuum of light wavelengths, it appears to the eye as a set of distinct ribbons of concentrated hues, with less intense areas of transition in between. In the same way, we will suggest, the rainbow of human individual differences consists of a few distinct types (three in this instance), to which most people belong, with some individuals falling in transition areas between. Thus we will use the rainbow as the visual symbol for the *neurotypology* of Neural Rainbow Theory, a new way of looking at human beings, describing on the one hand, the biochemical origins of the categories, and on the other, the ethological 'reasons' for them, in humans as well as other animals.

The Handshaking Model of Brain Function
A new approach to brain connectivity

Before proceeding further with our discussion of human types, we need to talk a little more about dynamic aspects of brain organization – especially those features that Neural Rainbow Theory suggests are most importantly affected by different degrees of prenatal hormone exposure.

The three axes

The first of these features has to do with basic dimensions of the brain and body. The body, including the brain contained within the skull, is clearly a three-dimensional structure. These three dimensions can be described as three axes: 1) the *long axis* from head to toe, what scientists call rostro- (meaning head) caudal (meaning tail); 2) the *front-back axis*, from back to belly (the scientific term is dorso- [back] ventral [belly-side]; and 3) the *right-left axis*.

These three body/brain axes are established at the very earliest stages of prenatal development: even before the organism has turned from a disk into a cylinder, there is a clear head-end vs. a tail-end (rostro-caudal axis), a back- and a belly-side (dorso-ventral) – which together define right and left sides. This basic architecture (a kind of design 'scaffolding') provides the framework within which all parts of the body and brain grow and develop – cells are formed, migrate along these axes to where they are supposed to go, sometimes undergo additional changes once they get into place, and in general prepare to undertake the functions they will support lifelong.

To appreciate the importance of this architecture for both neural and body function, it's helpful to remember that throughout the central nervous system (CNS: the brain and spinal cord), certain basic categories of *function* are associated with each of the three axes.

1. The dorso-ventral axis. This axis represents a division between *sensory vs. motor function*. That is, sensory signals coming in from the surface of the body tend to be processed in areas on the back (dorsal) side of the CNS, such as the back half of the spinal cord, or in the parts of the brain that are toward the back half of the head. Outgoing signals, such as those destined for controlling the muscles, tend to originate in brain areas more toward the front (ventral portion) of the head, and leave the spinal cord from its front half.

2. The rostro-caudal axis. The second axis does not involve a simple two-part distinction. Instead, it is associated with *functional staging* – it is the axis along which neural signals are passed, in 'pathways,' along series of relay centers, flowing either from the body periphery toward the top of the brain (the cerebral cortex), or in the reverse direction, from the top of the brain out to structures near the surface of the body.

Interestingly enough, the rule of *two-way signal flow* holds for all neural control systems, whether they are primarily motor (involved in moving muscles or managing glands), or primarily sensory – designed to gather input information from around the body. This two-way flow means that in motor systems, there is constant sensory feedback coming into the brain to help it make online adjustments in output; while in sensory systems, there is constant, ongoing 'top-down' modulation by the brain, which not only helps upper levels of the brain govern how the eye, ear, and skin respond to stimulation, but also to manage the ways in which this information is passed up through the nervous system.

The rostro-caudal axis is additionally important since it is along this axis that the nervous system develops over time, both in the case of the individual and across species – older functions are more caudal, newer functions more rostral. Thus the very oldest neural functions are housed in the spinal cord, somewhat newer processing is supported by the part of the brain at the bottom of the skull (the 'brainstem'), and so on. (The way the different levels interact with each other along the rostral-caudal axis is the focus of the 'Triune Brain' model developed by MacLean and Papez – see chapter bibliography – which addresses several issues of interest to Neural Rainbow Theory.)

The cerebral cortex located at the top of the brain is the newest of all, and is most developed in mammals. Sometimes it is said that the most recently evolved brain functions are located in the *frontal lobes* of the cortex – these are certainly the latest developing in a human child – but interestingly, a large part of the function of this part of the frontal lobes is to serve as an *integrator*, providing links between older functions (primarily from a lower part of the brain called the limbic system, that we'll discuss later) and neural activity in newer areas.

3. The right-left axis. The organization of the right-left axis arose as a means of managing *how the two sides of the nervous system control the two sides of the body* (at least, in those animals who are organized bilaterally, across a midline, not radially, like a starfish). For invertebrate animals, this control is arranged so that the right side of the brain is specialized to run the right side of the body, and vice versa. For vertebrates, this is flipped, so that the right side of the brain oversees the left side of the body, and vice versa.

The exclusivity of these specializations becomes very clear in cases of unilateral brain damage (injury to only one side). For example, if motor cortex on the right side of a person's brain is damaged by trauma or a stroke, function will be impaired on the left side of the body – muscles in the left hand or arm or leg, etc. may be affected, depending on exactly which specific region within right-side cortex was involved.

Researchers have also suggested that as animals have become more complex, a second level of right/left specialization has developed. This level of right/left specialization is associated with different categories of sensory signals and motor gestures, most often summarized as 'functional asymmetries.' For instance, we often hear about 'right brain skills' such as emotional intelligence, or 'left-brain skills' such as verbal ability.

The concept of handedness is related to this newer level of R/L specialization, not the older one, since the term refers to the answer to the question, "Which hand do you use to write with?" Writing is an example of 'fine motor control,' which we will discuss later as a left-brain skill. Thus the conventional use of the term "handedness" is an instance of the left-brain-bias that can be found in many areas of research on human brain function. (To reveal this bias, consider the opposite case – if "handedness" meant, "Which hand and arm do you use to confidently hold and carry a child?" [a right-brain skill, as we will see], just about everyone would be designated left-handed!)

Later we'll talk more about right-brain vs. left-brain skills, and explain how the details of this second level of right/left organization may provide a useful bridge between brain and behavior, to help us better appreciate the significance of individual differences in *brain connectivity* associated with sex hormones.

How the axes work

Before doing that, though, we need to step back and consider one more fact about all three axes that is crucial for understanding brain and body function. This has to do with the 'dynamic relations' along all three axes – that is, relationships that involve a fourth dimension, that of time.

When studying and thinking about brain and behavior, it's easy to focus just on brain structure, its anatomy: which part is connected to what, and where does a particular pathway go? A great deal of medical education, for instance, is fixated on anatomy, asking students to memorize the names of hundreds of brain parts, often with little insight into how they actually do their job.

A much more difficult concept is how different parts of the brain *work*, and most importantly, how they *work together over time*, in a *dynamic way* – that is, their function, their physiology. Often this is addressed in a very static manner, that is, by identifying the particular role of each brain part as though it works in isolation, like parts of a car – a carburetor is a carburetor, with a particular function, whether or not it is actually installed in a car, interacting with other parts. But in the brain those interactions are everything – the rule is that for brain functionality, 'everything is *dynamically* connected to everything else,' and we can't expect to have a very sophisticated appreciation of brain function if we fail to appreciate this.

How are these 'fourth-dimensional' relations linking different brain parts important, and what do they have to do with behavior? To answer this, we will first describe the relations in a general way, and then give examples showing how these relations affect the three axes. We will talk about relations in the form of three modes – teamwork, rigid hierarchy, and disconnection. They are not often described as such by psychologists or neurologists, but some researchers and clinicians are clearly aware that the brain has the three modes, and the modes are certainly reflected in behavior. It's possible that describing brain/behavior relations in this way could help us appreciate not only how the brain works in general, but understand how individual differences in sex-hormone exposure could impact these dynamic relations in fundamental ways.

1. Teamwork relations. First, let's assume that the ideal for relations among brain parts is the same as relations between people, that is, working in a flexible 'teamwork' way – for example, each individual (person/part) should have its own 'job description,' with a unique contribution to make to an overall goal. The style of working together should be that of a sensible type of democracy; there may be a coordinator who can be counted on to oversee things in a very general way, but from task to task, the choice of exactly which one takes the lead depends on what needs to be done and who is best at it – sometimes one part will take the lead, sometimes another, but in all cases, every contribution is valued, and all work together in a harmonious, efficient way.

This may sound more like human beings interacting, than like medical descriptions of how the body and brain work, but I don't think it's a coincidence. After all, as biological beings, every aspect of our life reflects the same basic principles – we can only do what we are, which is to be biological. It makes perfect sense that relations among individual parts of the brain resemble relations among individual human organisms.

Just as with people, this type of 'handshaking' teamwork relation among brain parts should ensure the most resilient type of function – that is, with a basis grounded in specialization (each region can be counted on to play its part well), but also reaping the benefits of combined skills, in an approach that is synergistic – that is, more can be done, and with greater sophistication, by the group working together in this harmonious way, than by one or two working alone. (The term 'handshaking' is borrowed from the early days of computer modems, when different models of modems installed on different computers were said to successfully 'handshake' if their connection allowed the computers to communicate with each other.)

The idea of a 'teamwork' brain is the model that helps us understand how the brain can be so flexible, changing responses on a minute-by-minute basis, adjusting to new situations and new contexts, able to create what seems to be an infinite number of new reactions out of the same component parts. Linguists are fond of talking about language in this way, as though it were unique in this aspect, but language is just one of many behaviors that show the brain working according to a coordinated, teamwork model.

This happens to an almost miraculous extent – scientists designing robots know all too well that even the simplest animals have many more 'degrees of freedom' than the best robot they can build. The brains of animals do this all the time, when approaching almost every task – if they did not, the animal would not be 'adaptive' (because not *adaptable*) and wouldn't last very long. Sometimes it's said that such behavioral flexibility is true only for primates, or perhaps mammals in general, but researchers have described amazing flexibility in many organisms, not only animals, a tribute to biology's tenacity and determination for organisms to persevere in a changing world. Individuals need to have not only a repertoire of adjustable behaviors, but a biologically-based repertoire of links between input, integration, and output supporting many levels of adjustment and gradation – and this becomes more true, the more complex an organism's daily life.

One of the best examples of neural teamwork happens along the right-left axis. We will see in the Brain Asymmetries section below, that the right and left sides of the brain have areas of specialization that are quite specific – not vaguely defined areas of function, like 'music vs. speech,' but categories based on *physical characteristics* of sensory stimuli and motor gestures. By combining the specializations, with both sides working in tandem, it becomes possible for very complex tasks to be accomplished. Virtually all everyday behaviors (listening to someone talk, speaking yourself, opening a jar, reading a book, etc.) depend on such coordination, where *both sides of the brain work together at the same time*. If you try to do these same tasks with only one side contributing (e.g., through a failure in connection, as described later), performance is degraded. In some cases, only the internal quality of the experience of the task may be reduced, but in others, the failure of teamwork might be expressed in a way noticeable by others, such as losses associated with traumatic brain injury, or distinctions between types of reading problems (also discussed under Brain Asymmetries).

2. Hierarchical relations. Then, consider what would happen if these 'teamwork' relations were transformed to become much more rigid and hierarchical. In this case, one and only one part becomes the leader, making part B do its thing, which in turn forces part C to do its function, etc. In such a situation there is never any opportunity for changing response to a new situation – all the parts work in the same way every time, with no adjustments for different situations, and no tolerance for a difference in response. The resemblance to human social relations is obvious – this is the kind of structure used in military organizations, or in the worst of workplace (or family) structures, where the Boss is always the Boss, and there is no appeal from lower levels.

Of course, such organizational styles are very primitive – they may work well in a life-or-death situation ("all for one and one for all"), but we know from experience they are a terrible way to function on a day-to-day basis. If the component parts are complex themselves (whether brain parts, or human individuals) – for instance, if they have skills other than the single one fitting the rigid chain of command, or capabilities for graded responses or a range of responses – being forced to work within the rules of a rigid hierarchy is an extremely wasteful way of making use of their abilities. What a hierarchy demands is component parts that are individually simple, mechanical, interchangeable, 'cogs in a wheel.' It is interesting to observe how military training is designed specifically to transform recruits from complicated individualistic human beings into the simple, knee-jerk, almost non-biological robotic units required for such a primitive social structure.

The idea of a hierarchy is not at all foreign to the brain. As noted by the neurologist Hughlings Jackson in the 19th century, there are many instances in the nervous system which clearly involve hierarchical control. Jackson focused on those in which newer parts of the nervous system (such as the cortex) seem to exert *repressive* control on older, lower ones (this was the feature of Jackson's idea that appealed to Freud as a model for the psyche). Thus when Jackson saw a person such as we mentioned above, with limp muscles due to 'flaccid paralysis,' he noted that the injury always involved *the nerve* going from the spinal cord to the muscle – but when the symptom was 'spastic paralysis' (with muscles clenched and too tight to move), he found that the damage was usually in *the cortex*.

From this, he reasoned that the role of the motor nerve (and its cells of origin in the spinal cord) was to provide an ongoing flow of neural energy to the muscle, while the role of the motor cortex was to *control* the amount of activity sent to the muscle. Thus if motor cortex was damaged, this 'brake' was removed, and with the nerve 'released' from top-down control, it sent so much activity to the muscle that the muscle became hyper-contracted – 'over-working,' thus useless.

The nervous system has other instances of hierarchical control that we experience every day, but may not recognize as this style of function. For example, the autonomic nervous system, which manages many basic aspects of our biological and emotional life, is made of two components, the sympathetic nervous system (SNS: the "fight/flight" system) and the parasympathetic nervous system (PSNS: important for keeping a calm heart, good digestion, quiet breathing).

The parasympathetic component seems to be organized according to the teamwork model we described above – it has separate components sited at different organs around the body, that can work alone or in concert with others, as needed, and there is evidence that control of PSNS extends into the cortex.

In contrast, the sympathetic nervous system (SNS) is organized hierarchically, with something very like a military structure. (Its name means that everything it controls responds together, like soldiers marching in step.) The SNS consists of a 'chain' of ganglia (groups of cell bodies) lined up from top to bottom of the spinal cord which when activated, always do the same thing at the same time, so that all the organs affected by SNS follow its staccato drum – this is truly an 'all for one' type of system. The SNS responds in an all-or-nothing way to stress – it sends the body into overdrive, racing the heart, speeding up breathing, shutting down digestion. There do not seem to be any SNS centers per se above the spinal cord – it is a very old, very primitive system compared to the modulated, distributed structure of the PSNS.

Looking at these two parts of the autonomic nervous system, it would seem to be sensible given our present stress-filled world if people had adapted to have the PSNS predominate – to "maximize para" – but unfortunately many individuals have the type of nervous system where the SNS is extremely active and reactive – they are said to have "high sympathetic tone." This does not mean they are 'sympathetic' with other people – almost the opposite, they are anxious, competitive, always in crisis mode, with heart rate and other basic body functions a hair-trigger away from going ballistic. (These are the "Type A" personality types well-known to physicians.)

Because of the over-activity of their rigidly hierarchical SNS, these individuals have troubles with digestion, etc., and find everyday life very stressful, with that ancient fight/flight system kicking off at the least provocation. They may even have trouble with their sphincters, since it is the PSNS that keeps the sphincters closed (PSNS in its 'wisdom' knows you don't want to eliminate where you eat!), and thus too much SNS activation can override that control, resulting in embarrassment. Such troubles (bedwetting, etc.) occurring in boys of school age may signal a system that is being subjected to extreme SNS stimulation, such as physical or psychological abuse at school or at home.

Another example of a failure in hierarchical control has to do with hyperactivity. There is evidence that there is a 'normal' degree of relative activity at the level of the cortex compared with subcortical areas such as the limbic system and brainstem, such that a certain amount of activity in cortex ensures that it will be able to manage and modulate function at lower levels, including responses to incoming sensory signals. However, in some individuals, perhaps as a result of prenatal conditions we will describe later, the relative levels of cortical/subcortical activity may be out of balance, with the cortex showing a level that is too low, like the idle of a car set too low. As a natural result, just as in Hughlings Jackson's description of 'spastic paralysis' in the motor system, the lower centers are allowed to over-respond.

This may be the case in some hyperactive children, who can appear to be almost possessed by something (perhaps sensory centers in their brainstem!). When these children are given treatments designed to activate the cortex (and *not* lower levels) – such as Ritalin-type medications, or special types of training such as biofeedback – the cortex can be returned to 'normal' levels of activity, which in turn will regain control of lower parts of the brain. As a result, the child becomes calm and attentive, with the balance of activity restored.

These features of cortex and lower centers such as the brainstem can be readily measured with quite inexpensive devices, offering a way to distinguish such children, for whom a cortical/brainstem imbalance indicates a need for cortical stimulants, vs. those whose cortical/brainstem balance is OK, and for whom another approach for managing behavior is needed.

Currently there is a great deal of interest in the hierarchies of processing from body periphery into cortex that are represented in the sensory nervous systems – eye, ear, and skin. Some of the newest and most exciting human brain research focuses on the 'top-down' management of sensory input accomplished in these systems. We are finding that the brain constantly monitors and modulates its own pathways, extending all the way out to actual structures in the eye, ear, and skin. This type of *neurological capability for self-modulation* can be crucial for many skills needed in everyday life, that we tend to take for granted until they break down.

Top-down sensory modulation makes it possible to: selectively attend to one signal or another (the failure is 'attention deficit'); tolerate a wide range of stimulus levels, from quiet to loud (failures are called 'photophobia,' 'hyperacusis,' etc.); self-manage signals coming from inside the body (some types of chronic pain may be an example); and control overall level of arousal (what the hyperactive child cannot do).

3. Disconnected relations. Finally, what would happen to neural function if the parts of a teamwork or hierarchy should become anatomically (or physiologically) separated from each other, if the lines of communication between them, their *connectivity*, should be compromised in some way? (This is like human beings competing with each other, or in the extreme, ceasing to communicate – pulling their phone lines, refusing to read their email.) In that case, each part might still be able to achieve its own limited function, and behavior might be 'successful' to the extent that some isolated expressions of very specific skills might occur – but the 'normal,' beautifully coordinated, repertoire of multisite modulated performance would be lost.

We have already seen examples of disconnection. Perhaps the most obvious examples have to do with actual neural injury. For instance, disconnection between motor neurons of the spinal cord and the muscles they serve (as might happen in spinal-cord trauma, or if a nerve is injured) leads to flaccid paralysis where an arm or other limb hangs useless. Another example of disconnection can result from damage to pathways within the brain connecting areas for hearing with those for speaking. In this case, a person cannot repeat what is said – they might be able to talk, but not self-correct when errors are made, because the connections providing sensory feedback are lost.

Disconnection might be behind less obvious sorts of problems. For instance, adults with special skills (being able to memorize a telephone book, or remember thousands of license-plate numbers) often exhibit such skills in isolation from other types of more 'normal' everyday behaviors. These people are often said to have 'islanded' function – this is predictably based on an 'islanded' situation in their nervous systems, where connection between parts that can do different types of tasks has been lost in some way. Another example is people who may be very good when they are working with one hand at a time (for instance, doing some fine-motor-control task), but are not very coordinated in two-hand tasks, or have problems with eye-hand coordination. It makes sense that these conditions reflect an underlying neural arrangement where the 'right hand doesn't know what the left hand is doing' – due to diminished connectivity between the left and right sides of the brain, or, for eye-hand coordination, there may be a breakdown in communication linking visual parts of the brain with those for controlling the hands.

Also, people with brains that differ in the quality of connectivity along one or another axis may neurologically perceive the world in different ways.

For instance, when we get exasperated enough to ask 'Can't you tell that I'm angry?' or 'Does he not see it?' the answer may actually be no. Different levels of ability in rostro-caudal axis functioning can lead to a type of failure in neural processing that no one would call damage, but which can result in definitely different 'styles' of function, that make certain people more or less deaf, blind, or numb to some types or features of signals. If we understand this, we may be able to change our expectations of their abilities, or find ways to improve their capabilities with training. You can't just tell someone to 'change their brain' – but certain training strategies can accomplish that, dramatically improving processing. We'll see later that the individual differences in skills based on brain connectivity might provide important clues to the origins of categories of individuals.

(The status of all these dynamic-processing, 'handshaking' relations in the brain, involving all three body/brain axes, and including changes with training or medication, can be studied using relatively inexpensive techniques, such as evoked potentials. Several of the references to my work in the Chapter 2 bibliography detail new developments and applications in this area.)

The EPIC Model of Functional Asymmetries
A new approach to brain asymmetries

In Chapter Three we will discuss how prenatal testosterone may work to adjust and radically alter relations linking parts of the brain and body, along all three axes of organization. Of these, perhaps the most important are relations along the right-left axis, which involve *brain asymmetries*, that is, specializations in which either the right or the left brain excels. (This discussion applies to the 'second level' of brain asymmetries discussed earlier – that is, over and above the simple rule linking side-of-brain to side-of-body, for muscle control, etc.) In order to appreciate the importance of changes created by testosterone, we need to know more about this second tier of right-left brain functions, which support complex interactions between the two sides.

Of course, differences in 'right-brain/left-brain' skills have been discussed by researchers, neurologists, and educators for many years, and several versions of the distinction have been popularized for explaining individual differences like learning styles. Most of these are presented as opposites, as though functions of the right and left brain can be classified as 'separate but equal.' Also, the distinctions referred to are typically vague and abstract – for example, the left brain is said to be specialized for speech, language, and analytical processing, while the right brain is better at music, emotions, and intuitive insights.

From a neurobiological point of view, it is extremely difficult to understand how such abstract distinctions could be put in place, cell by cell and region by region. For example, how can a brain be 'wired' to be able to identify an incoming signal as either 'speech' or 'music,' and then route the signals to the proper side?

However, the EPIC Model of Functional Asymmetries provides a new way to re-interpret virtually all of the research on brain asymmetries, using concepts and terms that are much more biological (taken from the sciences of sensory and motor psychophysics – more later), offering clues to how *specific* features of the right and left sides of the cortex could support even these general types of specialization. The biological basis of the EPIC model means that it can be applied not only to human behaviors but also to aspects of everyday life common to all animals (examples of functional asymmetries which have been observed in other animals are included in the chapter bibliography's reference to my paper in *Frontiers in Bioscience*).

"Separate and different"

Perhaps the most important feature of this new approach is the recognition that with regard to the two sides of the brain, it is not at all a case of 'separate but equal.'

As summarized in Table 2.1 (from the 2008 edition of my *Zebra* book), the EPIC model predicts that the right side of the brain is responsible for processing in three 'domains' of function: Extrapersonal space, Intrapersonal space, and Coordination, while the left brain specializes in only one, Peripersonal space, mostly providing 'content' skills for working in tandem with the 'frame' abilities of the right side. (The frame/content distinction was used by the linguist Peter MacNeilage to discuss similarities between language and bimanual coordination, but the EPIC model posits that a frame/content relation characterizes functional asymmetries in general.) Definitions of all four domains are listed in Table 2.1, and will be discussed in more detail later.

Because the right side is designated as having more responsibilities than the left, and is much more important for overseeing general health, physical as well as mental, the EPIC model refers to the right brain as 'polypotent,' that is, having *many powers*. In addition, because of its importance in health matters, the right brain is also identified by the model as 'the mother of the brain and body' – several anatomical and physiological features supporting that honorific title will be described below.

Table 2.1
The EPIC Model of Functional Asymmetries:
four domains of specialization

Left-Brain Specialties	*Right-Brain Specialties*
Peripersonal Space (processing of sensory stimuli and gestures made *near* the body surface or involving certain kinds of actions)	**Extrapersonal Space** (processing of sensory stimuli and gestures made *far* from the body surface or involving certain kinds of actions)
	Intrapersonal Space (physical and mental health – the space *within* the body)
	Coordination (keeping right- and left-side functions in sync)

(based on Table 2.1, p. 47, in How is Your Brain Like a Zebra? *Xlibris, 2008)*

Relevant to the division of labor regarding general health, we know that the right side of the brain is the first to start growing and differentiating during prenatal life, and seems to go on predominating for the first several months of life, perhaps extending well into the second year. This makes sense if the right side is primarily responsible for things like immune function, which is of life-and-death importance as the very young child is exposed to potential dangers on a daily basis. (We will see that for some fortunate individuals, this condition of the right-side predominance continues throughout life, assuring good health at all stages. Later we will discuss what gives these individuals such an advantage, and why others may not be so lucky.)

These differences in specialization for general health even show up in cases of brain damage. For instance, neurologists have known for a long time that people who suffer injury to the right side of the brain are more likely to contract infections or die of a heart attack afterwards than those with left-side damage. For heart attacks, the risk is increased even for individuals who have entirely healthy hearts, suggesting that the right side of the brain 'cares for' the heart in some crucial way that the left side does not, and that anything that interferes with this nurturance puts the heart at risk.

Special right/left functions

As suggested in Table 2.2, according to the EPIC model, there is one area where the two sides of the brain can be seen as specialized in *complementary* ways: the two domains of Peripersonal space (left brain) and Extrapersonal space (right brain). As shown in the table, this has to do with the very different demands for processing signals and gestures made very close to the surface of the body vs. those that occur at more of a distance.

If features of sensory signals and motor gestures are defined according to the terms used in sensory and motor psychophysics (research linking highly-specified *physical* characteristics of stimuli and gestures to the behavior and sometimes physiological state of a perceiver/performer) are employed, it becomes clear that one does not need to study the *cortex* on the right and left sides to find the rules for this type of distinction. Psycho-physical definitions of stimulus and gesture invoked in the EPIC model map very well onto properties already present in portions of sensory and motor systems *at the body surface*. Thus cortical functional asymmetries can be re-interpreted as *upward elaborations* of distinctions already present at the sensory and motor periphery.

To explain this, we will describe examples from each of the major systems – vision, hearing, touch, and motor control. Table 2.2 provides a summary of details, including examples of the peripheral sensory and motor organs of interest.

TABLE 2.2
EPIC model details of Peripersonal vs. Extrapersonal space
management for visual, auditory, somatosensory,
and motor processing

PERIPERSONAL SPACE << left brain >>	EXTRAPERSONAL SPACE << right brain >>
Vision	
high spatial frequency	low spatial frequency
static image	motion
color	light & dark
parvocellular elements	*magnocellular elements*
Audition	
high acoustic frequency	low acoustic frequency
rapid changes in time	slow changes over time
broadband listening	narrowband listening
basal cochlea	*apical cochlea*
Somatosensation	
local light touch	deep pressure
static event	motion over skin
Meissner's corpuscles	*Pacinian corpuscles*
Motor control	
small angles of movement	large angles of movement
a few muscle fibers	large groups of fibers
fine manipulation	postural control
small motor units	*large motor units*

(based on Table 2.2, p. 49, How is Your Brain Like a Zebra? *Xlibris, 2008)*

1. Visual asymmetries. In the visual system, the retina at the back of
the eye includes many types of cells – the rods and cones, which are the visual
'receptors,' and other cells which assist in visual processing, including cells
which send two basic modes of input separately to the brain.

One cell type is specialized for detecting light/dark differences occurring over relatively large areas of space ('low spatial resolution'), and for recognizing *movement* – this type of cell provides information to the 'magnocellular' visual system. The other type of cell, which supplies the 'parvocellular' visual system, is better at identifying tiny details (it has 'high spatial resolution') and distinguishing colors, for objects that are *stationary*. The outputs from these two types of retinal cells are kept separate as they are passed into the brain, and research on brain asymmetries suggests that these distinctions are also important at the level of the cortex. That is, the right brain specializes in magnocellular processing, while the left brain is better at parvocellular visual tasks.

To understand the difference, let's consider two examples of visual tasks. The first is watching a horse cantering along a horizon at twilight. This is a perfect magnocellular (right-brain) task: it requires distinguishing the darker shape of the horse against the lighter sky background, and recognizing that it is a horse by the overall shape and by the characteristic movements – the large, rhythmic gestures of the canter, and the flowing shapes of the mane and tail. The second example is reading a line of red numbers printed in 10-point type – a perfect parvocellular task, because it involves color processing and recognizing tiny details of visual objects that are static on a page, usually viewed in bright light.

2. Auditory asymmetries. For the auditory system, the distinctions are present within the inner ear, in the form of different responses along a strip of tissue called the basilar membrane, the 'receptor surface' of the auditory system, thus the ear's version of the retina. The basilar membrane is coiled up like a snail shell, about 4 cm long from the 'basal' end, nearest the middle ear, to the 'apical end,' at the center of the coil. The basilar membrane responds to sounds in ways that analyze the sound according to time and frequency, so that the auditory receptors called hair cells which are attached to the membrane can send the analyzed signal on to the brain.

In the case of sounds (or parts of sounds) that happen relatively slowly and are low in pitch, the membrane moves over a large part of its surface, and relatively more toward the apical end. For other sounds or parts of sounds which are shorter/faster and higher in pitch, less of the membrane moves and most of the movement occurs in the basal end. Research on brain asymmetries suggests that this difference in basilar membrane response may also be the basis for specializations of auditory cortex in the right vs. left side of the brain. That is, the right brain may specialize in processing slower, lower-pitched sounds, while cells on the left side should be good at handling shorter/faster, higher-pitched sounds.

To illustrate these distinctions for auditory asymmetries, a single task –

listening to speech – shows us how such auditory specializations sometimes have to work in parallel, at exactly the same time. First, to identify *how* something is said, the listener must keep track of changes in voice pitch (which carries cues as to whether the speaker is happy or sad or is being sarcastic). This is a perfect right-brain task, because it requires listening to the part of the speaker's production that is fairly low in pitch (even for a woman's or child's voice), forming an acoustic pattern that changes fairly slowly over time. In contrast, the task of telling *what* is being said means that a listener has to identify the actual speech sounds, the 'phonemes' being produced. This is generally a left-brain task, because the cues to phonemes are usually extremely short/fast acoustic events, and many involve pitches that are well above the pitch range used for the voice. This strategy of *combining* right- and left-brain skills to listen to (and to accurately produce) speech is an example of the 'frame/content' relationship mentioned earlier used by the linguist Peter MacNeilage to compare motor control of speech to bimanual coordination. As noted earlier, the EPIC model predicts that *all* the Peripersonal/ Extrapersonal combinations identified in Table 2.2, not just those related to motor control, are used in a frame/content way.

3. Asymmetries related to touch. The skin is not only the largest organ in the body, crucial for basic functions such as gas exchange and temperature and water regulation (sabotaging these protective functions of the skin, as deep burns may do, can be life-threatening), it also provides forms of communication that no other sensory system can. As the visual system tells us about how things look, and the auditory system how things sound, the skin is all about how things feel – that is, 'tactile' sensory information, ranging from temperature, to general texture, to large as well as tiny details of shape.

It does this by means of special nerve-endings embedded in different layers of the skin, which may directly stimulate the two sides of the brain in different ways. These nerve-endings are the receptors of the 'somatosensory' system (*soma = body*). Some situated very near the surface of the skin are designed to be extremely sensitive to small, light touches that occur briefly at just one location. These 'light touch' receptors (such as Meissner's corpuscles) are concentrated in those parts of the body which are (therefore) most sensitive to this type of contact, such as the fingertips, lips, and tip of the tongue. A very different type of skin receptor is located deep in the skin, and is designed to detect skin stimulations involving more pressure, and moving across the skin. These 'deep pressure' receptors (called Pacinian corpuscles) are not concentrated in any one place, but are found everywhere on (and inside) the body.

An example of a job for left-brain somatosensory processing occurs when a tiny splinter is detected in the skin, and the very fine 'high resolution' abilities associated with the light-touch receptors may be used to locate exactly where it is. An example of a right-brain somatosensory task is feeling someone hugging you or squeezing your arm (both deep pressure) or caressing the back of your hand (a moving stimulation). When we pet an animal like a dog or a cat, we are stimulating this right-brain touch system, not only for ourselves (as the fur slides beneath the palm of the hand) but also for the animal.

In animals who lick each other as a basic form of communication, whether between a mother and child, or between two adults, the stimulation is clearly targeting the deep-pressure receptors, and thus the right brain. We have noted that research indicates that the right brain is also important for immune function; in fact, there are studies of animals such as mice, which show that the mother's licking of newborn pups is very important for stimulating their immune systems (it also helps encourage peristalsis in the digestive tract). Without this type of activation, the mouse pups will sicken and die, even if they are given food and water and are kept warm. One researcher found that if he stroked newborn mice on a regular basis with a wet paintbrush, they flourished and grew – just as though they were enjoying the benefit of their mother's licking.

In general, stimulating the right brain by activating deep-pressure skin receptors may be one of the oldest and most important ways that two organisms can communicate mutual support. Everyday interpersonal gestures like hugs, one person looping an arm over another's, pressing body to body ('you can *lean* on me'), carrying a child, squeezing a shoulder, or even a firm handshake, can be an effective nonverbal communication that not only 'says' "I'm here, I support you," but may even be providing *actual neural support* by 'up-regulating' the right side of the brain and thus recruiting its many supports for physical as well as mental health – the objective physiological basis for the subjective sense of support.

(I've always thought hospitals should have trained professional 'huggers' on staff, whose job is to conduct 'hugging' rounds, visiting patients on a regular basis to reassuringly squeeze a hand, press a shoulder, lay a hand gently on a cheek, embrace the person if possible; the health benefits could be incalculable. It is already well-known that holding, carrying, and rocking premature babies (just like all babies) can improve their health, and many Neonatal Intensive Care Units are already using this very old and inexpensive way of recruiting the right brain to help babies grow and thrive. The same should work for any clinical patient of any age, even if they're sleeping – like the auditory system, the somatosensory system never sleeps, and even in a coma, those signals can still go straight to the 'mothering' right brain, with all the attendant benefits.)

For humans and other animals, there may even be an important right-brain somatosensory function involving the inner ear. Earlier I mentioned how important *licking* is for many animals, not only as support communication, but also in terms of the positive physiological effects derived from its stimulation of deep-pressure receptors in body tissues. Of course, humans don't lick their babies, nor do we as adults lick each other as a sign of affection and bonding, as so many other animals do. But it is possible that one of the reasons we find a calming human voice so effective – not only to listen to, but also to produce– is that we have learned to use the voice (and the anatomical structures that produce it) to 'stroke' the *auditory* parts of the right brain, just as a loving licking tongue would activate *somatosensory* areas, also on the brain's right side.

The process would start with the *physical* way that the sound of a calming vocal tone which is moving slightly up and down in pitch and loudness 'strokes' the surface of the inner ear's 'cochlear membrane,' the inner-ear auditory receptor surface embedded with cells that send their own signals to the brain. Many theories have been advanced for the origins of human speech, but it may not be coincidental that human verbal communication, so important for bonding between mother and child, extending even to before birth, and between children and adults of all ages, utilizes the same structures in and around the mouth and upper respiratory tract that other animals use for 'somatosensory support communication' with each other. For example, as horses lip and nibble each other's skin as a sign of friendship, we use our lips and teeth to make the clicks and lisps of speech sounds; and a human mother coos to her baby, and we 'sing' our emotions to each other, using rhythmic motions of our vocal folds and tongue, just as a mother cat licks her kittens with a long, wet tongue, stirring the answering purring in their own small throats.

4. Motor asymmetries. By this time, it should be obvious what the right-left brain distinction for the motor system is – the difference between gestures that are relatively slow, larger, involving whole structures like the tongue, whole limbs, or even larger areas of the body (all a right-brain domain), vs. movements that are very tiny, perhaps making only a small angle of movement in a single joint (predictably a left-brain specialization). The biological basis for these two types of movement exists in the connections between muscles and motor neurons: 'large motor units' where a single motor neuron controls many muscle fibers, vs. 'small motor units,' where the neuron/muscle fiber ratio is closer to one.

The production of speech is a good example of an instance where these two specializations *must work in parallel*. Right-brain skills for making larger 'frame' gestures are used to control the opening and closing of the jaw for the timing of syllables, along with managing long-term changes in voice pitch needed for vocal melody, and syllabic-length pulses of the muscles between the ribs, to provide the wind-energy that makes speech possible.

Within this frame, the left brain works to create very fast, very small movements of the tongue and lips, for articulating the different phonemes of speech, building words with amazing speed from millisecond to millisecond.

And finally, the right brain in its coordinator role pitches in to ensure that both sets of gestures, stretching from the lungs to the vocal folds to the lips, occur in the proper sequence. Given this description of the incredible synchronization over space and time needed for speech, it is not surprising that problems such as stuttering can occur. In fact, one original idea about the origins of stuttering suggested that this type of speech problem is due to a failed coordination of the right and left sides of the brain – the description given here certainly seems to support such a conclusion.

5. Brain asymmetries in action. We've seen that new research on the specializations of the right and left sides of the brain show that they affect multiple aspects of our lives, from general health to special skills. We've also described that many everyday tasks require teamwork combining the skilled contributions of both sides – for instance, as we listen to someone talk, we analyze the phonemes of speech with our left brains at the same time as we're interpreting their emotional tone with our right.

In summary, let's close this section with two images which capture the combination of skills and abilities we've described for each side of the brain in a single picture – the first, an image representing right-brain specializations, and the second, a cross-section of left-brain abilities.

For the right-brain picture, imagine a mother rocking in a rocking chair, cradling a baby in her left arm, and nursing the baby at her left breast, while another child plays quietly on the floor beside her. The mother is using her right brain's visual abilities as she runs her eyes up and down her baby's body, and from time to time glances at the other child to make sure all is well there, too. The auditory parts of her right brain are listening to the rhythmic creak of the chair, the gentle sounds the nursing baby makes, and the humming of the older child singing to herself as she plays.

The mother's right-brain somatosensory areas are activated as she caresses the baby's smooth legs and arms, holds the little hands and feet, and feels the warm weight of the baby pressing against her breast and side. Her right-brain motor skills are active, too, supporting the baby securely in that right-brain-managed left arm, helping her right hand and arm move gracefully and carefully as she caresses the child, and pressing her foot lightly against the floor, to keep the chair rocking in its heartbeat rhythm. She also draws on right-brain speech-motor skills as she talks in a low, cooing tone to the baby, moving the tone of her voice up and down in a slow, musical way that both calms and entertains the baby who listens and watches her with sleepy eyes.

We can't leave this picture without remembering that there are other right-brain skills at work that are not so easy to see, affecting the mother as well as the baby. First, the mother's right brain is not only responding to each of these sensory stimuli and accomplishing the motor gestures, but is also coordinating across all these different systems and is even bringing in left-brain skills as well, to touch lightly the tips of the baby's fingers, or study the fine details of her eyebrows and hair, or provide the fine-motor control to push against the floor just enough each time to keep the chair rocking with a minimum of effort. She is also using her right brain to attend to *everything* in her surroundings; the oversight of attention on *both sides of space* is definitely a hallmark of the right-brain's excellence for extrapersonal space processing.

Thus the mother's brain is working in a harmonious, 'whole-brain' way – she has equal access to special skills from the right *and* left sides, along with her right brain's capabilities related to coordination and nurturance. As a result, rocking in a chair, being with her baby, this woman achieves a remarkable degree of effortless multitasking, able at once to monitor the baby's comfort and her own, keep track of what the older child is doing, think about the experiment she'll work on tomorrow, while listening for the timer on the oven or the ring of the telephone, seamlessly connected to an even wider sphere beyond her immediate responsibilities in this room.

Second, as the mother's right brain processes all these sensations, the other systems it oversees are being stimulated in turn – her parasympathetic nervous system is active, ensuring that her heartbeat is calm and steady, and her immune system is not only being stimulated and strengthened for her own sake, but is actively producing ingredients for her breast milk that will protect her baby through the early months of life.

In addition, the baby's own right brain, still predominating as we've seen at this age, is being activated in every way by what the mother is doing – the slow gentle caresses over its skin, the rhythmic rocking, the melody of her voice, the warmth of her side, the slow surge of the warm milk, the good food stimulating the digestive system, and the baby's own immune system responding to the protection her mother is sharing with her.

In contrast, for our picture representing left-brain skills, imagine a watchmaker bent over his work. His left-brain visual skills for fine spatial resolution help him focus on the miniature gears and wheels that glisten in the bright light of the workbench. The auditory portions of his left brain are activated as he half-hears the confused clicking of multiple clocks around him, then focuses on the tiny, closer ticking made by the watch in his hands. He draws on his left-brain somatosensory skills to lightly touch and rearrange the myriad watch components, and depends on left-brain motor skills for the fine-motor-control tasks performed primarily by his right hand, crucial for working in this small space, with its microscopic margins for error.

For such a job, multitasking is not important – rather, focusing on the job at hand, shutting out all extraneous and potentially distracting stimuli, is the way to guarantee that the job will be done well. For this left-brain task, there is no wider sphere than the work on the bench, the minuscule sounds and visual patterns, the precise movement of the fingers on his right hand, the tiny motions of the watch's parts. In the next chapter, we will see it is not accidental that the watchmaker we've drawn here is a man – this type of focused, 'islanded function' that serves the watchmaker so well may be the very effect that prenatal testosterone is 'designed' to accomplish in a unique and powerful way.

Anatomical brain asymmetries and testosterone: overview

The last 50 years have seen a dramatic increase in the number of individuals from many professions who have become interested in the neurological bases of human behavior, including educators, psychologists, and neurologists. Many theories about how brain organization supports behavior have stressed the importance of brain asymmetries, the differences in the specializations of the two sides of the brain that we've described above. While many researchers have studied the behavioral and physiological characteristics of functional asymmetries (using methods such as presenting different types of visual patterns to the eyes, or different kinds of sounds to the ears), others have focused on features of the brain itself, including anatomical asymmetries in certain parts of the brain, with the suggestion that these might offer clues to brain organization underlying differences in functional asymmetries, and perhaps even provide insight into the developmental time course of these features.

'Perisylvian' asymmetries. In particular, certain portions of the brain surrounding the large groove on the side of the brain known as the Sylvian fissure have been identified as showing a systematic pattern of asymmetries from person to person. These perisylvian (pS) regions have been recognized for more than a century as crucial for many aspects of speech and language – they include auditory areas, regions important for motor control and sensory feedback for the face and vocal folds, and areas needed for language perception and production. The same regions have also been a focus of interest in functional asymmetries, for instance, it is known that damage to these areas on the right side of the brain does not always give the same results as left-sided damage.

Early studies of pS anatomical asymmetries, based on dissected brains, provided evidence for three types of patterns: 1) cases where one or more of the pS areas was larger in volume on the right side (a 'right-brain advantage');

2) brains in which those same areas were larger in volume on the left side ('left-brain advantage'); and 3) instances where the volume of those areas was approximately the same on both sides (the 'symmetrical' brain). Soon it was reported that the same patterns seen in dissected brains could also be measured noninvasively in living subjects, using magnetic resonance imaging (MRI).

In the research on these anatomical asymmetries, it has been noted that for most of the groups of individuals studied, the pattern most frequently observed was the one where the volume of the region was larger on the left side. In fact, some of the brains were very much larger on the left. The repeated observations of a majority of left-favoring brains, seen from experiment to experiment, has led most researchers in this area to conclude that the 'left-favoring' pattern is the standard ('normal'), and that the other two types (symmetrical and right-favoring) should be considered as nonstandard and predictably associated with disordered function (thus 'abnormal'). (Note that researchers drawing these conclusions did not settle on actual numbers regarding their predicted proportions of standard vs. nonstandard. Results reported in one early paper showed a distribution of: 63% left-favoring, 33% symmetric, and 4% right-favoring.)

It is not at all clear why such conclusions arose from this research, since most of the brains that were the subject of these earlier studies represented *biased samples*. Specifically, they were either autopsy brains (for example, adult brains from a hospital morgue, or spontaneously aborted fetuses – both questionable with regard to their "standard" nature), or from groups of individuals for whom the 'volunteer bias' may be crucial – people who volunteer to take part in scientific experiments are recognized to represent a sub-set of the general population, with predictably common characteristics such as a willingness to take risks. As we will see later, it may not be at all surprising that such individuals (the risk-taking volunteers as well as those whose brains ended up in autopsy series) included a majority of left-favoring brains.

It is also difficult to understand the conclusions we've cited regarding "normal" and "abnormal" asymmetry patterns, since few of the early reports in this literature documented any other features from the owners of the brains studied, such as handedness, gender, personality, etc. – and such contexts continue to be poorly represented even in later studies. Most surprisingly (and perhaps most tellingly), there are few reports of pS asymmetries studied in women, and none at all that attempt to sample people who might represent a broad spectrum of entirely normal individual differences, such as different categories of handedness, choice of profession, or areas of excellence which might be associated with differences in neural organization. (The interpretation of research results on pS asymmetries is also hampered by *methodological differences across experiments*, the same difficulty that has led some researchers to declare that functional asymmetries in general do not exist. In pS research, those differences include the choice of specific anatomical regions used from study to study, and the criteria governing how the measurements are done.)

Those caveats aside (for now – we will return to them later), researchers immediately posed three obvious questions regarding the nature of pS asymmetries: 1) When does the pattern of asymmetry/symmetry first appear – is it created after or before birth? 2) What controls which asymmetry/symmetry pattern develops in a particular individual? and 3) How are these anatomical differences related to other types of features in the same individuals, such as general health, aspects of behavior, or clinical conditions?

The answer to the first question was provided by the research as it progressed – the same three patterns of anatomical asymmetry found in adults could also be found in human fetuses (from terminated pregnancies), establishing that this aspect of brain structure was definitely created prenatally. Such results also led researchers to conclude that this type of brain anatomy was fixed by birth, and did not change, barring neurological injury, throughout life. This led to the very exciting concept that one might be able to measure such patterns, using a noninvasive method such as magnetic resonance imaging, at any time in a person's life, and derive clues about how that brain grew before birth.

The GBG Model of perisylvian asymmetries. With relation to the second two questions, a group of collaborators (Geschwind, Behan, and Galaburda) offered some tentative answers, framed in their (GBG) model first described in detail in 1985, and summarized in book form in 1987 (see under Galaburda in the chapter bibliography). These scientists had conducted some of the early anatomical studies on pS asymmetries, working with adult brains from a hospital morgue. To create their model, they combined these findings with results from other laboratories, plus their own extensive clinical observations of adults with neurological disorders, and children with learning disorders.

The authors began by noting that these clinical populations were notable for a predominance of males. They also pointed out that many boys with learning disorders also had immune problems, such as allergies, and that left-handedness or ambidexterity was more common among this group than in the general population. They noted further, that for those neurological patients who had most difficulty recovering from brain damage, the majority were males – even when suffering comparable damage, women seemed to recover more quickly and more completely.

To explain these differences, and to put them in the context of the anatomical pS asymmetries which they and others had measured, the GBG group turned to experimental findings from the same set of multidisciplinary sciences known as psychoimmunoneuroendocrinology (PINE) that we've reviewed in this chapter. As we've said, these sciences emphasize the importance of sex hormones as organizational agents for shaping the brain and influencing immune function, during prenatal as well as postnatal life. The GBG model took two observations from this literature: 1) while estrogens serve as 'growth hormones' in the brain, androgens (such as testosterone) have been shown to interfere with such effects; and 2) testosterone has also been shown to suppress immune function, including growth of the thymus gland, important for immune response during childhood.

Geschwind had already become famous for his theories about "disconnection syndromes" in the brain, in which certain types of neurological symptoms were attributed to breakdowns in the connections between different brain areas. The GBG model for pS asymmetries represented an extension of this idea, and suggested that high levels of prenatal testosterone could interfere with brain connectivity in such a way as to change the patterns of brain asymmetry.

The GBG model made some very specific predictions about these effects. It suggested: 1) under "normal" levels of testosterone (never really defined – we will address this in a moment), the brain of a developing fetus should grow to have the pS regions larger on the left; 2) high levels of testosterone during pregnancy would slow growth selectively on the left side; 3) as a result of this left-side slowing, regions on the right side were allowed to begin getting larger, eventually leading to a brain which was symmetrical, or even in rare instances, one which actually favored the right side.

In support of these predictions, the authors offered a wide range of observations from clinical populations, combined with data from the PINE literature regarding the effects of sex hormones on the brain. They acknowledged that while their model was based on a great deal of evidence, it was still highly speculative given the state of knowledge in these areas. They consistently pointed out its highly predictive nature, and encouraged other researchers to test its hypotheses through examination of a variety of populations using all the techniques currently available to students of brain and behavior.

The GBG model excited a great deal of interest and controversy, and also increased research activity of just the sort its authors called for. While there have been many proponents of the model, other researchers have expressed concern about some curious oversights. For example, in spite of its apparent breadth of scope, there is a notable lack of attention to many aspects of 'normal' human behavior which were targeted in earlier literature on individual differences – personality, special skills, susceptibility to disorders other than learning problems or those involving immune function.

Also, some of the clinical observations seem curious; for example, children with reading problems don't usually seem to be what one would call 'high-testosterone' people. On the contrary, these boys are often gentle and shy, with good social skills but slow in certain specific abilities related to reading (we will talk much more about this later). When considered from these points of view, the GBG model appears to be self-limiting to a rather surprising extent, given its invocation of such basic neurobiological mechanisms.

Another self-limiting factor, certainly in the early work, and one which is perhaps the most glaring and most difficult to understand, is the almost total lack of reference to women, either in the populations discussed by the GBG authors, or the mechanisms invoked. The active agent in the GBG model is prenatal testosterone, and the authors do posit that there is a continuum of prenatal exposure. But they never refer directly to the complete range of this continuum (from zero to high), only the distinction between 'normal' levels of testosterone vs. 'high' levels. They do not address the question of brains that develop in the relative absence of any testosterone at all – predictably the case for most females. This is disturbingly reminiscent of a basic flaw which has affected virtually all biomedical research for the past century, and has only recently been addressed by U.S. funding agencies, that is, the general and widespread practice of excluding girls and women as subjects in biomedical research.

It is possible that the authors might say in response to this objection, that the left-favoring brain pattern is so robust that any testosterone levels ranging from zero to moderate will allow the brain to assume its left-favoring 'standard' form, and that only at very high levels does testosterone act to slow down left-sided growth. They might say this, but to my knowledge, the question has never been raised and no such explanation has ever been given.

In fact, another curiosity is that subsequent research reports from other laboratories which took the correctness of the GBG model as a given, often failed to report the gender of experimental subjects – another cause for suspicion regarding the difficulty which the GBG model had with explaining "standard" female development. In spite of continuing interest in this area, and a variety of experiments designed either to follow up on the model's hypotheses in humans, or explore whether other primates exhibit the same type of asymmetry (some do), many of the predictions of the GBG model remain to be tested, and many questions regarding the significance of such asymmetries remain to be answered.

Chapter Two Summary: Taking stock

In this chapter, we have seen that: 1) during prenatal growth of the human brain, it is possible for the developing brain to be exposed to testosterone, with important consequences for multiple aspects of brain structure and function; 2) changes in the patterns of connectivity within the brain, such as those created by prenatal testosterone, can have dramatic effects on behavior; 3) specializations of the right vs. the left sides of the brain are quite different from each other, and are important in a wide variety of features of everyday life, ranging from general health to special skills; and 4) other researchers have recognized the possible link between brain asymmetries and prenatal testosterone.

In the next chapter, we will combine the areas of research reviewed here, to reveal a new way of describing (and accounting for) not only individual differences, but also three major categories of individuals.

Chapter Two Bibliography

[Note: As mentioned in the Preface, the following list is in no way intended as a complete representation of all the literatures relevant to the topics covered in this chapter, but only to provide references to: (1) works mentioned in the text, or from my personal library, representing sources of information used in my teaching (including anatomy and physiology; and development, including embryology) and for writing the chapter; and (2) citations from my own research that led to the theoretical models described. For understanding the latter, note that references to brain-imaging studies, using methods such as repeated evoked potentials (REPs), qEEG, and PET, are part of my research describing dynamic relations along the three organizational axes of the nervous system (the Handshaking Model); and references to my work on brain asymmetries – 'ear advantages,' etc. – are about the EPIC Model.]

Arey LB (1937) Developmental anatomy, 3rd ed. Philadelphia PA: WB Saunders Co.
Arnold AP, J Xu, W Grisham, X Chen, Y-H Kim, Y Itoh (2004) Minireview: Sex chromosomes and brain sexual differentiation. Endocrinology 145 (3): 1057-62.
Bosma JF, J Showacre (1976) Symposium on development of upper respiratory anatomy and function. Washington DC: National Institute of Child Health and Human Development.
Bryden MP, IC McManus, MB Bolman-Fleming (1994) Evaluating the empirical support for the Geschwind-Behan-Galaburda model of cerebral lateralization. Brain & Cognition 26: 103-167.
Davidson RJ & K Hugdahl (Eds) (1995) Brain asymmetry. Cambridge MA: MIT Press. [see especially: W Wittling, "Brain asymmetry in the control of autonomic-physiologic activity," pp. 305-357; and M Hiscock & M Kinsbourne, "Phylogeny and ontogeny of cerebral lateralization," pp. 535-578].
Davies J (1957) Embryology of the head and neck in relation to the practice of otolaryngology. San Francisco CA: American Academy of Ophthalmology & Otolaryngology.
De Kloet ER & W Sutanto (Eds) (1994) Neurobiology of steroids. San Diego CA: Academic Press.
DeGroot LJ (Ed) Endocrinology, 3rd ed. (1995) [3 volumes] Philadelphia PA: WB Saunders.

Edelman GM, VB Mountcastle (1978) The mindful brain; Cortical organization and the group-selective theory of higher brain function. Cambridge MA: MIT Press.

Efron R (1990) The decline and fall of hemispheric specialization. Hillsdale NJ: Lawrence Erlbaum Assoc, Pubs.

Finger S (1994) Origins of neuroscience: A history of explorations into brain function. Oxford: Oxford Univ. Press.

Galaburda AM & N Geschwind (1986) Cerebral lateralization; Biological mechanisms, associations, and pathology. Cambridge MA: MIT Press.

Griffin JE & SR Ojeda (Eds) (1996) Textbook of endocrinology, 3rd ed. NY: Oxford Univ. Press.

Hawkins LK, JL Lauter (1999) The effects of age upon ABR waveform latency stability. Tejas 23: 56-68.

Hugdahl K & RJ Davidson (Eds) (2003) The asymmetrical brain. Cambridge MA: MIT Press.

Jacobson M (1978) Developmental neurobiology, 2nd ed. NY: Plenum Press.

Kalthoff K (1996) Analysis of biological development. NY: McGraw-Hill, Inc.

Kalthoff K (2001) Analysis of biological development, 2nd ed. Boston: McGraw-Hill, Inc.

Kluge AG, BE Frye, K Johansen, KF Liem, CR Noback, ID Olsen, AJ Waterman. Chordate structure and function, 2nd ed. NY: Macmillan Pub. Co, Inc.

Lauter JL (1982) Dichotic identification of complex sounds: absolute and relative ear advantages. J Acoust Soc Amer 71: 701-707.

Lauter JL (1983) Stimulus characteristics and relative ear advantages: a new look at old data. J Acoust Soc Amer 74: 1-17.

Lauter JL (1984) Contralateral interference and ear advantages for identification of three element patterns. Brain & Cognition 3: 259-280.

Lauter JL, P Herscovitch, C Formby, ME Raichle (1985) Tonotopic organization in human auditory cortex revealed by positron emission tomography. Hearing Res 20: 199-205.

Lauter JL, IJ Hirsh (1985) Speech as temporal pattern: A psychoacoustical profile. Speech Communication 4: 41-54.

Lauter JL, RL Loomis (1986) Individual differences in auditory electric responses: comparisons of between-subject and within-subject variability. I. Absolute latencies of brainstem vertex-positive peaks. Scand Audiol 15: 167-172.

Lauter JL, RL Loomis (1988) Individual differences in auditory electric responses: comparisons of between-subject and within-subject variability. II. Amplitudes of brainstem vertex-positive peaks. Scand Audiol 17: 87-92.

Lauter JL, P Herscovitch, ME Raichle (1988) Human auditory physiology studied with positron emission tomography. *In* J Syka & RB Masterton (Eds) Auditory pathway. NY: Plenum; pp. 313-7.

Lauter JL (1990) Auditory system. *In* AL Perlman & RC Collins (Eds) The neurobiology of disease. NY: Oxford Univ. Press, pp. 101-123.

Lauter JL, RG Karzon (1990a) Individual differences in auditory electric responses: comparisons of between-subject and within-subject variability. III. A replication, and observations on individual vs. group characteristics. Scand Audiol 19: 67-72.

Lauter JL, RG Karzon (1990b) Individual differences in auditory electric responses: comparisons of between-subject and within-subject variability. IV. Latency variability comparisons in early, middle, and late responses. Scand Audiol 19: 175-182.

Lauter JL, RG Karzon (1990c) Individual differences in auditory electric responses: comparisons of between-subject and within-subject variability. V. Amplitude variability comparisons in early, middle, and late responses. Scand Audiol 19: 201-206.

Lauter JL (1992) Processing asymmetries for complex sounds: Comparisons between behavioral testing results and electroencephalography (qEEG). Brain & Cognition 19:1-20.

Lauter JL, RF Oyler (1992) Latency stability of auditory brainstem responses in children aged 10-12 years compared with younger children and adults. Brit J Audiol 26:245-253.

Lauter JL, RF Oyler, JM Lord-Maes (1993) Amplitude stability of auditory brainstem responses in two groups of children compared with adults. Brit J Audiol 27:263-271.

Lauter JL (1998) Neurophysiological self-control: Modulation in all things. J Comm Disord 31:543-549.

Lauter JL, JM Lord-Maes, C Baldwin (1999) Repeated evoked potentials (REPs) in multiple sclerosis: Demonstration of a new tool for individual neurological assessment. Tejas 23: 53-60.

Lauter JL (1999) The Handshaking Model of Brain Function: Notes toward a theory. Med Hypoth 52:435-445.

Lauter JL (2000) The AXS battery and neurological fingerprints: Meeting the challenge of individual differences in human brain/behavior relations. Behav Res Meth Instru Comput 32: 180-190.

Lauter JL (2004) New approaches to understanding the human brain: Three theoretical models and a test battery. In Lauter JL (Ed) All in good time: A tribute to Ira Hirsh. Sem Hearing 25:269-280.

Lauter JL (2007) The EPIC model of functional asymmetries: Implications for research on laterality in the auditory and other systems. Frontiers in Bioscience 12:3734-3756.

Levine JL, RL Kurtz, JL Lauter (1984) Hypnosis and its effect on left and right hemisphere activity. Biol Psychiat 19: 1461-1475.

McEwen BS (1994) Steroid hormone effects on brain: Novel insights connecting cellular and molecular features of brain cells to behavior. In ER De Kloet, W Sutanto (Eds), Neurobiology of steroids. San Diego CA: Academic Press, pp. 525-542.

McKittrick CR & BS McEwen (1996) Regulation of serotonergic function in the CNS by steroid hormones and stress. In TW Stone (Ed) CNS neurotransmitters and neuromodulators; Neuroactive steroids. Boca Raton: CRC Press, pp. 37-76.

MacLean PD (1973) A triune concept of the brain and behavior. Toronto: Univ. of Toronto Press..

MacLean PD (1990) The triune brain in evolution; Role in paleocerebral functions. NY: Plenum.

McCulloch WS (1965) Embodiments of mind. Cambridge MA: MIT Press. [see especially: J Lettvin, HR Maturana, WS McCulloch, WH Pitts, "What the frog's eye tells the frog's brain," pp. 230-255].

Montagu A (1986) Touching; The human significance of the skin. 3rd ed. NY: Harper & Row.

Moore KL (1977) The developing human; Clinically oriented embryology, 2nd ed. Philadelphia PA: WB Saunders Co.

Nishimura H, R Semba, T Tanimura, O Tanaka (1977) Prenatal development of the human with special reference to craniofacial structures: An atlas. Washington DC: National Institutes of Health.

Oyler RF, JL Lauter, ND Matkin (1990) Intrasubject variability in the absolute latency of the auditory brainstem response. J Amer Acad Aud 2: 206-213.

Palfai T, H Jankiewicz (1997) Drugs and human behavior, 2nd ed. Madison WI: Brown & Benchmark, Pubs.

Papalia DE, SW Olds, RD Feldman (9th ed) Human development. Boston: McGraw-Hill.

Patten BM, BM Carlson (1974) Foundations of embryology, 3rd ed. NY: McGraw-Hill.

Payne AP (1996) Gonadal hormones and the sexual differentiation of the nervous system: Mechanisms and interactions. In TW Stone (Ed) CNS neurotransmitters and neuromodulators; Neuroactive steroids. Boca Raton: CRC Press, pp. 163 175.

Rao MS, M Jacobson (Eds) (2005) Developmental neurobiology; 4th ed. NY: Kluwer Academic / Plenum Pubs.

Ridley M (1999) Genome; The autobiography of a species in 23 chapters. NY: HarperCollins Pubs., Inc.

Ridley M (2003) Nature via nurture; Genes, experience, and what makes us human. NY: HarperCollins Pubs., Inc.

Segalowitz SJ (1983) Two sides of the brain; Brain lateralization explored. Englewood Cliffs NJ: Prentice-Hall, Inc.

Sergent J, MC Corballis (1991). 10 ups and downs in cerebral lateralization. In FL Kitterle (Ed), Cerebral laterality: Theory & research. Mahwah NJ: Lawrence Erlbaum Associates, Inc. [for an opposing view, cf. TenHouten entry]

Sexton E (2001) Dawkins and the selfish gene. Cambridge: Icon Books.

Steinberg R (Ed) Music and the mind machine; The psychophysiology and psychopathology of the sense of music. Berlin: Springer-Verlag.

Taylor J (Ed) (1958) Selected writings of John Hughlings Jackson (2 vols). London: Staples Press.

TenHouten WD (1992) Cerebral lateralization: A scientific paradigm in crisis? Critique of Efron and Corballis. J Social Evolutionary Sys I-5(3):319-326.

Torrey TW (1971) Morphogenesis of the vertebrates, 3rd ed. NY: John Wiley & Sons.

Woolley CS, E Gould (1994) Steroid action on neuronal structure. In ER De Kloet, W Sutanto (Eds), Neurobiology of steroids. San Diego CA: Academic Press, pp. 83-402.

* * *

Chapter Two Tables
(titles abbreviated; for full versions, see originals in the text)

❧

◈ Chapter Three ◈

THE TRIMODAL MODEL OF BRAIN ORGANIZATION:
THREE BRAIN TYPES, SIX GENDERS

In the last chapter, we saw that sex hormones can influence the brain during early development, including impacting connectivity, and we discussed the different patterns of connections linking different parts of the brain, summarized in a new approach to specializations of the right vs. the left sides. We also reviewed one previous attempt to explain certain aspects of individual differences as the effects of prenatal testosterone.

This chapter will introduce a new set of conclusions known as the *Trimodal Model of Brain Organization*, which forms a fundamental part of Neural Rainbow Theory. The Trimodal Model (TM) draws on both the Handshaking Model of Brain Function, and the EPIC Model of Brain Asymmetries (both discussed in Chapter Two) to describe how individual differences in prenatal exposure to sex hormones may influence all the versions of brain connectivity discussed in Chapter Two, to create: 1) a *continuum* (a 'rainbow') of individual differences involving *clusters of features*, including general health, gender behavior, social behavior, and special skills; 2) *three major divisions* of that continuum (*three 'brain types'*), just as the continuous spectrum of a rainbow can be divided into a few main colors; and 3) because sex hormones are identified as the active agents, this process is said to result in a total of *six genders* – that is, the three brain types as expressed (to different degrees) in each of the two chromosomal genders. (Although much of our discussion will focus on humans, the general principles of TM are considered to apply to all animals, to be further explained in Chapter Four.)

Sex hormones and the developing brain

Although the Trimodal Model (TM) component of Neural Rainbow Theory takes its departure from the work on perisylvian (pS) anatomical asymmetries described at the end of Chapter Two, it interprets those data in very different ways, and addresses a much wider range of behavior in humans (and other animals) than did most previous studies of brain asymmetries. To do this, the Trimodal Model utilizes the descriptions of four domains of *functional* (i.e., physiological and behavioral) asymmetries provided by the EPIC model outlined in Chapter Two.

Brain connectivity and asymmetries

To see what the Trimodal Model predicts, and prepare to understand how it contributes to the broader conclusions of Neural Rainbow Theory, let's recall what we discussed in Chapter Two about the relation between brain connectivity and the right/left specializations of the EPIC model. First, it was noted that the right brain starts developing before birth earlier than the left side, and seems to predominate in overall brain and body control until well into the second year of life.

Second, regarding the EPIC specializations, we described the right side as 'polypotent,' with a larger 'job description' than the left side – not only is the right side uniquely responsible for three of the four EPIC domains (one of which is general health), it also oversees the coordination between its three domains, and the single domain for which the left brain is responsible.

Third, we described body/brain connectivity in terms of dynamic links affecting all three body/brain axes: head-to-tail, right-to-left, and back-to-front, and suggested that the right side of the brain seems to be important for coordinating these types of connectivity, as well. Specifically, it was predicted that if the right brain is predominant in a person, all three axes of connection will be able to work in a resilient, 'teamwork' manner, and all skills will be available, whether based on the left or the right side of the brain. Given this arrangement – all depending on nurturing oversight and coordination by the right brain – the body and brain are assured maximum flexibility of response to different situations, combined with maximum accuracy of all types of sensory perception and motor performance.

From this overview, it is clear that there are several ways the Trimodal Model differs from the GBG model reviewed in Chapter Two, and other previous interpretations of asymmetries. First and perhaps most importantly, TM places a *much higher value on the right side of the brain* than did earlier approaches (which tended to privilege left-side abilities as more 'advanced' and thus more important than the those of the 'primitive' right side). Because of the right brain's polypotent responsibilities, and especially its roles in coordination and general health, TM sees the right brain as the 'mother' of the brain and body, overseeing a much wider range of functions than the left, making it a fundamental component of the nervous system, crucial for survival. In this, the right brain is seen as analogous to the X sex chromosome – not only is the presence of two X chromosomes necessary for a female embryo to be healthy, but even in males, at least one X is required if the fetus is to survive – it can grow without the y chromosome, but if the X is missing, it will die.

Second, TM uses the Handshaking and EPIC models introduced in Chapter Two to *broaden the significance of brain asymmetries* into a *global picture* of right/left relations affecting many more individual characteristics than the few mentioned in previous research. (With specific reference to pS anatomical asymmetries – whatever the final consensus as to their nature and significance – TM interprets these as simply one index of how the two *complete* halves of the brain develop and are related.)

Third, while the GBG model invoked a range of testosterone exposure from the 'naturally low' value predicted to be typical of 'normal' *males*, to very high in individuals with disorders, TM again expands the concept of a continuum of hormone exposure to include (actually, beginning with) a *hormone-free state*, predictably typical of a large number of *females*.

Related to this, the only 'normal' brain type in the GBG model was the 'typical male' one created with 'naturally low (but still male)' levels of T exposure – where the sole definition of 'normal' was 'disorder-free.' In contrast, TM provides a way of including all brains, XX and well as Xy, no matter their functional profiles, within the same generative model, all shaped by variations in prenatal hormonal exposure.

'Gendering the brain'

For TM, chromosomal sex is important only as an index of *absolute levels* of hormone exposure (because of prenatal testes action, male embryos are *all* exposed to much higher T overall than female embryos can be). Of greater significance, however, is the *relative level* of exposure within the two categories of absolute level (that is, +/- testes), based on the prediction that the *patterns of relative exposure* – the 'three modes' of 'Trimodal,' the 'three brain types' we've mentioned – are *exactly analogous in both chromosomal genders*.

This point is most easily visualized in the form of a 'periodic chart' (see Figure 3.1) with two rows based on chromosomal identity (representing the bimodal distribution of *absolute* levels of testosterone – i.e., higher overall in Xys than in XXs), and three columns representing the *relative* levels of T exposure, from lower to moderate to higher (as we'll see in a moment, the three categories of relative levels of T will become the basis for the three TM brain types). [The analogy here is the periodic chart of the elements, where the rows are based on ranges of atomic weights, and the columns refer to 'families' of elements where members of the same 'family' are similar in physical appearance and chemical 'behavior' because they have the same number of electrons on their outer shells. On that analogy, one might refer to the value which in Fig. 3.1 increases from right to left, and from upper row to lower, as the 'testosterone weight' experienced by an individual during development.]

Perhaps the best way to think about this process is that these brain adjustments, because they are based on sex hormones, are *all* related to 'gender.' And once we see, in the next section, how distinctive brain types can be, how they are expressed in a whole host of individual characteristics – some with life-and-death consequences – we can recognize this process as a crucial part of the development of every individual.

Figure 3.1
Periodic chart of 6 levels of prenatal testosterone (T)

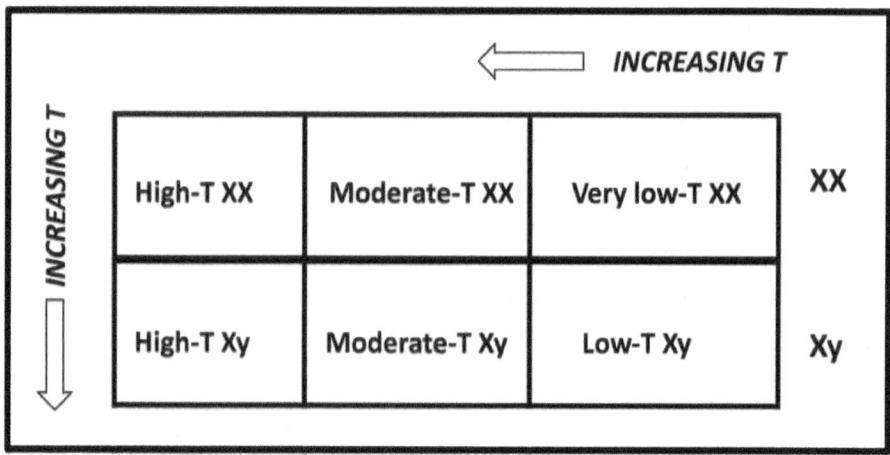

Thus TM frees the concept of 'gender' from being limited to (and determined by) the static 'sexual identity' of sex chromosomes, and suggests instead that it should be recognized as the result of a *dynamic, epigenetic process* in which a range of hormonal exposures is used *in a slightly different way in every embryo* to shape versions of the three brain types, for *both* chromosomal identities. TM calls this hormonally-based process of interactions between absolute and relative levels of sex hormones (ranging from zero to high) 'gendering the brain,' with the result that, at least for those species (such as most modern-day humans) which make all three brain types, *there are not just two genders, but six.*

The idea of 'six genders' may sound radical, but we need to remember the baby mice treated with the 'opposite' sex hormone (see Chapter Two). And we will see later in this chapter that brain types can be so distinctive in terms of individual features of health, psychology, and behavior that individuals often 'cross the chromosomal line' – i.e., some chromosomal females can be more like certain types of chromosomal males than they are like certain other females, and vice versa.

As a result, the six categories of individuals described by TM are as real as chromosomal genders – in fact, more functionally 'real' or 'distinct,' in that they are internally consistent in a way that chromosomal genders alone are not (as the chart reminds us, there are [at least] *three versions of XX* individuals, and [at least] *three versions of Xy*, a fact that may have been largely responsible for much of the confusion characterizing studies of 'sex differences in the brain,' etc.).

Of course, the most obvious manifestation of the variation within chromosomal gender is the 'gender rainbow' that the LGBTQ+ community has been working to raise consciousness about for decades now. It is to be hoped that the many details involved in TM's three brain types, as an aid for identifying 'clusters' of individuals along the continuum, will serve as yet another a source of evidence corroborating the biological fact that brains which develop in diverse hormonal environments will naturally be diverse.

In talking about 'six genders,' it is crucial to remember that, as with the six iconic colors in a rainbow, this focus on a *few categories* should still be understood as representing a *continuum* – TM simply uses *three* brain types and *six* genders to denote 'targets' of the process, not limits to the possibilities. Even the two categories of 'chromosomal gender' – XX and Xy – do not exhaust all the possibilities of genetic variation involving sex chromosomes, especially not when applied to non-human animals (for example, in birds, the individuals who lay eggs are ZW and their partners are ZZ – and we can expect there are variations within those as well).

[The concepts of TM and the supporting research are in their very earliest stages, and the epigenetics of individual variation – the domain of TM – are only just beginning to be studied. In no way can one say that any of these things is well enough understood to draw any kind of final conclusions – and yet, a distinction between two chromosomal genders *does* seem to be important to biology (for animals who use sexual reproduction, a large segment of the population makes eggs, and an equally large segment makes sperm), and we'll see that there *do* seem to be many details about the way that humans as well as other animals develop, behave, and organize themselves in space that, when viewed in the right way – and when considered *together* instead of being studied in isolation from each other – suggest that something like the three 'brain types' does indeed exist.

People DO resemble each other in the ways TM talks about, in addition to being individually unique. TM and Neural Rainbow Theory are simply my own attempts to make a best guess about this fascinating topic, a guess based on the data I've collected in my laboratories, my observations in labs, clinics, classrooms and life in general, and what I've learned about what has been reported by others – whether in the humanities, the social sciences (which to me include the psychology and 'sociology' of other animals), and biology in general. I hope as a scientist I am always humble, and remain open-minded about how future knowledge may transform anything we conclude now; but, like Darwin, I still want to 'make a beginning' – to put down what I think about what I know, inadequate as it might be, to try to figure out what it all might mean.]

To illustrate the TM concept of 'six genders,' Figure 3.2 adds to Fig. 3.1 by providing brain-type labels (one for each column – names will be explained later) and gender numbers (inside the cells: #s1-6, numbered in order from lowest to highest T), showing how the format is indeed like a periodic chart: 3 brain-type columns x 2 chromosomal-gender rows, with the progression from column to column, and from row to row, *based on the same underlying variable*: increasing amounts of T exposure – both from individual to individual, and within one individual over time.

Figure 3.2
Periodic chart of 6 levels of prenatal testosterone (T):
3 brain types x 2 chromosomal genders =
6 genders

	Focal	Middle	Polytropic	
INCREASING T	High-T XX *Gender 3*	Moderate-T XX *Gender 2*	Very low-T XX *Gender 1*	**XX**
	High-T Xy *Gender 6*	Moderate-T Xy *Gender 5*	Low-T Xy *Gender 4*	**Xy**

⇐ **INCREASING T**

Figure 3.3 (next page) is essentially the same chart as Figs. 3.1 & 3.2, but with even more information – this version is essentially the Trimodal Model in a nutshell. As in Fig. 3.2, the two rows are labelled for XX and Xy, the arrows indicate changes in absolute T, increasing from right to left, and from top (XXs in row 1) to bottom (Xys in row 2). The columns now have two sets of labels, both useful for discussing the TM concept of brain types. The lower labels – *left-favoring, symmetric, right-favoring* – refer to the vocabulary of asymmetry patterns as used in the earlier literature (such as for pS asymmetries). The upper labels – *focal, middle, polytropic* – are the new terms developed for TM, summarizing the characteristic 'style' of each brain type.

The trapezoid shapes that now fill the six cells add even more detail. They are designed as 'fingerprints' of each brain type, to indicate the pattern of *degree of access* each brain type has to the capabilities described in the EPIC model: right-side triangles refer to right-brain abilities, left-side triangles are for left-brain skills, and the middle triangles represent a particular set of skills TM associates with moderate T exposure, for XX as well as Xy individuals (more later). Note that although each chromosomal gender has its own versions of the three brain types, the crucial outcome is the *analogies in the brain types shared across chromosomal genders*. We will return to this figure later, as we talk more about how the six genders are made, and exactly what representative individuals are like, as we further develop the argument that there truly are six categories of individuals.

Figure 3.3
Skill 'fingerprints' for 3 brain types
and 2 chromosomal genders,
based on differential access to right/left specializations
as described by the EPIC Model

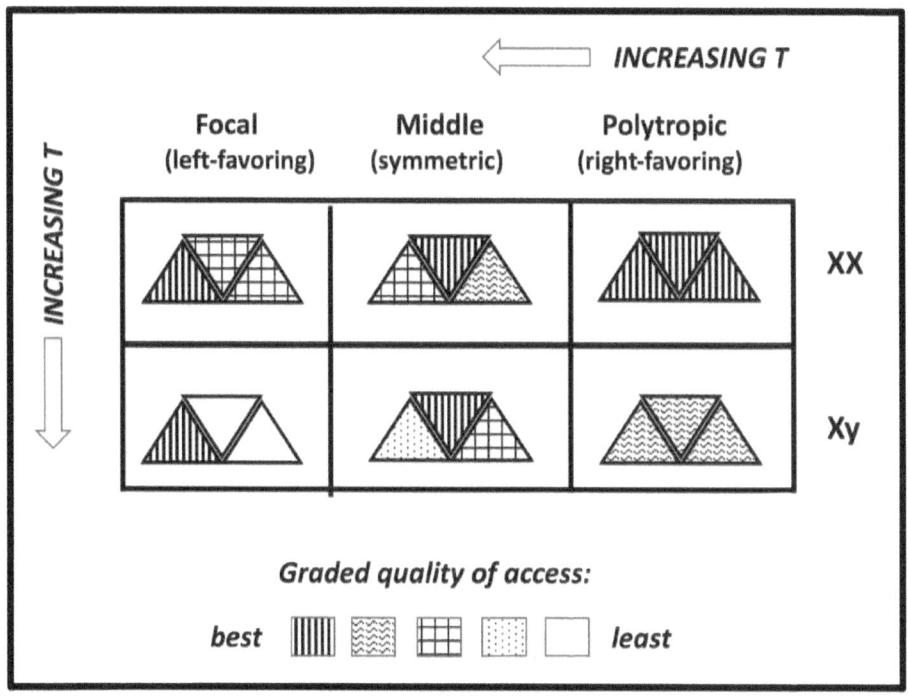

The pattern of variation illustrated in Figs. 3.1, 3.2, and 3.3 that is new is *not* the two rows – given the information that brains in both XX and Xy fetuses are protected from exposure to estrogens, but Xy fetal testes can produce high levels of T, anyone could predict there would be two rows.

The pattern of variation that *is* new is the columns – the brain types – and especially the prediction that brain types *cut across the rows* – that is, analogues of each brain type can be found in both chromosomal genders – and also that for each row, the same three brain types are *created by the same mechanism* (lower vs. middle vs. higher levels of T exposure), with analogous results in terms of individual anatomical, physiological, and behavioral profiles.

Finally, TM predicts that these patterns of variation have population distributions that vary from species to species (discussed further in Chapter Four). For most modern *human* societies, the distribution of brain types overall (collapsed over the two chromosomal genders) is predicted to be as shown in Figure 3.4, with each brain type represented in approximately 1/3 of the population.

Figure 3.4
Proportions of the 3 'iconic' brain types
in the general population

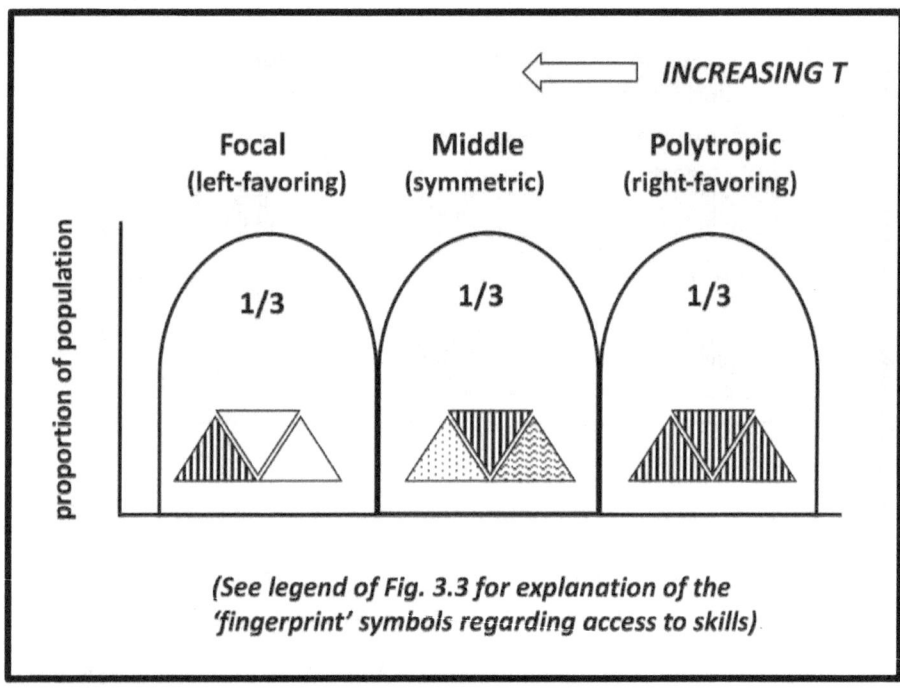

(See legend of Fig. 3.3 for explanation of the
'fingerprint' symbols regarding access to skills)

And Figure 3.5 (next page) displays the predicted relative proportions of brain types (the 'fingerprint' symbols now omitted for clarity) within separate populations of the two chromosomal genders:

Figure 3.5
Predicted relative proportions of 3 brain types
in XX vs. Xy populations

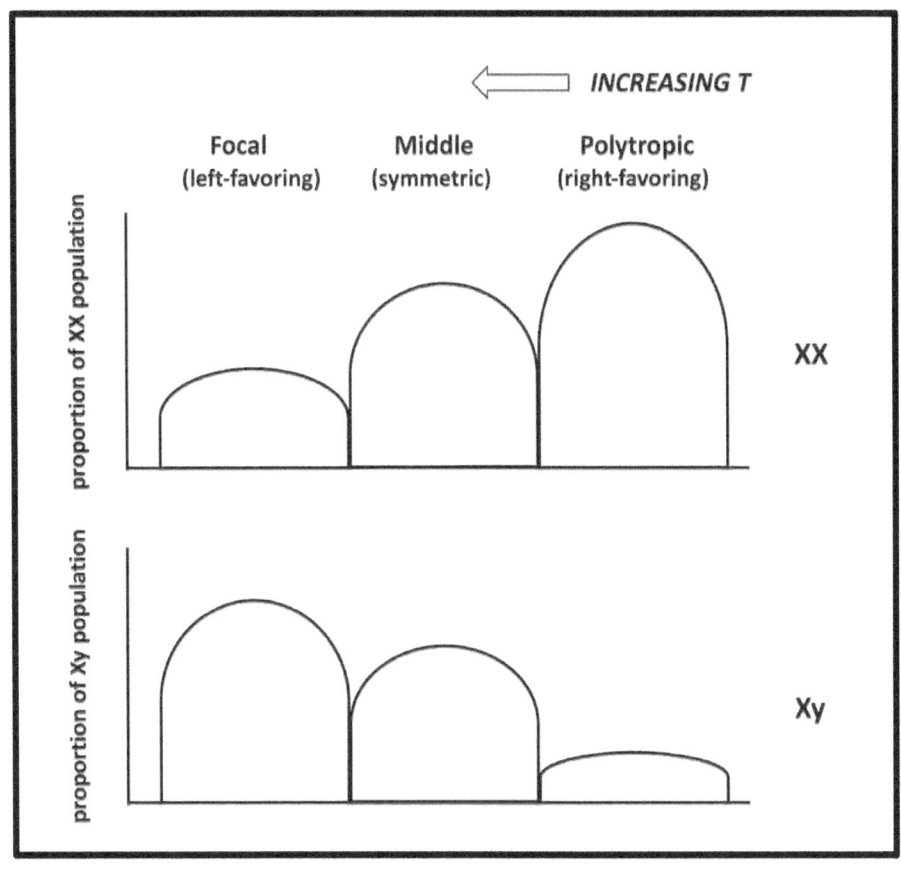

Making three brain types, shaping six genders

Now in order to see how TM describes the *development of the three brain types/six genders complex*, let's go more slowly through the process, following what happens to a developing organism exposed to different hormonal environments: either hormone-free, moderate T exposure, or high T exposure. Following that, we will describe in some detail how the 'balance of power' between the polypotent right brain vs. the left side (based on *the degree of access* to the two sides), can affect many, many aspects of anatomy, physiology, and behavior, creating the individual differences basic to TM.

It must be emphasized again at this point that the categories of individuals we will be describing – the three 'brain types,' the 'six genders' –

are ultimately based on *brain connectivity*. About this, TM makes two assumptions: 1) the original 'blueprint' for all brains calls for essentially the same *neurological modules* supporting the right/left specializations to be distributed in essentially the same way to the right and left sides of the brain, but 2) it is the difference in the *degree of access* to the different modules that accounts for the rainbow of expression of the skills and capabilities involved.

Thus if an individual has difficulty in a particular skill area (e.g., reading problems based on undeveloped phonemic awareness, or spelling errors due to incomplete mental imagery), it is not because one or another module is actually missing, but because *access* to the module, the *connectivity* that would make it available for use, has been compromised in some way (in TM, this is attributed to testosterone).

Our discussions about brain types in the rest of this chapter will emphasize *prenatal* hormonal effects on brain connectivity, primarily because TM predicts that what happens prenatally is for the most part permanent – at least regarding an individual's overall brain-type, which by the time of birth is essentially fixed. At the same time, it is helpful to think about brain types as clusters of *tendencies* – an in-born 'center of gravity' for each person, with a certain amount of *fine-tuning* yet to be made – and that 'fine-turning' can have significant consequences for personality, health, and behavior. Descriptions of the 'tendencies' of a particular brain type should be read in that way, not as something fated and final.

The hopeful thing about this approach is that: 1) it is based on *connectivity*, rather than anatomically present vs. anatomically missing abilities; and 2) brain connectivity remains *to some extent* plastic (changeable) throughout life. (After all, all forms of learning, at any age, change how parts of the brain talk to each other, and the process is the same no matter the brain type involved.)

Many things about a person's environment (education, nutrition, emotional support, hormonal events from decade to decade, etc.) can affect brain connectivity, and whether those changes are positive or negative depends on exactly what happens and when. But knowing more about the details offers the promise of objective guidelines for how to take care of ourselves and other people, for achieving and maintaining good physical and mental health, and for enjoying a full and meaningful life. If it's true that a person's basic (biological) identity – their brain type – is more or less established by birth, *and* there are still pixels in that portrait that remain to be filled in – then it is clearly left for a combination of postnatal environment, experience, and the members of the 'village that raises' each and every one of us to finish the job.

[Note that in the following discussion, I will use 'woman' and 'man' to refer to the two chromosomal genders, even though I don't believe those terms are ultimately very useful given the diversity of 'gender' described by

TM. However, until we can all agree on appropriate names for each of the six gender categories the model suggests, these will have to do. Also, in Chapter Four we will discuss the six genders further, to explore the 'why' of the process as a whole.]

1. 'Hormone-free' prenatal development (XX only): Gender One. As the nervous system begins growing in the human embryo, there are many kinds of activity that proceed in the same way no matter what the sex chromosomes of the embryo are. Nerve cells and supporting cells called glia are formed at the core of the developing nervous system, and begin migrating to their destinations, where they will take their various final forms, and help build all the different parts of the nervous system, including the brain itself. Some cells will form parts of the peripheral nervous system (PNS: nerves going to different places in the body, including the sensory organs and muscles), while others will take their places in different parts of the central nervous system (CNS: the spinal cord, and the different levels of the brain within the skull).

These cells not only gather together as particular parts of the brain, but also reach out to make connections with each other and with cells in other parts, 'wiring' the CNS, PNS, and body together. The result is a seamless web of interconnections, in which it is hard to say where the 'body' stops and the 'nervous system' begins. Body and nervous system are so highly integrated from a functional standpoint that most non-neural parts of the body would find it extremely difficult to do their job if something happened to their supply of neural energy and control.

This dependence extends well beyond parts of the body associated with sensation and muscle management, to include the major systems for survival such as digestion, cardiovascular function, respiration, reproduction, and immune response. Thus development of the brain and nervous system is intimately related to the quality and nature of development in every part of the body, and any agent which influences the nature of neural connectivity may have dramatic impacts on many basic body systems.

In shaping an XX embryo, the developmental process, left to its own devices (if there is no perturbation in the chemical environment within the uterus, including no testosterone), will create a fetus with a highly integrated brain and body, characterized by the capabilities for flexible, elastic, resilient behavior we have described above. If the process continues on without interference, the mother can expect the pregnancy to be as comfortable as possible, and culminate in a successful delivery with no complications, and the arrival of a healthy, happy baby who has every physiological resource needed to grow up into a happy, healthy human adult, with excellent access to all right- and left-brain skills.

Under the Trimodal Model, the most important agent of 'interference' in this process is prenatal testosterone, and also remember what the PINE sciences tell us about sex chromosomes vs. prenatal sex hormones – *that it is hormones not chromosomes that determine gender in the largest sense (as used by TM)*. With these in mind, we can also conclude that the individual whose development we've just described will be a woman.

Free of any interference from T, she will have the type of brain that grows to favor the right side (pS areas larger on the right, etc.), with all that implies. This type of brain, developing in a hormone-free environment, is referred to for obvious reasons by TM as 'polytropic' (meaning 'many-skilled') and also as a 'right-brain/whole-brain,' in recognition of the whole-brain coordination and oversight provided by the right side.

An individual with this type of brain will have good physical and mental health, and excellent access to all the specializations of both sides of the brain. Also, because of the very good cooperation between right and left sides of the body ensured by the coordinating influence of the right brain, she will also have good athletic skills, although she will probably not be as much of a specialist at this as other brain types can be, discussed below.

Later we will talk more about this type of brain, and the features characterizing the lucky person born a 'polytropic.' But to appreciate the nature of the polytropic brain, we need to see how other brain types are made. To do that, we need to consider what happens during development if conditions are not maintained 'hormone-free' – that is, if testosterone does in fact enter the developmental picture. For our review, we will need to keep track of whether the sex chromosomes are XX or Xy, because Xys are much more at risk regarding extremes of exposure.

2. Testosterone exposure in other XX individuals: moderate & high – Genders Two and Three. In Chapter Two, we said that one possible source of testosterone during prenatal development is the mother's adrenal cortex. The extent of adrenal-cortex testosterone production depends on the individual woman and also on her psychological environment. Some women tend to produce little or no testosterone in this way, while others seem to be very active producers – they are 'high-T women.' In some, the levels produced are fairly consistent over time (usually true for very low levels), while for other women, there can be a wide fluctuation, involving peaks of markedly elevated production (though nowhere near what testes can do). A woman's psychological environment is important since stress can affect both the adrenal gland and the adrenal cortex, and in certain cases, can result in the release of a mix of substances such as adrenalin and testosterone into her bloodstream.

Thus a developing embryo and fetus can be exposed to low to moderate amounts of testosterone from the mother's adrenal cortex. If the developing child has XX chromosomes, such exposure may result in different degrees of masculinization of both her body and brain. ('Masculinize' is only a relative term here – an XX cannot be transformed by these means into a fully-featured male, because this requires much higher levels of testosterone than can be produced by a mother's adrenal cortex; also, functional testes depend on the presence of the SRy gene, typically carried only on the y chromosome.)

However, particularly in the case of a mother whose T levels fluctuate during a pregnancy, adrenal-cortex testosterone can change the appearance of external organs such as genitals, and alter brain development. It is important to note at this point that because different body systems develop at different rates, the timing of fluctuating testosterone (whether from the mother's adrenal cortex or a fetus's own testes) during pregnancy can be very important as to which features are affected. For example, TM predicts that it's the *timing* of prenatal T exposure that creates the variation highlighted in the LGBTQ+ movement, providing a vivid expression of the within-chromosomal gender continuum. Thus all combinations along the continuum may be possible – a very male brain in a feminine body, a very feminine ('polytropic') brain in a masculine body, and everything in between.

Since the determining agent here is graded (that is, *degrees* of exposure to testosterone), not an absolute 'either-or,' the results will also be graded. As a result of this 'gendering the brain' process, there are not two genders, but many – a biological 'gender rainbow' – though, as suggested earlier, this rainbow is most helpfully summarized as a basic set of six 'colors' – the six cells of Figs. 3.1 and 3.2. (Later we will see how this same exposure continuum is reflected in many additional features of individuals.)

Before continuing to consider Xy embryos, let's review how testosterone acts to alter brain development. As outlined in Chapter Two, the PINE sciences suggest that as estrogens support brain connections and communication, androgens such as testosterone can serve as agents of disconnection. We have just described all the work of making connections between brain parts and between body and brain that go on during prenatal development (and continue being made across the life span). Testosterone can interfere with any and all of this – depending on the timing, it may prevent connections from forming before the fact, or destroy those that had already been put in place.

If the degree of testosterone exposure is low to moderate, as in the XX exposed to maternal T described above, such effects may be minimal or at least limited. The effect of moderate amounts of T may be to interfere to at least some extent with the right brain's oversight of ongoing development in the rest of the brain and body – including growth of pS regions on the left side of the brain (since the left side begins growing later than the right). If this particular aspect of right-brain control is somehow degraded by testosterone, that may allow left-side pS regions to go on growing beyond the time when (under low-T conditions) they would have stopped, so that instead of remaining smaller than on the right side, they go on enlarging.

With sufficient prenatal testosterone, left-side pS regions may come to be the same size as the right (this is predicted to happen in at least some female fetuses). These women should retain good access to right-brain skills, especially social skills, and they may have such good coordination between the two sides of the body that they are very athletic. However, the problems with connectivity introduced by their moderate levels of prenatal T might block access to at least some left-side skills, so that they may have somewhat more trouble with certain aspects of reading, for example, than the polytropic right-favoring brains.

With even higher T, pS areas on the left side may grow larger than the right (perhaps possible in a few female fetuses). These women may be good at fine-motor-control sports such as tennis, but socially somewhat less comfortable than their right-brained or symmetrical-brained sisters. Due to the lessened general-health participation of the right brain in these women, they may be the ones most at risk for cardiac problems, sleep and eating disorders, pain conditions such as migraine, temporomandibular joint pain, and premenstrual syndrome. They may also be prone to immune-system problems of several types, including autoimmune disorders and cancer.

To create either symmetrical or left-favoring brain types in XX fetuses may take less absolute testosterone than if the fetus were a male; research is needed to determine if this is true. However, it is known that there are 'moderate-T' type women, who have the feature profile we've suggested is associated with symmetrical brains (more details about this later), and there are also 'high-T' women, with features compatible with left-favoring brains.

TM also identifies an intermediate step between symmetrical and left-favoring brains, the 'left-middle' brain, found in both XX and Xys, predictably created over a certain zone of prenatal T levels, and characterized by a diverse combination of pluses and minuses regarding right-brain vs. left-brain skills (as with all brain types, those 'pluses and minuses' are to a certain extent adjustable based on events that occur after birth; more about that later). Because the features of left-middles are more marked in Xys (due to the higher overall levels of T), we will wait to discuss more about left-middles in the next section.

3. Testosterone exposure in Xy individuals: low, moderate, high – Genders Four, Five, Six. Everything we've said so far about T from the mother's adrenal cortex holds for Xys as well. But something else happens in Xys that can radically overshadow those relatively limited effects.

Around the middle of the second month of gestation (about 6 weeks PCA) in humans, the top end of the embryo's nervous system is starting to form into what will eventually become the brain. At this point, the nervous system in general is quite primitive, and the head end is just a rounded bump. (By the end of the second month, when the embryo has the external form of a tiny one-inch doll, its nervous system will still be extremely primitive relative to a full-term mammal, at about the stage of a snake or chicken. During prenatal development, the external form of the body matures fairly quickly, but in a moderate-sized mammal such as a human, the nervous system is very slow-growing.)

At the sixth week, all the structures in the embryo that will eventually be used to make genitals, gonads (ovaries or testes) and other internal structures for reproduction are in their beginning, 'primordial' stages of growth. In the absence of testosterone, all of these will go ahead to take their female forms. However, if the embryo has a y sex chromosome (with its SRy gene intact), the SRy gene (perhaps triggered by adrenal-cortex testosterone in the mother's bloodstream) shifts the developmental path of the gonads away from becoming ovaries, toward becoming testes.

Since we've had ultrasound to help us monitor pregnancy, many people are aware that fetal testes form well before birth. But what may not be generally known is that they not only achieve a recognizable form, but begin producing testosterone on their own – and continue producing it throughout the rest of gestation, over the period of time when major stages in brain growth and organization are going forward. If we remember the concept that testosterone interferes with the growth of brain structures and connections, we see that the fact and amount of production of testosterone by fetal testes is extremely important.

Of course, as with maternal testosterone, testosterone production by the fetus is of a graded nature – that is, in some individuals, the testes make very low levels of testosterone, in others it is moderate, and in still others, fetal T fluctuates wildly throughout gestation in a 'roller coaster' fashion, sometimes reaching levels in the bloodstream as higher or higher than they will be at puberty! (Any woman who has carried both a girl and a boy in separate pregnancies will not be surprised at this – she knows there is a dramatic difference between these two experiences, and that the fantasy of girls and boys being 'the same' at birth – and even well before birth – is just that.)

Effects of low to moderate prenatal T on Xys. These gradations in prenatal T production predictably create graded effects on brain connectivity as well. For those male fetuses exposed to low to moderate levels of T, it is expected that the developing brain will be able to retain much of its connectivity, and thus continue to benefit from the nurturing guidance of the right side of the brain. At lower levels, a very few of these boys may be born with a right-favoring brain, with all the associated benefits. However, as more and more testosterone comes into play during prenatal growth, the alterations in connectivity which it creates tend to interfere with the right side's guidance of growth of the left, and this allows the left side to grow a little more. As a result, many boys, particularly those with moderate exposure, will have brains in which the left-side pS regions approach symmetry with the right.

Over a fairly wide range of this type of right/left 'balance,' brains should continue to have fairly good access to right-brain skills such as imagery and social skills, and most of them will also enjoy the good general health that right-brain access ensures. However, throughout the zone of relative brain symmetry, due to the interference with right-brain control of left-brain growth, they may have relatively poorer access to left-brain skills such as phonemic awareness, which we've described as crucial for learning to read.

The type of right/left balance in brains with more or less symmetrical pS regions may provide extremely good skills for coordinating the two sides of the body, so these boys may be athletic to an advanced degree. Their choice of sport, however, may reflect their particular type of athleticism – good right/left coordination, but relatively poor fine motor control (a left-brain skill). As a result, they will probably self-select into sports and positions within sports that do not place such a high premium on fine-motor control – for example, football rather than tennis; football linemen rather than defensive backs, etc.

If these low-to-moderate-T boys have the choice (or are forced to change as many young athletes do because of early injury), their considerable social skills may lead them to avoid competitive sports altogether and express their athleticism in other activities where an excellence in 'choreography of the body in space' is prized, such as acting or professional dance.

We should note the similarity in this description with the one we gave for the XX individuals earlier. This underlines the idea that it is prenatal sex hormones, not chromosomes, that are primarily responsible for determining gender behavior and many other aspects of individuals, such as athleticism, arising from the right/left relations described above. We will return to this idea later.

Effects of high prenatal T on Xys. Finally, we need to consider those male fetuses whose testes produce high levels of testosterone. In these cases, as levels of testosterone fluctuate, rising sometimes to puberty-high levels then falling and rising again, neural connectivity along all three body/brain axes can be seriously affected. Increasing interference with right-brain guidance of brain growth may begin to impact the right side itself, and pS regions on the right may actually start to shrink. The brain may enter the early stages of a switch in balance of power overall, from right-side dominance to left.

94

Given the dramatic differences in right-brain/left-brain oversight summarized in the EPIC model (see Table 2.1) , this change may not be about 'balance' at all, but more a case of a catastrophic loss of the crucial competencies of the right side, leaving *only* what the left side can do. For a person in this situation, 'left-side dominance' may simply amount to 'that's all I have.' Thus the islanded state of the high-T-exposed brain is reflected in the person's behavior, 'islanded' to the limited skill set associated with the left side. As a result, that person might be called 'left-dominant'– but only because it's all they have to work with.

Boys whose brains stop in the very early stage of such a switch (that is, with only moderately-high T exposure) may excel in a very different kind of athletics than those with truly symmetrical brains. (As noted above for XX individuals, TM calls this a 'left-middle' brain type – an intermediate step between symmetric and left-favoring.) This kind of athlete is one who combines general athleticism (skills for coordination provided by their still fairly symmetrical brain), with fine-motor control (via 'dawning' prominence of left-brain skills provided in these early stages of the loss of access to the right side). As a result, they may self-select into sports and positions within sports that put a premium on fine-motor skills – for example, tennis or gymnastics, quarterback or defensive back in football, guard in basketball.

The fact that they have good fine-motor control is a sign that their brains have good access to other left-brain skills, such as phonemic awareness. Thus these boys may generally do well in school. Their lack of some right-brain skills such as eye-movement coordination and some types of mental imagery may make them somewhat labored readers, particularly with regard to comprehension. However, this is more subtle, and may not be noticed as much as the types of reading problems that plague the more symmetrical brains we described above. In support of this prediction is the fact that college athletes specializing in gymnastics and tennis tend to have higher grade-point averages than do their colleagues in football and basketball.

Interestingly, these moderately-high-T boys may do quite well at kinds of imagery which involve a more static (left-brain-type) visual task – such as 'picture this gymnastic pose in your mind' or perform a 'mental rotation of images' as a series of static pictures, much like a film slowed down to focus on frame by frame. Yet 'speeding up' the film to arrive at a real-time impression of flowing movements may be a virtually impossible imagery feat.

These boys may also have 'eidetic imagery,' in which images stay in the mind (and may be difficult to ignore). This is a neural-based skill (remember the parvocellular visual system from Table 2.2?) which may be of benefit in some pastimes (such as for an artist who needs to recall the details of a natural scene from memory) but a real detriment in others (such as rapid reading, where the visual system has to 'erase' letters in the brain almost as soon as they are captured, to get ready as the eyes move to the next point on the page).

Unfortunately, in many boys, prenatal testosterone does not stop here. Even higher amounts produced over the course of gestation may diminish brain connectivity even further, leading to an actual shrinking of the pS region on the right side, and explosive growth on the left. The result is different degrees of a marked 'left-hemisphere symmetry' in pS regions – much like those reported in the earlier literature in adult brains from hospital morgues, or spontaneously-aborted fetuses.

Shrinking of right-brain areas and over-growth on the left side may be a sign that left-brain skills are coming into prominence, while connections to right-brain skills are being lost to these brains. Thus abilities for fluent mental imagery will disappear, 'social intelligence' will diminish, the ability to use any type of right-brain skill (such as being able to perceive the emotional tone of voices or facial expressions) will decrease. (Note that these left-favoring brains may excel in verbal skills depending on a 'glib' use of vocabulary and rapid delivery, but the type of 'sociability' that goes with this manipulative, 'sales pitch' use of language does not have the depth of the true social intelligence that depends on intact access to the right brain.)

Along with loss of the right brain's skills, its 'mothering' management of general health may also be lost, making individuals with left-favoring brains prone to many types of health-related problems. Losing the nurturing parasympathetic (right-brain) management of several brain/body systems may mean these individuals face higher risks of heart problems, digestive disorders, sleep disorders, and immune-system dysfunction than other types of brains. Diminished parasympathetic control may even be associated with very specific problems, such as urinary incontinence including bedwetting (without good PSNS control, sphincters for elimination will open more easily, often at inappropriate times).

These types of physical difficulties with general body management could be the biological basis for more general psychological features of individuals. such as some types of personality. For example, the elevated ('released') sympathetic tone of left-favoring brains should result in their exhibiting aggressive, competitive, heart-attack-risk-prone Type A behavior. The loss of PSNS management could lead naturally to an anal type of personality, with its origins in the fact that its body's sphincters may seem to have a life of their own, requiring a constant, near-conscious effort to control them if they are to be kept behaving in a socially acceptable way. (Of course, the right-favoring and symmetrical brains should not have such difficulties, or such personality problems, since they can depend on their 'mothering' right brain to take care of all such things 'behind the scenes,' where they belong.)

In fact, the overall breakdown between conscious awareness (located for these focal individuals on the left side) and the rest of the brain and body could easily be seen as the basis for a general distrust of body function – perhaps in extreme cases leading to an actual fear and hatred of the body and of physicality in general. Many instances of such attitudes, including dislike of being hugged or even touched. such as shown by autistic individuals, or the hyper-cleanly habits seen in many forms of obsessive-compulsive disorder, may all be attributes of brains in which the left side has become isolated from the right brain and the body, and has lost a sense of kinship with them, as the necessary neural connections were attacked by prenatal T.

Summary of the origins of the three brain types/six genders complex

To summarize what has been predicted here: 1) there is a continuum of individual differences in exposure to prenatal testosterone, ranging from zero to very high; 2) because Xy individuals but not XX can make their own prenatal T, the two chromosomal genders experience a difference in *absolute levels* of exposure – XXs overall lower than XYs; 3) in spite of the differences in the absolute values of XX vs. Xy exposure, the continuum of *relative levels* for each will give rise to the *same three categories* of *brain types* – right-favoring (least prenatal T, found mostly in XX), symmetrical (relatively moderate exposure, found in both XX and Xy) and left-favoring (relatively highest exposure, found in both XX and Xy, but most common – and most extreme – in Xy, due to the absolute-level difference); 4) thus the result is a 'rainbow' of six genders – two chromosomal genders x three brain types.

In Chapter Four we will return to the idea of designating these six profiles as 'genders,' and discuss how NRT applies that conclusion of TM to larger questions about social organization in humans and among animals in general. However, for the rest of this chapter, we will describe each of the three major brain types in more detail, to gain a better appreciation of the many individual characteristics involved.

Trimodal Model catalog of individual features by brain type

In the previous discussion we mentioned a few features associated with each of the three major brain types. In this next section, we will review a larger catalog of features, beginning with 'Brain hallmarks,' to see in each case how they compare and contrast individuals exposed to relatively less or more testosterone during prenatal life. (The discussion will be summarized in Table 3.1, found toward the end of the chapter.)

Brain hallmarks: polytropic, middle, focal

We have already said that the hallmark of the right-favoring brain is its complete access to all brain skills and abilities – it is truly the 'right-brain/whole-brain' type. Thus TM refers to it as "*polytropic*," that is, 'many-skilled' – an epithet used by Homer to describe Odysseus, meaning 'jack of all trades and master of all.'

The hallmark of the symmetric, or "*middle*" brain, is its athleticism, its advanced abilities for 'choreography of the body in space' – equally useful for professions and hobbies such as athletics, acting, and dance. The designation of 'middle' refers to its intermediate position along the T-exposure continuum, its intermediate status regarding access to the skills of the two sides, and the symmetrical condition of pS regions on the two sides of the brain.

The hallmark of the left-favoring, or "*focal*" brain is its tendency to focus on one task at a time, neither distracted nor helped by contributions from other parts of the brain. This tendency arises in its neurologically 'islanded' nature, having undergone rather severe disconnections from the rest of the brain and body as a result of high levels of exposure to prenatal testosterone.

Handedness

Handedness has long been an issue in studies of brain asymmetry and individual differences, and it was a focus of the GBG model discussed earlier. 'Handedness' is a biased term – as typically used, it means "which hand is used for fine-motor control." (If it meant "which hand and arm are confidently used to hold and carry a child," most humans would be labelled left-handed.) But given the usual definition, the three brain categories would fall out this way: both the polytropic (right-brain/whole-brain) and the focal (left-favoring) would be right-handed, since by definition, both have good access to left-brain skills such as fine-motor control.

In contrast, individuals with middle (symmetrical) brains should represent a rainbow of ambidexterity/left-handedness. This is based on TM's prediction that all brains are built with the same assignments of the different skill modules to the same sides of the brain in essentially the same way – fine-motor control and phonemic awareness on the left, mental imagery and social skills on the right, etc.

Thus TM, as part of Neural Rainbow Theory, does not predict that the brain of left-handed individuals is flipped in some way, but rather that their hand preference for fine-motor tasks shows that they have either found a roundabout way of getting access to left-brain fine-motor abilities, or are maximizing a certain level of ability of their right brains to support this type of motor performance.

In any case, TM predicts that no person who is ambidextrous or left-handed for tasks requiring fine-motor control will exhibit such skills at a level comparable to that seen in a truly right-handed person. (Note that this is quite different from other approaches, including the GBG model, which posit that most left-handers have their brain modules for fine-motor control located on the right instead of the left side, just as some people are born with the heart on the right rather than the left side of the body.)

Birth order

TM predicts that the amount of adrenal testosterone that a particular woman tends to make during pregnancy will decrease from pregnancy to pregnancy for her. The effect must be judged for each woman (and it may change if she changes partners), but in general, babies earlier in her series will have relatively higher prenatal T, while those later will have lower levels. TM also predicts that children of the same parents will not bridge between extremes, such as a focal brain followed by middle then polytropic; rather, siblings from the same parents will predictably occupy a relatively limited 'sibling range,' a set of neighboring points along the brain-type continuum, separated from each other by only a few units.

In fact, as we'll see in the next chapter, this 'sibling range' might also be a good guide for choosing a lifelong mate – predictably someone with a brain type that is not exactly like yours, but close – like a sibling. Many people who have long and happy marriages report that they have always felt psychologically like siblings, with compatible personalities, common interests, etc. Apparently when combined with a healthy non-sibling sexual attraction, this is the ideal neurological basis for a lasting pair-bond. Birth-order differences from child to child should be reflected in all the individual features covered by TM, including the items mentioned in this catalog.

Body type

In Chapter One we reviewed suggestions made by Sheldon during the 1940s regarding a systematic approach to individual differences based on body type. TM predicts that bodies and brains created under the continuum of prenatal testosterone exposure described here would map fairly well onto Sheldon's three-component 'mix' of body-type components. In general, individuals with either the polytropic brain or middle-brain type should have mesomorphic bodies, since these are predictably the most healthy style, with the best combination of efficient food use and storage capacity.

In contrast, individuals with left-favoring brains will predictably have a body which is either ectomorphic or endomorphic, body styles which betray basic problems with food-use efficiency, which can be life-threatening in survival situations. The ectomorphic body type is a 'gas-guzzler,' burning food quickly without much capacity for storing it ('spending without saving' – not adaptive for coping with occasional food shortages); while the endomorphic body type represents the opposite disadvantage, storing ('hoarding') all too well, leading to increased body mass and thus decreased mobility, a life-and-death deficit around predators.

Age of puberty

The polytropic brain will come to puberty at a 'normal' age (polytropics will be the 'standard' for many of the aspects listed here). One of the actions of prenatal testosterone is to 'prime' parts of the brain, such as the hypothalamus, important for timing the onset of puberty (as discussed in detail by Nyborg, mentioned in Chapter Two). As a result, the amount of prenatal testosterone will be reflected in the timing of puberty – moderate levels of T will result in somewhat delayed puberty (compared with polytropics) for both XX and Xy, while high levels will bring about somewhat earlier puberty than in polytropics, for both XX and Xy.

Height

Maximum height predicted for different individuals follows from the predictions above regarding onset of puberty, since initiation of hormone production by the gonads around puberty acts to stop developmental bone growth, and thus 'freeze' height. As a result, polytropics will be of 'medium' height (of course this will be relative within a gene pool, interacting with genetic and nutritional contributions to height), middle brains will be relatively taller (since their puberty is delayed and growth continues), and focal brains will be relatively shorter (earlier puberty means growth stops sooner).

Coloration

Pigmentation throughout the human body is achieved primarily by concentrations of melanin, produced by special cells in the skin, eyes, hair, and parts of the brain. One area of the brain that contains melanin-producing cells is the substantia nigra (SN), a tiny center in the brainstem which has become famous for its role in Parkinson's Disease, attributed to a loss of SN capacity to make dopamine, a neurotransmitter important for motor control. The SN in Parkinson's Disease also can be shown to be abnormally pale when dissected – apparently failure in the ability to make dopamine is paralleled by a failure to make melanin.

The metabolism of melanin is associated not only with the biosynthesis and metabolism of dopamine, but also the neurotransmitter norepinephrine (related to adrenalin), important in the sympathetic nervous system. For instance, the same chemical ('dopa') is used in the synthesis of both melanin and norepinephrine (the more melanin, the less norepinephrine, and vice versa), as well as to synthesize dopamine. And very high levels of dopamine can repress the release of melanin-stimulating hormone (MSH) by the hypothalamus, leading to decreased melanin production (high levels of dopamine also repress hypothalamic release of prolactin, the hormone needed for producing breast milk – suggesting a possible biochemical connection between very pale skin and trouble with breast feeding!). Both dopamine and norepinephrine are found in higher levels on the left side of the brain as opposed to the right, and both can have different effects on the brain and body depending on overall levels – there is a 'normal' value, compared with levels which are either too high or too low, which can be dangerous in different ways.

The specific prediction of TM, then, is that individuals with polytropic and middle brains (with their moderate levels of dopamine and norepinephrine) will tend to have relatively more melanin, while those with left-favoring brains should have relatively less (again, this will be relative within gene pools). Thus polytropics and middles will tend to be brunettes, with darker eyes, hair, and skin. Increasing levels of prenatal testosterone will be associated with lighter-colored eyes, hair, and skin, as brain type shifts toward the left. (There may be a special form of the left-middle brain type mentioned earlier, which has a 'contradictory' pattern of coloration, combining very pale skin with dark eyes and hair. Informal observations suggest that these individuals may be at particular risk for stuttering and some types of emotional disorders, but as with all TM concepts, more research is needed to verify these predictions.)

The effects of prenatal T on general coloration may provide a way to account for the frequent observation of anomalous coloration in an individual compared to siblings from a series of children produced by the same parents. Thus, perhaps because of that child's place in the birth order (discussed earlier in this catalog), or a special situation pertaining during the pregnancy (more or less stress, use of a relevant medication, etc.), the 'recipe' for coloration encoded in that family's genes may be over-ridden to some extent, resulting in instances such as a blonde child in the middle of a series of brunettes. (In former years, the production of a blonde child by two brunette parents was taken as a sign of infidelity by the mother, but if these predictions about prenatal testosterone are correct, blame might more accurately be placed on a biochemical rather than a sociological event.)

Autonomic emphasis

We've just mentioned norephinephrine and its predicted difference in concentration across the brain types. Polytropics should have a predominance of modulated, advanced, parasympathetic management over the autonomic nervous system; middles should be intermediate between PSNS and SNS, tending toward more PSNS; and focal brains may have very poor PSNS access. As a result individuals with focal brains should have elevated 'sympathetic tone,' that is, higher blood pressure and heart rate, problems with digestion (since the PSNS manages digestion), trouble with sphincters, etc. – all the ills that come with losing touch with your right-brain 'mother' and her caring PSNS interface with the body as a whole.

Handshaking relations

This term refers to the connectivity patterns described in Chapter Two, where we concluded that the most advanced brain was the one characterized by the most elastic, resilient, flexible type of connectivity along all three body/brain axes. Because TM considers that testosterone is the principal disconnection agent working before (and after) birth, it is by definition the polytropic brain type, developing in a 'hormone-free' prenatal environment, that will have the most flexible and 'many-skilled' type of connectivity linking parts of the brain with each other and with the body (the access to good PSNS management mentioned in the previous item is part of this picture). Middle brains should have an intermediate degree of connectivity and thus elasticity of function, while focal brains should have to cope with fairly primitive connectivity patterns, becoming rigidly hierarchical in some cases (a brain and body working like a military organization instead of a coordinated democracy), and completely unconnected in others (extremely poor access to right-brain skills for general health, etc.).

Skills

1. Phonemic Awareness (PA). Phonemic awareness is the ability to hear-out (be consciously aware of) speech sounds ('phonemes' such as *b, s, a,* etc.) *inside syllables.* PA does *not* refer to the ability to match visual letters to speech sounds heard in isolation, which is properly called 'sound/symbol correspondence' – a critical distinction which has led to much confusion among educators over the past few decades. PA is crucial for accurate speech articulation, learning to read and spell, and listening to verbal instructions, and as such it is a must for success in conventional classrooms (and perhaps for everyday listening to speech in many situations, including noisy backgrounds, or when using a hearing aid). [There is an excellent test for PA, useable for ages five and older, which avoids the confusion with sound-symbol correspondence, and provides a direct way of assessing this important skill; for more, see references under Lindamood in the bibliography at the end of this chapter.]

Yet in spite of PA's importance, research has shown that approximately 1/3 of all humans are born *without* intact phonemic awareness, and that this substantial proportion of the population does *not* develop this skill on their own, or as a result of standard methods of instruction in schools. Such a large number suggests that the lack of PA is not a 'disorder,' but simply a normal statistical variant of human brain organization (e.g., one of the three TM brain types). Although the educational system often uses the term PA, it is usually taken to mean sound/symbol correspondence, and as a result, significant numbers of children lacking PA are being missed (and thus mis-taught) by the system.

To my knowledge, there is only one effective training program for PA, but though that program has been offered since the 1970s by a group of specialized clinics, it is not taught in schools of education, and is only used in a handful of public schools which have found it can improve academic performance in children of all ages. The results of this specialized training can be amazing – PA in those individuals lacking it can be 'waked up,' and thus added to a child's (or adult's) repertoire of skills – the program can be effective at any age. Our interpretation of the strategy employed by this training program is that it re-establishes the brain connectivity supporting this important skill, originally perturbed due to testosterone exposure at some time during prenatal development.

The Trimodal Model agrees with the research on PA, and assigns PA as a left-brain skill (for the reasons discussed in Chapter Two), thus predicting that only 2/3 of humans (those with polytropic and focal brains) will have good access to PA. The one-third of humans whom the theory predicts will have middle-type brains should have relatively poor access to left-brain PA – a good numerical match to the previous research on the incidence of PA problems in the general population.

2. Eye-movement coordination. As we use our eyes to follow a moving object, or slide them along a line of text, the right and left eyes must be coordinated with each other, much like two dancers who move together in step and in time. However, research has shown that in many children of school age, the eyes do not 'dance well' together – the right may go off in one direction, and the left in another, then they may cross and go off again – all while the child is trying to read a paragraph. (A simple device called the Visagraph – sadly no longer available – can demonstrate this in dramatic detail.)

It is not surprising that such children dislike reading – they complain of headaches when reading, and say that the "letters move around on the page, and sometimes even fall off." Of course the letters don't move – this is an illusion arising from uncoordinated eye-movement. Just as is the case with PA, eye-movement coordination is not assessed in the schools, and is not trained for in the schools – though again, there are effective training programs for improving eye movements, which have been shown to make a dramatic difference in children's ability to read.

The Trimodal Model considers coordination between right and left eyes, as with any type of right/left motor coordination, a right-brain skill. Thus the prediction is that polytropics and middle-brain individuals will naturally have better eye-movement coordination (at least initially – see next paragraph) than will those with focal brains.

In some middle-brain children, initially good eye movements may actually *degrade* over time as they continue in school. This can happen in the many middles with poor PA, as they have more and more trouble with longer and longer words, and start literally casting [their eyes] around for help – and their increasingly erratic eye movements testify to their confusion. This is a good example of the unintended effects of an educational system (like ours) which seems to be as ignorant of the severity of problems caused by an inborn lack of PA as it is regarding the potential effect of a lack of PA on eye-movement control.

3. Fine-motor control. As discussed in Chapter Two, fine-motor control is another left-brain skill, depending on the 'small motor units' within muscles of the body. As such, it should work in the most advanced way in both polytropics and focal brains, but generally be less accessible to middle-brain types. Because 'handedness' is actually a fine-motor-control concept, individual differences in the degree of fine-motor control should follow the patterns described under that item (see above).

4. Mental imagery. When we read or hear the sentences, "The boy chased the dog" and "The dog chased the boy," some of us see pictures or movies in our heads of those actions, while others do not. This is called 'mental imagery,' and is extremely important for comprehending verbal material that is read or heard. (It also seems related to arithmetic skills, at least in the early grades, where children with reduced reading comprehension due to poor mental imagery often also have trouble handling the spatial 'pictures' used in teaching addition, subtraction, etc.)

Imagery helps us understand even things that are more abstract (sometimes called 'concept imagery'). For example, as a child is learning vocabulary items such as "ambition" and "duty," he may spontaneously see a picture in his mind representing "ambition" as a man in a suit rushing along carrying a briefcase, and for the second, a soldier standing at attention under a flapping flag. Individuals who do not make such images may find reading very labored, even if they have excellent PA. Such children (and adults) may be able to read aloud in a way that *sounds* accurate, but if they do not at the same time 'picture' what they read, they may have to go over something several times to figure out what is meant. This is the type of child who may enjoy reading in the very early grades, but begins having trouble as soon as the pictures start disappearing from books used in school. Again, mental imagery is not assessed in the schools, and is not trained for, even though effective programs are available.

And as with PA and eye movements, the numbers of children and adults impacted by the lack of imagery – so fundamental to reading and learning – is daunting. Because TM assigns comprehension-related mental imagery as a right-brain skill (see Chapter Two), it predicts that polytropics will have the best mental imagery, while many middle- and focal brains will have problems.

This might help explain why some individuals called 'hyperlexic' ('really good at reading') can read aloud with perfect articulation, yet have problems understanding what they've read. TM predicts this combination is a clear sign of a focal brain, with good access to left-brain skills such as PA but poor access to right-brain capabilities such as mental imagery. Thus the use of the label 'hyperlexic' is yet another instance of left-brain-bias – as though, if (left-brain) PA is good, that's all that matters – and comprehension (right-brain) is considered less important.

5. Cortical visual acuity. As the name suggests, this refers not to *retinal* acuity, but a type of ability provided by the 'high spatial resolution' skills of the left brain (see Chapter Two). Thus polytropics and focal brains should have excellent cortical visual acuity (assuming intact retinas), while middles may have some trouble with this. A lack of access to cortical visual acuity (also not addressed in schools – the educational system does not even seem to be aware of such a possibility) may account for the fact that many children begin having reading problems as the *size of type* decreases in texts used across the early grades. Yet teachers know by observation that even a child who does not 'need glasses' (i.e., correction directed to the eye itself) may improve in reading scores if material originally printed in a size typical for adults (e.g., 10-pt is used in most newspapers) is simply increased to 18 or 24.

6. Emotional intelligence. As we've suggested in Chapter Two, this rather abstract concept can be biologically defined as the direct result of the types of physical stimuli that the right brain is specialized for handling – moving visual patterns of facial expressions, slow and low-pitched vocal melody, the preference for receiving and giving hugs and caresses (activating deep-pressure skin receptors) rather than light, static touches (via light-touch receptors). Even language as a vehicle for the expression of emotional states, needs, and general bonding between individuals is in this same way a right-brain activity.

Thus polytropics and middles with their good access to such right- brain skills will have a deep confidence about dealing with other people, and an 'intuitive' ability to express and perceive emotions. To those with focal brains, being able to do such things may appear almost magical and prescient – picking up on, and using, physical cues that to them essentially do not exist. In fact, focal brains may dismiss emotional intelligence as 'soft' and useless – after all, since they lack it, can it really exist, and even if it does, who needs it?

Many individuals with focal brains (particularly those Xys with advanced states of disconnection) will not even 'be in touch' with their own emotions, and thus resent polytropics or middles if they dare to mention (the fact) that *they* understand a focal better than he knows himself.

7. Social skills. The ability to be comfortable with people, to perceive subliminal clues about how they're feeling and reacting, and be able to respond in a way that keeps relationships elastic and flexible, depends on a cluster of interpersonal skills that polytropics and middles should have, based on their access to right-brain abilities. It is not an accident that this description is reminiscent of the type of internal connectivity we've described as true for these types of brains – as we said before, it's natural to think of relations between human individuals as reflecting the relations within our nervous system, the basis for all our behavior.

Along the same lines, then, our description of what prenatal (and postnatal) testosterone does to brain connectivity, offers a metaphor for the types of social relations that will be most 'natural' for focal brains. They will feel most comfortable (if that is the right word) in groups where a clear line of command, or pecking order, is established. Individuals with these types of brains will feel completely at home in the type of rigid social hierarchy that polytropics and middles would find imprisoning. If focals are put in a leadership position (or their aggressive tendencies make them seek it out), they will approach it in a primitive, egotistical way – they will be autocratic, punitive, narcissistic 'leaders.'

Some focals will not find even this primitive a social structure congenial, but seek to be essentially asocial, and prefer to live and work alone, with little contact with other humans or even other biological entities such as pets. They may be content with the 'society' of inanimate, mechanical things such as cars, computers, or video games.

(Chapter Four will explore further how these differences in the social profiles of the different brain types can be seen as the 'building blocks' of the social organization of all animal species, including humans.)

8. Athletic intelligence. We've said that athleticism draws primarily on two general areas of brain skills: coordination between the two sides of the body (a right-brain specialty), and fine-motor control (a left-brain skill). Thus polytropics will have both sets of abilities (though they may not have two-sided coordination to the advanced degree that middle-brains do), middle-brains will excel at two-sided coordination, and left-middles may combine this with good fine-motor control, for a somewhat different kind of advanced athletic ability.

Such details regarding degrees of fine-motor control should be important for coaching individuals who want to play one sport or another, or one position or another within a sport – something coaches already know, possibly without recognizing the specific neural basis for their insights. And as noted earlier, 'athleticism' by this definition also fits individuals for doing many more things than just competitive sports. Being able to move well in space, with physical confidence, presence, and grace, is a basic requirement for professions such as acting and professional dance. (Many actors report a history of athletics, where injury side-tracked them into theater, which turned out for them to be a neurologically-compatible Plan B.)

A final note about athletic *participation* is the *personality* associated with each brain type (we'll talk more about this below). Although polytropics have substantial athleticism and deeply enjoy physical activity, they will probably tend to do this for its own, whole-brain sake, and not have the driving personality needed to perform in the top rung of competitive sports.

Middle-brains may be attracted to sports in a carrot-and-stick way – the carrot is that they are good at it, the stick is that because they find their lack of phonemic awareness hurts them in school, participating in sports gives them a chance to 'play to a strength' and thus gain self-esteem. Finally, left-middle brains (those with enough middle qualities to have good coordination, supplemented with left-brain fine-motor skills) will predictably be those who go the furthest in competitive participation, particularly in sports and positions demanding fine-motor control (tennis and ice skating come to mind). And some individuals with left-middle brains may also have the obsessive-compulsive personality, the 'killer instinct,' required to put all other life concerns and priorities aside, to focus only on perfecting their sport.

Finally, individuals with extremely left-favoring brains may recognize themselves colloquially as 'spastic,' 'can't dance,' who are not at all coordinated (lacking good connections with the Great Coordinator the right brain), and so feel no attraction at all to sports or to any pastime that requires them to get up and walk across a space. They would prefer to sit still in one static position and move their fingers in small repetitive arcs over the miniature works of a watch, or the keys of a computer keyboard or a cellphone.

9. Artistic ability. This is another category of skill that has often been discussed in terms of brain asymmetries ('drawing with the right side of the brain,' etc.), but usually in confusing ways. Artistic ability actually covers a variety of skills, and depending on the genre, needs to be considered on an individual basis. The concept of 'creativity' in most cases predictably refers to the ability to make new connections, which may depend on being able to exploit a certain degree of disconnection in the brain. There is a fine line, however, between describing 'new connections' that others can appreciate, and reporting on those that only the artist can see.

Art is about communication, and if an audience cannot 'see with the artist's eyes' (or 'hear with the artist's ears,' etc.), it is an exercise in self-stimulation only. Polytropics will be creative, in their combination of right-brain 'big picture' skills with a left-brain knack for finding new connections. However, they will predictably not have the degree of obsessiveness needed to hone a craft to the exclusion of other life activities, and may not have the ambition and self-promotional skills to ensure their art comes to the public eye.

Individuals with middle-brains may be good performers of art created by others, but a lack of access to left-brain 'separation' skills may keep them from being good originators. Those having what we've called left-middle brains may be the best candidates as artists, since they will combine at least some right-brain skills for emotional expression and response, with left-brain abilities which are basic for artistic endeavors such as: mentally 'recording' a static scene for use in a later painting or verbal description; building a mathematical musical pattern and holding it 'frozen' in the mind for recording; fine-motor skills for painting and sculpting; and perhaps most importantly for becoming an 'accomplished' artist in any venue, the tolerance for highly repetitive practice and drill. Rembrandt painted the same self-portrait over and over; Mozart could shut out all distractions while composing; it is a commonplace that well-known artists often have limited if not aberrant social lives and pour all their energy and time into their work.

Health

1. Immune function. The next few items deal with general health, and the predictions are based on TM's assignment of general health as a right-brain domain. With regard to immune function, it is predicted that polytropics will have good 'immune-response balance,' with an immune system that is neither under- nor over-reactive. They might experience occasional upper-respiratory events as their immune system responds to challenges, but no serious immune conditions – neither AIDS nor allergies nor any type of cancer. During childhood they will have very few middle-ear episodes, and in adulthood, they will be fairly resistant to infections that can bring other brain types low.

Individuals with middle-brains will have an intermediate degree of immune response, tending to be fairly healthy and resistant to infections. Left-brain types should be most vulnerable to a range of immune-system problems, ranging from asthma and allergies, to autoimmune (hyper-reactive) immune disorders such as lupus and multiple sclerosis, to a variety of cancers. Left-brain women should be those most at-risk for breast cancer; it is not surprising to find that breast cancer most often affects the left breast, suggesting that even in these women, there is some lingering protection from the right brain over the right side of the body, that becomes marginal – thus the left brain 'fails' first) if there is an immune challenge such as environmental estrogens or hormone-affecting radiation from living near nuclear reactors.

Recall that the GBG model stressed allergies in learning-disordered children. TM predicts that allergies do indeed affect a subset of individuals with learning disorders, specifically those where left-brain skills such as phonemic awareness out-shine right-brain abilities like mental imagery. It is well-known that children and adults with autistic spectrum disorders typically have problems with hyper-reactive immune response, leading to allergies. TM predicts that for a number of reasons, these individuals represent cases of brains exposed to high levels of prenatal testosterone. (We will talk more about autism under the Developmental and Learning disorders section below, including TM's neural explanation for the onset of autism in the middle of a child's second year.)

2. Cardiac function. We've already suggested that any condition which reflects a predominance of sympathetic over the parasympathetic nervous system should be associated with increasing levels of prenatal testosterone. Thus polytropics should have the best cardiac health, middles should have an intermediate degree, with some risk for certain types of health and vascular problems, and focal brains should be most at risk for heart attacks, as their predominating SNS is left free to 'hammer' the heart in a very non-nurturing way.

3. Eating habits. Again, access to parasympathetic 'body wisdom' involved in selecting and storing food, including conscious attitudes regarding a healthy body size and shape should ensure polytropics the best instincts about eating. Middle-brain types may be intermediate in this; they may tend to eat too much, and be fooled by quasi-foods (such as junk foods or alcohol) and thus get into difficulty with nutrition; but they will eat for joy as part of a general positive attitude toward physical life.

Individuals with left-favoring brains will predictably be those whose reduced access to right-brain management of health keeps them not only from knowing what is good for them to eat, but also from having intact feedback connections regarding how much food is needed by their brains and bodies. Individuals with bulimia may be left-middles, with a somewhat different combination of problems than those with anorexia, predictably those exposed to higher levels of prenatal T. Again, autism identifies itself as a left-brain condition by the fascination with non-nutritive junk foods often seen in these children.

4. Sleep habits. Relations between the cerebral cortex and brainstem are important for 'shifting gears' between waking and sleep, and for cycling through different stages of sleep, to ensure that the body and brain are restored in the proper ways. Polytropics, with their more elastic connectivity linking different levels of the brain, will have the best luck with sleeping – able to fall asleep when ready, experience all cycles without waking, and wake up when they are refreshed. Middle-brains will be very good at sleeping and falling asleep – they may be able to nap almost at will, and fond of sleeping as a way of passing time.

Individuals with focal brains, with their rigid hierarchies for ordering different levels of the nervous system, will have a hard time trading control from cortex to brainstem. Thus they may have a hard time going to sleep, and often experience disabling insomnia. They may also be among the people who can get by on a very little sleep, which may attest to the islanded function of their waking life – at the end of the day, there is little whole-brain restoring to do.

5. Emotional health. We will talk more about details related to this category under 'Other conditions,' below, but from a very general standpoint, it will help to provide an overview here. First, polytropics should enjoy the best emotional health. They benefit from their whole-brain, whole-body connectivity that keeps the entire system working in harmony, with no sense of conflict between 'mind and body' or between 'self and body.' These people will be integrated in a very literal way, and will feel at one with their bodies. They enjoy all aspects of physical life, celebrate being with small groups of other people they care about, take delight in sharing the riches of biological life with other animals, and feel a kinship with the biosphere in general. They naturally see the earth as their 'mother' and are very much at home in the natural world.

Middle-brains will be much the same, though they may need human companionship, especially positive feedback, somewhat more than polytropics. They may 'use' loving interactions with other people to help them restore the connections in their brains that moderate exposure to testosterone removed during prenatal growth, but this will be done in a healthy way. That is, they will see other people as nurturing them, and seek to return the favor. Thus middles are loving and loyal, and depend on other people to a marked extent for their sense of self-worth.

The concept of 'focal-brain emotional health' in many cases is almost an oxymoron. Because these brains (particularly in Xys) lack good access to right-brain skills for emotional perception and expression, the whole idea of an emotional life may be foreign and almost distasteful to them, and many focal brains will scoff at emotions as 'weak' and a waste of time. Of course, this usually refers to positive emotions – focal brains (again, especially Xys) are masters of negative emotions, since these are integral to the fight/flight sympathetic nervous system which dominates in them – they can be quick to anger, quick to take offense, highly territorial, resentful and revengeful. These attributes make it difficult for them to live with any degree of harmony with other people, and they may actually seek out professions and lifestyles where their emotional inadequacy is not a handicap.

Group membership

1. Preferred structure. We will talk a great deal more in the next chapter about the sociology of brain types, and how the continuum we've described helps us understand many things about how human beings and other animals interact with each other. For a general summary, though, we can observe that the sociological expressions of the three principal brain types are direct reflections of the brain organization that we've described for each.

For example, polytropics will be attracted to life in smaller groups where they know and get along with everyone, and where the general organization is one that is at once respectful and nurturing. (The most basic model is a loving mother and child.) Such groups will take it for granted that there should be autonomy and integrity for each contributing part, and a flexible working arrangement that allows one or another contributor to take the lead, depending on the nature of the task at hand. Democracy is a natural social organization for polytropics, though tempered with the common sense realization that democracy is not synonymous with anarchy, that it's crucial to have an older, wiser coordinator around (modelled on the right-brain 'mother,' and embodied in the actual 'grandmother' role in natural societies) to watch over the whole enterprise from behind the scenes, and make sure the balance and harmony go on working. (Many of the problems of democracies in modern industrialized countries arise from the fact that there are no wise grandmothers overseeing and guiding the process – more on this later.)

Middle-brains like being in groups, also, but will be a little more gregarious than polytropics, and won't mind being in larger groups where some members are more or less strangers. They get energy from other people, and enjoy having interactions that span a range from very loving to somewhat competitive. They like being leaders and being recognized with some degree of fanfare for their contribution, but won't seek to lead in a hierarchical, dominating way. Middles lead to be loved, and are willing to make any changes required to keep that support coming. Many of the best politicians are middles – not all that great on phonemic awareness, maybe, but loving the limelight not as a path to power, but primarily for its testimony that a lot of folks care about them.

The sociology of focal brains (especially in Xys) is fairly simple, as we've suggested before. Their brains provide good models for a solitary life, or for living in rigidly stratified structures where everyone knows his place. They won't 'need' other people (except as unquestioning devotees), and will be happiest in professions where they are alone most of the time. They are not 'group people' (they prefer to be the one rooster on the dung heap), and shun advances from other people looking for any type of relationship other than what is absolutely required for monopolizing resources, dominating subordinates, or receiving homage as the Dear Leader.

Focals are terrible bosses, since they rule by domination and humiliation – they subscribe to the sympathetic nervous system school of leadership, where fight and flight are the only modes of action. They are predatory, and believe in the zero-sum-game model of social interaction – "somebody has always got to lose – and it isn't going to be me." Yet sadly, it is focals who most often end up in command positions, at least in most of the societies we know, simply because they are so ruthless in their insistence on always being The One, the guy who can brow-beat people with other types of brains into letting him seize control.

2. Choice of professions. Predictions under this heading follow naturally what we've already said about access to different brain skills combined with preferences regarding interactions with others. Polytropics, because of their whole-brain access, will be able to do almost anything they choose (after all, that's why TM refers to them with Odysseus' epithet of 'polytropic,' or 'many-skilled'). The exceptions involve types of behavior that are *not* natural to them: taking extreme risks, hurting people, long-term isolation from others, or jobs that demand repetitive, mindless obsessive-compulsive focusing on one or a few details out of context. (And that describes so many jobs!)

In fact, the feature that makes polytropics such a prize in small-group situations may be their major downfall in large, competitive societies that demand high levels of killer instinct to climb the career ladder. It will often be said of polytropics that they 'lack ambition.' Work is not their only priority, and so they may either choose professions where this is never an issue, or actually pursue a profession in a different way than the conventional practice.

Even if they enter a profession which is typically characterized by ruthlessness or obsessive-compulsive behavior, polytropics may transform and improve it, both as a way of life and as a means to an end – though of course such improvement may not be noticeable to the other brain types who define the conventional way of doing things. One example is women managing businesses in a nurturing way, seeing employees as members of a social group not cogs in a wheel, and doing all possible to make the workplace a true home-away-from-home, such as providing access to nutritious and diverse meals served in a comfortable natural setting, allowing flexible schedules to accommodate other areas of life, and providing on-site spaces for nursing and daycare facilities for those who need it.

Individuals with middle-brains will be best at professions where their skills can shine, and their lack of some left-brain abilities (such as phonemic awareness) will not be a hindrance. We've said that anything that demands graceful, whole-body movement through space will be a wonderful pastime for middles – acting, dancing, even modeling (though not if it requires starvation – not a middle-brain strong point!), and many (though not all) types of athletics.

The good social skills of individuals with middle-brains will attract them to any occupation where they can perform for others' approval (like the ones we've just mentioned), and/or interact with others in a nurturing way. Thus middle-brain women and men will be strongly drawn to service professions such as teaching, nursing, and human-oriented sciences (though middles will chafe under the hierarchical organizations often imposed on these professions by focal brains).

Finally, as with the others we've described, if given the choice, individuals with focal brains will seek out the occupation that provides the best fit to their brains. The recipe for an ideal focal-brain job should include: working alone for long periods of time, repetitive relatively mindless work, focus on tiny details whether defined physically or mentally, with no need for considering the big picture or the implications of what one is doing. It is striking how mechanical and robotic this sounds, and as impossible as this type of work would be for most polytropics and middles to tolerate, it is perfect for focals, just what the doctor ordered. We can see that industrialized societies have essentially been built on this type of 'anthill' work – designed by focals (because it is natural for them), and all too often imposed on middles and polytropics, as either the only jobs to be had (a form of economic blackmail), or the only jobs where one can be assured self-esteem in a world where the norms for value, advancement, and success almost all come from individuals with focal brains.

Of course, all of this has been known for a long time. For example, virtually all literary studies of utopias emphasize the mismatch between human nature (in our terms, the psychology and sociology of polytropics and middles) vs. the mechanical and dehumanizing nature of life in industrial states. However, these authors have seldom suggested that the origins of a robotic society lie in the robotic nature of the (focal) brains that design and rule over it – a topic which will be discussed at length later in this book.

3. Natural societies. The previous two items were about sociology, that is, behaviors related to humans behaving in human groups specifically. Of course, other animals live in groups, too, but as we've noted, the study of social organization in animals other than humans is typically not called 'sociology,' but is referred to as a sub-topic of 'ethology.' We'll talk more about this in the next chapter, but for now we can say again that the way many humans live now, particularly in the industrialized nations, is not at all 'natural' for our species. Cities are very strange objects (though they do have parallels in other animals, as we will see), and the type of daily life that many of us take for granted, where most of the people we see during the course of a day are complete strangers, is anomalous as a way for any animal to live.

In human societies that are more natural (and more adaptive) than this, the three brain types would be seen in a somewhat different light. The first thing we would notice is that extremely focal brains would be at a severe disadvantage, since no one would allow such bullies to take any position of power. Because they can be so disruptive (and so wasteful of metabolic resources), far-left-favoring brains may not even exist in many human societies where group solidarity based on mutual trust is crucial. (Because focal brains are not 'genetic,' but represent the result of an 'epigenetic adjustment' of prenatal testosterone, humans living in survival situations may actually have found ways to avoid creating such limited, disruptive types of brains, and we will also talk later about that.)

But polytropics and middles would be very much at home in such natural human groups. The polytropics would be the 'grandmother' managers, attending to the physical and emotional needs of everyone, and lending the model of their harmonious brains to the structure of the group as a whole. Middles would be embraced as well, as loyal, useful contributors. Middle-brain women would provide the diversity of yet other 'colors' of the female rainbow (besides the polytropics), and could offer special levels of strength and perhaps some degree of restlessness for encouraging change when needed. Middle-brain men would be wonderful companions in such a group, as their good social skills give them a natural basis for interacting with women and children, and their strength and size render them good protectors against outside threats. Because their self-esteem is founded in the affection and respect of other group members, they will be loyal in fulfilling their brain-based roles as nurturers and defenders.

Developmental and learning disorders (DLDs)

One of the most puzzling and exasperating issues confronting today's industrial societies is the set of problems this phrase is used to describe. The phrase does not refer to middle-ear disease, or measles, or the need for glasses for reading – all these are taken for granted as features of childhood, or basic aspects of physical differences between individuals. Rather, "DLDs" include conditions such as hyperactivity, attention deficit, autistic spectrum disorder, stuttering, the variety of allergies – and a maze of difficulties centered on learning and reading.

Lacking insights into how the brain is built, and how the brain and body interact, these conditions are (and will remain) mysterious. However, a new approach to the most basic aspects of brain organization and function, such as offered by TM, may show us the way not only to a better understanding of the origins of these conditions, but also ideas for resolving them, to ensure that every child and adult can achieve their greatest potential.

1. DLDs and polytropics. Let's start by sorting the conditions by brain type. For polytropics, there are no known DLDs – these types of brains have access to all categories of learning skills, and enjoy good mental and physical health, at all stages of life.

2. DLDs and middle-brains. For middle-brains, however, we have already suggested that poor access to left-brain skills such as phonemic awareness may give them problems with reading – they may be good at imagery, but poor at 'word-attack' skills, that is, being able to 'sound out' and recognize words whether familiar or new. Some middles who lack good access to both left- and right-side skills may be at a serious disadvantage in reading, with neither phonemic awareness nor imagery to help them. These and other middle-brain individuals may have problems referred to as 'central auditory processing disorder' or 'auditory-only attention deficit' which in many cases is predictably due to an underlying lack of phonemic awareness, which makes it hard for them to listen to speech in a noisy background, where they may have to recognize words on the basis of a few sounds only, which they find hard to do.

Problems with phonemic awareness may also lead to certain types of speech and language problems, such as articulation disorders and language delays – simply because the children are not consciously aware of the tiny sounds inside syllables and words, that can guide their own production of the words, or help them solve the grammatical 'puzzle' of a sentence.

Children born with the type of brain we've called left-middle are predictably those who were of most interest to the authors of the GBG model discussed in Chapter Two. The 'middle-ness' of these children should make them left-handed to ambidextrous, while their 'leftness' may give them problems with immune function. And we would predict that their 'learning disorders' would be of a specific kind, different from those seen in right-middle or middle-middle brains (e.g., a lack of phonemic awareness), or those which plague focal-brain children (difficulty with imagery, etc.).

These left-middle children may also be those most at risk for stuttering – not 'developmental stuttering,' which probably affects several types of middle brains, but the kinds of chronic fluency problems that persist into adulthood. (It's been observed that many chronic stutterers tend to have light coloration – recall that item discussed above – perhaps particularly the 'paradoxical' combination of very pale skin with darker eyes and hair.)

Without going into the features of stuttering in more detail, it may be enough to recall our suggestion that the right brain manages the vocal folds' creation of 'vocal melody' over *long* periods of time, while the left brain controls their function in making very *short* speech sounds such as *b* and *z*. If the two sides of the brain are in conflict (which we've suggested may occur at a particular, left-middle dose of prenatal T), this might result in a neuromuscular 'stumbling' during speech, centered on the vocal folds.

This is not a new suggestion about stuttering – either as a 'conflict' between left and right brain, or focusing on the vocal folds – but it is new with regard to what TM suggests puts the two sides of the brain into conflict in the first place (prenatal T), and knowing this may help us identify exactly which of the children who begin stuttering in early childhood are most at risk for a continuing problem, and thus guide designs for therapy based on individual variation in brain type.

The fact that in some children, stuttering clears around age eight or nine may be further evidence that sex hormones are implicated in at least some fluency problems – as explained earlier, this is the age of adrenarche. If a younger child's brain is teetering on a threshold of conflict between right vs. left-side control, with resulting dysfluency (perhaps the case for some left-middle brain types), the additional hormonal dosage at adrenarche may serve to push the balance toward one side or the other (via changes in neural connectivity), which resolves the neural conflict and corrects the dysfluency. (Hormonal changes that *temporarily* perturb relations between right and left brain may also be behind anecdotal reports of occasional dysfluencies, along with minor balance problems, which some women experience during menopause.)

3. DLDs and focal-brains. Children born with focal brains are at risk for a very different set of problems than middles. In reading, they may be 'hyperlexic,' great at sounding out words, but poor at comprehension, which depends on imagery provided by the right brain. They may be good at fairly abstract arithmetic and mathematics, but at a loss when it comes to 'story problems' – again, due to a lack of dynamic imagery. (This is another example of the pitfalls of considering tasks in terms of global concepts such as 'language' or 'math' – one has to dissect the tasks in terms of the *component* skills required, before analyzing how one person or another performs.)

For focal-brain children, attention is a difficulty in *all* sensory modalities, originating in a very different underlying neural cause than the auditory-only attention deficit we described for middle-brain children. A focal brain's general inability to maintain sensory attention in fact comes from the same source as motor hyperactivity, that is, in the disordered relation between cortex and brainstem described in Chapter Two as a basic feature of focal brains.

There we explained how, if the cortex is not sufficiently active, the brainstem will tend to be hyper-active and hyper-reactive. A combination of frequent attention lapses plus constant motor restlessness indicates that the brainstem is 'released' and 'free-running' – which also means that these people will be hypersensitive to stimuli in all modalities (sounds, lights, touch to the skin), as their brainstem passes on incoming signals in an uncontrolled and unmodulated way to an overwhelmed cortex. (Note that sensory hypersensitivity in other situations, such as during migraine attacks, or when a person is under the influence of certain types of drugs, can be traced to the same disturbance in 'handshaking' relations we outlined in Chapter Two – in this case, an imbalance of activity comparing cortex and brainstem.)

The concept of a disrupted cortex/brainstem relation, in fact, helps us understand why medications that stimulate the cortex only (such as Ritalin, Cylert, and even nicotine) are said to have a 'paradoxical effect' – that is, they calm down hyperactive individuals, but stimulate people who do not have the underlying physiological problem. In the case of a hyperactive person, as the 'low-idle' cortex is stimulated by the drug, it 'wakes up' sufficiently to do its real job, which is to down-regulate the brainstem – as a result, these two levels of the brain are brought into a normal relation, and like magic, the hyperactive child or adult is able again to control motor activity, and also to turn the 'searchlight' of attention where it is needed.

In turn, the 'paradoxical' effect of Ritalin is explained as a case where the same cortical activator turns up an already normally active cortex, and the person either experiences a 'buzz' or feels 'druggy,' because he is experiencing a level of cortical activity that is too high for him – unusual and non-functional. Those individuals who have this response to Ritalin clearly should not be treated with a cortical stimulant, and a simple physiological assessment (see references to my AXS test battery in the bibliography at the end of this chapter) might help us learn more about these types of individual differences in children and adults.

Finally, conditions currently known as autistic spectrum disorders can be understood in similar terms. First, TM predicts that these are children made under conditions of high prenatal testosterone, thus creating a focal brain. The prenatal exposure may include an early burst of T (presumably from the mother, since evidence has been seen in girls as well as boys), that among other things, 'freezes' parts of the brainstem developing in these early stages in such a way that they never recover. Evidence for this comes both from autopsy studies of the anatomy of these areas (observed in individuals who died in their 40s), and from physiological responses which can reveal a brainstem that is behaving in a very primitive way.

Interpreting autism as a focal-brain condition makes it possible to accommodate all the features of this condition that otherwise seem only coincidental: immune system problems; unusual eating habits; a tendency to engage in repetitive 'self-stimulation' such as rocking or tapping; obsessive-compulsive characteristics such as insisting that objects be kept in the same place and things be done in exactly the same way time after time, day after day; failure to engage in social communication with others; failure to express positive emotions; tendency to extreme and primitive negative emotions such as hostility and temper tantrums.

A final puzzling feature of autism that can be explained by TM is the occasional onset of autistic symptoms as a type of 'regression' seen in a child during the 2nd year, after 18 months or so of what appears to be normal development. At about this same time, the corpus callosum, a large band of fibers that is the principal connector between right and left sides of the cortex, finally reaches its mature form. TM explains 'regression' in the following way: 1) high levels of prenatal testosterone created a left-favoring brain in these children before birth; 2) during gestation and during the first 12-18 months of postnatal life, the right hemisphere continues to predominate as in all children – which we've said is very helpful in ensuring good immune response during those early months; 3) but once the corpus callosum becomes mature, around 18 months, this allows the 'hidden,' pre-wired dominance of the left brain to be expressed, and right-brain skills such as desire for physical contact and affection, are repressed.

It is remarkable how this explanation also accounts for the types of treatment which have been found to be most effective in these children. All of these treatments, without exception, can be seen as directed to 'waking up' the repressed right brain in such children. Some of the strategies (all of them targeting right-brain specialties as described in the EPIC model – Chapter Two) include: encouraging the child to engage in whole-body gestures and actions; working on range-of-motion gestures to increase flexibility; stimulating deep-pressure receptors in the skin by tightly wrapping the child in clothing, or hanging a heavy object on the chest or back; gradually getting the child to accept hugging (also based on deep-pressure receptors); and interactively developing positive emotions and discouraging negative ones.

Even observations linking the first appearance of autistic behavior with the timing of immunization shots may be explicable using TM concepts. (Other researchers have taken the observation to mean there is an autism-causing toxin of some sort in the medium used for the shots.) TM suggests that it is simply a case of the right brain (already challenged regarding control in these left-brain individuals) being suddenly overloaded by having to mount an immune response to the mix of components – a 'drug cocktail' – administered in the shot. As a result, the 'hidden' left-brain dominance pre-programmed by prenatal T in these children, reveals itself in the form of autistic symptoms.

Other conditions

Hopefully it is obvious from the discussions in Chapter Two, and the TM catalog of features given in this chapter, that there are many, many aspects of human personality, behavior, and health which are impacted by prenatal brain development and the different degrees of testosterone exposure we've described. We have time here only to hint at this broad spectrum of implications, and will limit ourselves to a few clinical conditions which have caused great confusion in the past.

1. Psychiatric conditions. For instance, psychiatrists recognize that there seem to be several varieties of depression, and at least some of these (for example, post-partum depression) have been linked directly to hormones. TM suggests there are three categories of depression, one affecting each of the three main brain types. Because we've seen that biochemistry and neural connectivity are very different in the three types, it's possible that some of the confusion about diagnosis and treatment of depression could be resolved if individuals were 'neurotyped' as a first step, and then observed in terms of symptoms and response to different therapies, not only with reference to different drugs but also strategies such as biofeedback, exercise, and counselling. (Suggestions about how to neurotype an individual are included in my Zebra book – this was done routinely in my laboratories using an evaluation that took from 1-2 hrs, depending on the amount of detail requested.)

Besides depression, the symptoms associated with virtually all other psychiatric diagnostic categories suggest that they too are features of brains exposed to relatively high levels of prenatal testosterone. This includes: schizophrenia, obsessive-compulsive disorder, eating disorders, stimulant addiction, paranoia, anxiety attacks, chronic pain (migraines, temporomandibular joint pain, premenstrual syndrome, difficulty with menopause, etc.), neurosis, psychosis, and sociopathology.

Footnotes that TM suggests to this catalog of psychiatric ills include distinctions within diagnostic categories, such as the prediction that paranoid schizophrenia will be found more in left-favoring brains, while schizophrenia with hallucinations occurs in left-middles. (The idea is that auditory hallucinations reflect a lingering but 'static-filled' connection between the conscious left side and the (prenatally) repressed right, such that the intermittent activity from right-side auditory cortex is 'heard' as 'voices.')

2. Substance abuse. TM predicts that while focal-brains will be prone to stimulant addiction (seeking to increase their too-low cortical activity – recall our discussion of hyperactive children), middle-brains will look to depressants, such as alcohol, to console them when they are unhappy (and thus they will be more prone than focal-brains to alcoholism). In fact, radically different responses to alcohol (the 'crying drunk' vs. the 'mean drunk') could signal different brain types with different levels of cortical/brainstem activity. For example, in a focal-brain, with its already 'low-idle' cortex, when alcohol turns down the cortex even more, it releases their basic dependence on the *sympathetic* nervous system, making them angry and destructive, whereas for middles, turning down the cortex reveals their *parasympathetic* center of gravity, and they become weepy and regretful.

3. Violence. The final observation in this chapter regarding the behavioral characteristics of different brain types has to do with violence – in particular, some distinctions that TM predicts are also due to differences between middle vs. focal brains. In later chapters we will talk about violence in more general terms, and show how the larger issues considered by Neural Rainbow Theory help us understand the many paradoxes regarding violence that have long troubled humans.

But for now we will use 'violence' to refer to the very specific behaviors studied by psychologists and sociologists, such as children who set fires and hurt animals, boys who shoot other children in school, adolescents and adults who 'fly off the handle' and hurt other people, spouse batterers, the 'cold-blooded killer,' serial killers, etc.

TM predicts that: 1) individuals with polytropic brains will rarely if ever show these kinds of behaviors; 2) individuals with middle or focal brains can be violent, but only if – 3) the individual experienced violence as a child, whether the abuse was sexual, physical, or psychological. These predictions lead to the very hopeful conclusions that: 1) one-third of human beings (those with polytropic brains) are *not* at risk for these types of violence – due to the resilient nature of their brains; and 2) if we ensure that all children are given unqualified love, none of our children will be violent, either as children or adults. (If a 'well-loved' child becomes violent, we should suspect something happening behind the scenes, or there is actual brain damage.)

Child abuse does not just have vague, cognitive 'behavioral' effects – the transformations it makes in the brain are as biochemical and concrete as those resulting from prenatal testosterone: it 'turns up' the fight-or-flight sympathetic nervous system, and the chemicals released as a result can change the brain in basic and radical ways.

If the child is a middle-brain, abuse can create a person who shows a paradoxical combination of features. That is, he may show violent behavior, but in the context of many 'good' features associated with middle-brains, including strong, positive emotional ties to other people. Thus a middle-brain boy abused as a child may grow up to be a batterer, but he will be the type who genuinely needs the affection of the woman (or child or pet animal) he hurts, who follows each violent episode with weeping, regret, and self-recrimination. But again, because of the strength of his emotional attachment, the middle-brain batterer is also the type who will become a stalker, since his self-esteem is dependent on the emotional support of the woman. (Two clinical psychologists who specialized in domestic violence, Jacobson and Gottman [see bibliography at the end of this chapter] refer to this type of batterer as a 'pit bull' – a potentially kind and loving individual who has somehow been turned into an attacker. They suggested that a 'pit bull' has a better chance of successfully responding to rehabilitation than another type of batterer – see below.)

On the other hand, abuse of a left-brain child makes something else entirely – someone who may be equally violent, but with a very different context. Recall that we predicted focal brains can be asocial, even anti-social, with few emotional ties to other people. Thus if a left-brain person is hurt as a child, the additive effects of the abuse plus the high prenatal T don't leave much neural margin for supporting any type of positive human interaction, certainly not any type of intimacy, and his brain and behavior can become very primitive. If this man's 'violence of choice' is wife-battering, he will be the type who never asks for forgiveness – he considers the woman to be his property, like a car, and will not turn to her (or anyone) for emotional support. (Jacobson and Gottman call this type of batterer a 'cobra' – a solitary, who needs no one else, and may view other people more as prey than companions. Jacobson and Gottman suggested that for this type of man, 'out of sight is out of mind' – they say if a woman can get away for three days, he will forget her.)

The difference between these two types of batterers is not just interesting from an academic standpoint, but can be of life-and-death importance. First, it can provide a basis for counselling the women who are affected, to give them advice about how to get away from these relationships. (That was the motive behind Jacobson and Gottman writing their book – as a self-help manual, with descriptions and recommendations relevant not only to the problem of men-who-batter-women, but also women-who-batter-men, other individuals committing elder abuse, etc.) Second, the difference may give clinicians and partners guidelines for predicting which type of man is most amenable to being *treated* for his violence (based on the distinctive patterns of behavior as described above).

To assist their readers in making such predictions, Jacobson and Gottman not only provided excellent *behavioral* descriptions of the two types of men – which align beautifully with our TM profiles of an abused middle-brain ('pit bull') vs. an abused left-brain ('cobra') – they also reported some of their physiological work comparing and contrasting the two categories of men and their partners. To do this, they made simple measurements of autonomic nervous system (ANS) reactions (heart rate, blood pressure, etc.), while couples were engaged in (controlled) arguments in a supervised clinical setting.

Results showed that, as the women and the 'pit-bull' batterers became angrier, the more the ANS values went *up,* documenting increased SNS activation: higher heart rate, high BP. But for the 'cobra' batterers, the numbers went *down* – they were showing 'cold anger' – they were, like natural predators, 'cold-blooded' in their response. TM might say that for these men, the toxic combination of high prenatal T plus postnatal abuse essentially erased the 'mammalian' from their mind, and made them resemble reptiles in their most basic physiological nature, far below the realms of conscious awareness and control. (Thus the clinicians' term of 'cobra' seems accurate, and we will have more to say in later chapters about the biological reasons for why *mammal vs. reptile* is the appropriate contrast here.)

* * *

Finally, to overview the many features we've covered in this catalog, (and some not discussed here in detail – for more, see the 'Zebra book'), Table 3.1 provides a comparison of the three brain types in terms of many of the characteristics identified by TM as contributing to the 'fingerprint' profiles (cf. Fig. 3.3) distinguishing the three categories of individuals. The list is by no means complete, but the items that are included serve to illustrate the breadth and depth of this new approach to human typology.

Table 3.1
Features of the three iconic brain types

	left-favoring *"Focal"*	symmetric *"Middle"*	right-favoring *"Polytropic"*
Hallmark	focus on details	athletic ability	many-skilled
Handedness	right	ambidext/left	right
Body type	ecto/endomorph	mesomorph	mesomorph
Autonomic	sympathetic	PSNS	PSNS
Height	shorter	taller	medium
Coloration	paler	medium	darker
Handshaking	stiff/uncoupled	medium	elastic

Skills

1. phonemic awrns	good	poor	good
2. eye coordination	poor	medium	good
3. fine-motor contrl	good	poor to good	good
4. visual acuity	good to poor	poor to good	good
5. social skills	poor	good	good
6. emotional intelligence	poor	good	good

Health

1. immune	poor	medium	good
2. cardiac	poor	medium	good
3. food habits	poor	medium	good
4. sleep habits	poor	medium	good
5. emotional	poor	medium	good

"Season of birth"	Nov-Feb	July-Oct	Mar-June

Group membership

1. preferred form	hierarchies	partnership	partnership
2. natural societies	asocial (Perimeter)	loyal helper (Center)	grandmother leader (Center)
3. industrial soc's	professions	athlete, actor, model, dancer	all options

Developmental and learning disorders

visual dyslexia	vis/aud dyslexia	none known
attention deficit	central auditory disorder	
hyperactivity	specific language impairment	
cleft palate & lip	stuttering (left-middle)	
autistic spectrum	articulation disorders	

Recovery from brain injury

difficult	moderately hard	easier

Other conditions

depression-1	depression-2	depression-3
schizophrenia-1	schizophrenia-2	
'cobra' batterer	'pit bull' batterer	
chronic pain	(some chronic pain)	
heart failure	(some heart problems)	
alcoholism (mean drunk)	alcoholism (crying drunk)	
stimulant addict'n		
hyper/hypoactive immune (incl. autoimmune)		
eating disorders		
sleeping disorders		
epilepsy		
cerebral palsy		
Tourette's		
Alzheimer's		
Parkinson's		
ALS		
OCD		
anxiety disorder		
narcissism		
paranoia		
psychosis		
sociopathology		

'

Chapter Three Summary: Taking stock

In this chapter we've discussed details of the Trimodal Model of Brain Organization as it relates to prenatal development and the creation of a 'rainbow' of human brain types and genders. First, we reviewed how developing embryos and fetuses can be exposed to different levels of prenatal testosterone (ranging from zero to very high), where testosterone can come from either the mother's adrenal cortex or the testes in a male fetus (or both). Second, we considered how these different degrees of hormone exposure might affect brain connectivity (as discussed in Chapter Two) in very basic ways to create a continuum of individual differences, which we referred to as 'gendering the brain,' in the largest sense. Third, we suggested that, just as with a rainbow, this graded continuum of individual differences can be described as divided into distinct categories, three 'brain types,' expressed in clusters of individual features related to behavior, special skills, and general health. Fourth, we concluded that since all three brain types can be found in both chromosomal genders, the six cells of the brain type x chromosomal gender 'periodic chart' (Figs. 3.1, 3.2, 3.3, and 3.5, all outcomes of absolute x relative levels of hormonal exposure) should properly be considered a set of six genders.

In the next chapter, we will address the 'why' of these types of individual differences and categories, and see how they may be important not only for understanding more about individual humans, but also reveal the neurological bases of social organization in all animals, and suggest clues to the most 'natural' type of human social organization. In that chapter, we will be building on the Trimodal Model discussed here, and its myriad direct applications to individual psychology and health, to explore the wider implications of Neural Rainbow Theory, especially concerning topics in sociology and 'neuroethology.' The result will be new answers regarding how the organization of the nervous system is related to the organization of societies, for humans and for other animals.

Chapter Three Bibliography

Baron-Cohen S (2003) The essential difference; The truth about the male and female brain. NY: Basic Books.

Beavan C (2001) Fingerprints. NY: Hyperion.

Blum D (1997) Sex on the brain; The biological differences between men and women. NY: Viking Penguin.

Borysenko J (1996) A woman's book of life; The biology, psychology, and spirituality of the feminine life cycle. NY: GP Putnam's Sons.

Brizendine L (2006) The female brain. NY: Random House, Inc.

Bullough B, VL Bullough, J Elias (Eds) (1997) Gender blending. Amherst NY: Prometheus Books.

Burr C (1996) A separate creation; The search for the biological origins of sexual orientation. NY: Hyperion.

Cherfas J, J Gribbin (1984) The redundant male; Is sex irrelevant in the modern world? NY: Pantheon Books.

Colapinto J (2001) As nature made him; The boy who was raised as a girl. NY: HarperCollins.

Cronin H (2005) Getting human nature right. *In* Brockman J (Ed) The new humanists; Science at the edge, pp. 53-65. NY: Barnes & Noble Books.

Fausto-Sterling A (1992) Myths of gender; Biological theories about women and men, 2nd ed. NY: Basic Books.

Fox R (1980) The red lamp of incest. Notre Dame IN: Univ. of Notre Dame Press.

Gardner H (1983) Frames of mind; The theory of multiple intelligences. NY: Basic Books.

Henry JP (1992) Instincts, archetypes and symbols. Dayton OH: College Press.

Hird MJ (2000) Sex, gender, and science. NY: Palgrave Macmillan.

Jacobson N & J Gottman (1998) When men batter women; New insights into ending abusive relationships. NY: Simon & Schuster.

Jastreboff PJ, WC Gray, SL Gold (1996) Neurophysiological approach to tinnitus patients. Amer J Otol 17: 236-240.

Lauter JL (1992) Imaging techniques and auditory processing. *In* J Katz, N Stecker, D Henderson (Eds) Central auditory processing: A transdisciplinary view. NY: Mosby, pp. 93-115.

Lauter JL, SB Wood (1993) Auditory-brainstem synchronicity in dyslexia measured using the REPs/ABR protocol. Ann NY Acad Sci 682: 377-379.

Lauter JL (1995) Visions of speech and language: Noninvasive imaging techniques and their applications to the study of human communication. *In* H Winitz (Ed) Human communication and its disorders, Vol. IV. Timonium MD: York Press, pp. 277-389.

Lauter JL (1997) Noninvasive brain imaging in speech motor control and stuttering: Choices and challenges. *In* W Hulstijn, HFM Peters, P Van Lieshout (Eds) Speech production: Motor control, brain research, and fluency disorders. Amsterdam: Elsevier, pp. 233-258.

Lauter JL (1998) Neuroimaging and the Trimodal Brain: Applications in developmental communication neuroscience. Folia Phoniatr Logoped 50: 118-145.

Lauter JL, H Richey, S Gilmore, O Lynch (1998) Putting the 'central' back in Central Auditory Processing. J Develop Learn Disord 2: 51-106.

Lauter JL (1999a) Neuroimaging in developmental speech and language pathology. *In* P Dejonkere, HFM Peters (Eds) Communication and its disorders: A science in progress. Nijmegen: Nijmegen Univ. Press, pp. 499-502.

Lauter JL (1999b) Central auditory processing. Curr Opin Otolaryngol Head Neck Surg 7: 274-281.

Lauter JL (1999c) Functional asymmetries and the Trimodal Brain: Dimensions and individual differences. J Develop Learn Disord 3: 181-260.

Lauter JL, SB Wood, O Lynch, L Schoeffler (1999) Physiological and behavioral effects of an antivertigo antihistamine in adults. Percep Motor Skills 88:707 732.

Lauter JL (2000a) The brain and reading: Neural bases for a new perspective on reading skills assessment, and training. Invited presentation to Idaho State Conference on Reading and Learning. Boise ID.

Lauter JL (2000b) A new approach to CAP and CAPD. (1) Putting central auditory processing at your fingertips: The AXS Test Battery. (2) Neuro-audiological rehabilitation: Expanding your scope of practice. (3) 21st-century CAPD: Throwing away the crutches. Invited 3-hr presentation to Symposium on Central Auditory Processing in Children: Perspectives on Assessment and Management. Cleveland Clinic Foundation, Cleveland OH.

Lauter JL (2001a) Is reading 'unnatural' for 2/3 of our children? – Right brain, left brain, and the 'missing link' skills for reading and learning. Invited keynote presentation to SouthWest and Rocky Mountain (SWARM) division of American Association for the Advancement of Science, Denton TX.

Lauter JL (2001b) Neuroimaging: How understanding individual differences can improve your clinical practice. [3-hr educational video with manual] Rockville MD: American Speech-Language-Hearing Association.

Lauter JL (2002) Is reading 'unnatural' for 2/3 of children and adults? Presented to American Speech-Language-Hearing Association, Atlanta GA.

Lauter JL (2003) The Trimodal Brain and reading I: A new synthesis and some predictions. J Develop Learn Disord 7: 65-84.

Lauter JL, PF McKane (2003) The Trimodal Brain and reading II: Preliminary data on the co-occurrence of problems in phonemic awareness and eye-movement coordination. J Develop Learn Disord 7:85-96.

Lauter JL (2005) How is your brain like a zebra? Invited inaugural lecture in the SFA Regents Lecture Series. Stephen F. Austin State University, Nacogdoches TX.

Lauter JL (2007) The Trimodal Brain: A new neurotypology and its implications for Multiple Intelligences, hyperactivity, brain imaging, and education. Presented to First International Conference on Mind, Brain, and Education. Ft. Worth TX.

Lauter JL (2008a) How is your brain like a zebra? A new human neurotypology. Bloomington IN: Xlibris.

Lauter JL (2008b) The Zebra Brain: A new approach to understanding individual differences in children and adults. Presented to 16th Annual Parent Education Conference, Denton TX.

Lindamood P, N Bell, P Lindamood (1992) Issues in phonological awareness assessment. Annals of Dyslexia 42: 242-259.

Lindamood P, N Bell, P Lindamood (1997) Achieving competence in language and literacy by training in phonemic awareness, concept imagery, and comparator function. *In* C Hulme, M Snowling (Eds) Dyslexia: Biology, cognition, and intervention. London: Whurr Pubs., pp. 212-234.

Lindamood P, N Bell, P Lindamood (1997) Sensory-cognitive factors in the controversy over reading instruction. J Develop Learn Disord 1: 143-182.

MacNeilage PF, MG Studdert-Kennedy, B Lindblom (1983) Planning and production of speech; an overview. *In* JL Lauter (Ed) Proceedings of the conference on the planning and production of speech in normal and hearing impaired individuals: A seminar in honor of S Richard Silverman, pp. 15-21. ASHA Reports #15. American Speech-Language Hearing Association.

Mead M (1949) Male and female; A study of the sexes in a changing world. NY: Dell Pub. Co.

Miller JR (1990) X-linked traits; A catalog of loci in nonhuman animals. NY: Cambridge Univ. Press.

Moir A, D Jessel (1991) Brain sex; The real difference between men and women, NY: Dell Publishing Group.

Montagu A (1974) The natural superiority of women, 4th ed. NY: Macmillan Pub. Co.

Morbeck ME, A Calloway, A Zihlman (Eds) (1997) The evolving female; A life history perspective. Princeton NJ: Princeton Univ. Press.

Morgan E (1972) The descent of woman. NY: Stein & Day.

Nanda S (1999) Neither man nor woman; The hijras of India, 2nd ed. Belmont CA: Wadsworth Pub. Co.

Olson P (1981) Sons and mothers; Why men behave as they do. NY: M. Evans & Co.

Pfaff DW, AP Arnold, AM Etgen, SE Fahrbach, RT Rubin (Eds) (2002) Hormones, brain and behavior [5 volumes]. Amsterdam: Academic Press.

Pool R (1994) Eve's rib; Searching for the biological roots of sex differences. NY: Crown Pubs. Inc.

Rogers L (2001) Sexing the brain. NY: Columbia Univ. Press.

Sapolsky RM (1997) The trouble with testosterone; And other essays on the human predicament. NY: Simon & Schuster.

* * *

Chapter Three Figures & Tables
(titles here are summaries; for full titles, see text)

⤳ Chapter Four ⤳

SOCIAL ORGANIZATION –
NICHES, CHOICES, SOCIAL ROLES,
BRAIN TYPES, GENDERS

In many ways, undertaking a scientific approach to understanding the world is like being a reporter – you have to find out 'who, how, what, why, when, and where,' in order to reconstruct what happened and why (or at least, come up with a story). In Chapter One we talked about the *who* in our story – namely, ourselves, and our fellow humans. There we briefly recalled the long history of intense and continuing interest in the individual differences and similarities that are such striking features of human beings, and the general lack of consensus regarding whether such categories even exist – or if the question should be raised at all.

In Chapter Two we reviewed some new suggestions about *how* these individual characteristics as well as categories might be created. We discussed new approaches to thinking about features of the brain that create behavior, and how recent research shows that the brain is shaped in basic ways during prenatal life by a 'third factor' in addition to genetics and postnatal environment – namely, the degree of prenatal exposure to sex hormones (as mentioned earlier, sex hormones are only one of many epigenetic factors at work during development, but NRT considers gender shaping to be of such basic importance to the survival of species that it merits a special category). We also saw there for the first time that the principles we are developing may apply to other animals besides humans.

In Chapter Three, we described the results of this prenatal shaping – the *what* of our story. This is the continuum or 'rainbow' of brain/body characteristics that can be classified in terms of *clusters* of individual features that take the form of three categories, or 'brain types' that can be found in both chromosomal genders, creating a 'periodic chart' of a three-brain-type/six-gender complex. Finally, we concluded that this hormonally-based 'neural rainbow' is not just a neurological curiosity, but may in fact represent a fundamental process reflected in all aspects and spheres of human behavior.

In the current chapter, we consider the *why* of the rainbow of brain types (Chapter Five will address *When* and *Where*.) We will see that: 1) the brain's sensitivity to hormonal exposure is a powerful means of creating individuals who are thus adapted to fulfill certain *roles within the social organization of a species*; 2) successful performance of these roles is an absolute requirement for any species that propagates itself through sexual reproduction; and 3) as a result, a good fit between the three-brain-types/six-genders complex, and social organization, is crucial if a species hopes to have a future.

The big picture: Why brains and social roles are linked

Scientists are not always comfortable talking about 'why.' But doing so is absolutely basic to this chapter and this book. (Eventually we will go beyond 'why' and ask 'what do we think about it?')

Social organization: Why it's important

We said before that the fulcrum, the crux, the essential ingredient, of the way any species survives over time is the nature of the individual and the 'recipe' of genes and tendencies characterizing it that are passed on to the next generation. In very rare cases (in some plants and a few animals), the individual can do this just as single-cell organisms do, all alone, via asexual reproduction – either binary fission, budding, fragmentation, or parthenogenesis. But ever since biology 'invented' sexual reproduction, practically all animals and plants have seized on the advantages of this type of propagation (other comments on the issue are included in my *First Things* essay in the Volume Three Appendix).

This book won't review yet again the advantages of sexual reproduction – that has been discussed at length elsewhere. Suffice it to say that sexual reproduction provides the basis for a 'mix and match' process from one generation to the next, a mechanism that ensures homeostasis – that is, a dynamic balance between 'what to sell and what to keep' – retaining what seems to be working, plus also having the capacity to try something slightly new, especially if and when change seems to be called for.

As developed by biology on this planet, sexual reproduction means that at least two separate individuals are needed to propagate a species. (This doesn't seem to be strictly necessary – for instance, a science-fiction scenario might suggest the possibility of plants or animals who developed organs of special cells on the surface of their bodies with the capacity for making slight variations in their own genome, which they could then use to blend with their own original cells to grow new and slightly different individuals. But no such example is known to us on earth.) As a result, for all species that reproduce sexually, the nature of relations between individuals, *their social interaction*, is as basic a determinant of the future of a species as the recipe of individual genes. (We will see later that the biological importance of social organization goes well beyond chromosomal identity, which in a sense is just a simplistic 'Noah's ark' dyad of XX and Xy.)

We also need to remember that social relationships are not 'abstract,' somehow removed from the realm of biology and physics. For instance, in Chapter Two, we saw how social influences such as stress on the mother during pregnancy can change chemicals that change genes. So 'social interactions' should be seen as very concrete, biological phenomena, with biological consequences.

Social organization: five basic categories, three social roles

1. Five social organization categories (SOCs). There are millions of animal species on earth, living in all kinds of ways in all kinds of environments. These millions of species seem to differ in every way imaginable (and some almost unimaginable until we see it!). They vary in thousands of ways – in body size, shape and type of covering; number of legs; their nervous system; whether they breathe water or air; how they move around; what kinds of food they eat, etc., etc.

Yet in spite of this overwhelming, 'blooming, buzzing confusion' (to borrow a phrase from psychologist William James) of the diversity across species, there is only a handful of options for how a species arranges individuals in space – that is, its form of *social organization*. In fact, NRT suggests that in spite of many variations, there are only five primary Social Organization Categories (SOCs).

Which of the five SOCs is used by any given species at any given time depends primarily on their *basic reproductive economics*, that is, how each individual of a species obtains resources from the environment (one definition of 'economics'), resources that enable it to help *produce the next generation in a way that contributes to the continuation of the species*.

The final phrase of that last sentence is crucial. Just 'reproducing' does not guarantee 'continuation' – reproducing in the *wrong* way can lead a species in exactly the opposite direction, as we'll see. Biology has a set of rules or guidelines for how to reproduce in the *right* way, that is, aiming at continuation rather than extinction, and only those species which follow the guidelines can hope for a long and successful future. Neural Rainbow Theory summarizes this set of reproductive rules as QRS, standing for Quality/Replacement/Sustainable. Taken together, these three relatively self-explanatory terms highlight the evolutionary importance of producing a next generation of *quality* individuals at *replacement* levels in a *sustainable* way.

At the end of this chapter, we'll discuss more about the details of the three components of QRS, but for now it is enough to say that social organization is an important tool that helps a group or a species follow the QRS rules to achieve adaptive population management. The future of a group or species depends on their being able to do that, whether they seek to *maintain zero population growth* (as long as supportive environmental conditions remain stable), *increase population* slightly to counteract losses such as deaths from a disease outbreak or reduced food supply due to drought, etc., or *decrease population* somewhat if group numbers begin to overmatch resources. If conditions change, either in a more supportive or a more challenging direction, each SOC offers a certain degree of inherent flexibility to absorb small changes like the ones described here, or, if the changes are larger, a species or group may need to change their SOC in order to adapt to the novel situation.

One or another of the QRS rules may be broken as a short-term emergency measure to help a species (or a local group) survive a temporary environmental crisis – an unusually severe drought, brief failure of a particular food source, etc. – but continuing to break the rules even after the crisis has passed, particularly if the new version becomes permanent, puts the species or group at risk.

The way SOCs function as a tool for achieving QRS is based on the 'waterfall' set of *four levels of linked niches-and-adaptations* shown in Figure 4.1. This figure suggests that the environment-as-a-source-of-resources (Level One, 'economics') serves as a niche for which social organization categories (Level Two) are an adaptation, which in turn serves as a niche for social roles (Level Three) as an adaptation, which in turn serves as a niche for gender/brain types (Level Four) as an adaptation.

Figure 4.1

Waterfall series of 'lock-and-key' niches and adaptations linking economics *(generally, 'the environment,' shown at the top) downward through* Social Organization Categories (SOCs) *and their supporting* social roles, *to the* gender/brain type *categories of individuals described in Chapter Three. The diagram, a kind of 'niche-and-adaptation ladder,' illustrates that: economics (Level 1) serves as a niche for which SOCs (Level 2) are an adaptation; in turn, SOCs are a niche for which social roles (Level 3) are an adaptation; and in turn, social roles provide a niche for which gender/brain types (Level 4) are an adaptation.*

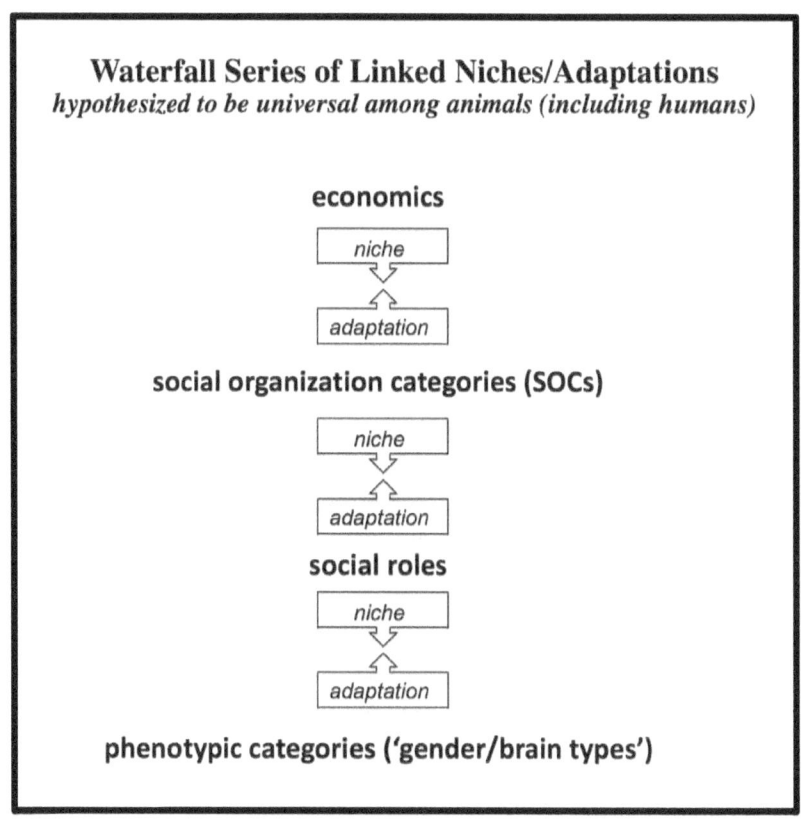

* * *

This might be a surprising thing to hear – first, across the millions of animal species, there are only five basic designs for social organization, and second, that these designs derive primarily from economics. Surely, one might say, there have to be many more options given the incredible variety of animals –

insects and fish and amphibians and reptiles and birds and mammals and ... primates and the species that surely breaks all the rules, (or is beyond the rules?) – *Homo sapiens*. After all, one might object, things such as the volume of cerebral cortex or the complexity of everyday life must be equally – if not more – important than such survival questions as how difficult it is to get food. Surely the same handful of options can't account for all animals?

Yet NRT suggests they do. Details from the science of ethology, the study of animal behavior including social organization (we'll highlight our social focus by using the term *socioethology*) show that virtually all animals employing sexual reproduction organize themselves in one of the following five ways (following the list is a set of 'SOC maps' illustrating how individuals living in each of the SOCs are arranged in space):

1) Solitaries – all individuals spend the vast majority of their time alone, except breeding-season interludes when one XX meets briefly with one Xy in order to mate, and the few months when mothers gestate and raise their young;
2) Pair-bonds – a brief (breeding season only), or year-round, sometimes lifelong, version of the minimum 'society' for making and caring for babies;
3) Center/Perimeter (C/P) – the NRT term for a *combination* of: a) small stable groups consisting of females and sub-adults (the 'Center'), each of which may be accompanied by a single male either seasonally or year-round; *plus* b) small unstable male-only groups, and solitary males, who live in the spaces between Center groups (the 'Perimeter'); the Perimeter functions as a sink for 'surplus' males not immediately needed by the Center groups;
4) 'Eusocial' – groups which may range from 25 to thousands, depending on the size of the animal, composed of one or two females, a few males, and a majority of individuals who are *functionally* sexless;
5) 50:50 – small to moderate-sized groups with a ratio of half females and half males living in fairly close proximity to each other; NRT sees 50:50 as the transformation of an original C/P arrangement in which some version of habitat loss has reduced the space that would have supported a Perimeter, forcing the surplus males to 'invade' the Center groups.

Figure 4.2

Maps of the five Social Organization Categories (SOCs). (Circles are females, triangles males; smaller symbols are children; for eusocial, the larger circle is the queen. Space is not to scale – that is, the territory for one solitary animal may cover hundreds of acres, while at the other extreme, thousands of eusocial individuals may live in a single nest of a few cubic feet.)

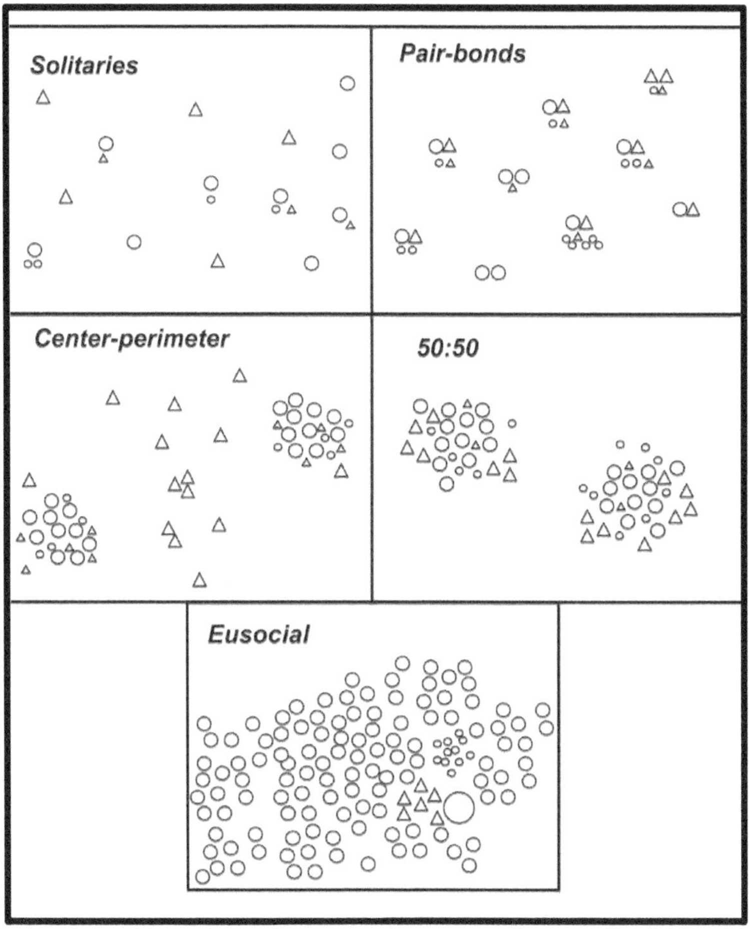

* * *

Examples of each of these illustrate that, while most animals (at least other than 'eusocial' insects such as ants and bees), if given the choice, seem to prefer option #3 (Center/Perimeter), one or more of these options is represented in every category of animal, from insects to mammals. For instance, option #1 (solitaries) is the primary lifestyle of bears as well as snakes; option #2 (pair-bonds) is practiced by sea horses, Canada geese, and gibbons; option #3 (Center/Perimeter) is the way of life for almost all mammals – from ground-squirrels and elk to lions and whales – a few large birds such as wild turkeys, and even some fish; option #4 (eusocial) in its most typical form is found in insects such as ants, termites, bees, and even one group of spiders – and in one mammal, the naked mole rat (more later) – but we will suggest it also helps us understand the nature of some human groups; and option #5 (50:50), perhaps because of the complex social-management skills required to cope with the implicit problem of 'too many males,' has been observed primarily only in a few primates.

2. Three social roles. The secret to why all the different species of animals can make do with only five SOCs may depend on what NRT refers to as "social roles." Even though these roles are related both to social behaviors and gender issues, it is important to know that this term should *not* be confused with the kinds of 'social roles' or 'gender roles' defined in sociology or psychology, that is, forms of expected behaviors (based on cultural not biological origins) derived from interactions with other individuals in the social surround of each person, and which shift from situation to situation (for example, the same person can fill the roles of: *child, parent, spouse, teacher, client, boss, employee*, and more).

A more accurate term for the roles we will be talking about here would be 'socioethological roles,' that is, roles specifically related to the *structural aspects of social organization*, such as the five categories of SOCs described above; but for convenience, we'll use the abbreviated form 'social roles' for our discussions. *NRT suggests that there are only three such roles – Grandmother-Leader, Loyal-Helper, and Focal-Asocial – and that in different combinations, it is they which form the structural 'skeleton' of each of the five SOCs, the* infrastructure *that enables how the species lives and functions within its environment.*

The importance of identifying these roles is that they offer a window on how the SOCs actually work – it is not a case of a lot of individuals with the same capabilities magically sorting themselves out into performing different behaviors, but arrangements of *individuals distinguished by certain in-born properties* which specifically *fit each of them for fulfilling the different roles* required for each SOC.

The title of **Grandmother-Leader** (**GL**) refers to the job of the older wiser females of a species, who provide leadership skills and the wisdom of experience to help certain SOC groups maintain themselves in all aspects of everyday behavior. The role can only be filled by a female, but in spite of the name 'Grandmother,' age and reproductive status are less important than a cluster of mental and physical features which we'll see later are related to brain types.

With regard to age, a younger woman with the requisite abilities can be considered (and recognized by group members) as a 'grandmother type,' and contribute to the group in that role, either as an aide to the current GL, or on her own. The NRT prediction is that any group with a designated GL will also have a series of younger similar females who apprentice to the GL role as they are growing up, and assist the principal GL when needed. Also, a candidate GL does not have to be a literal grandmother – that is, she does not have to have had a daughter and grandchildren herself – her chromosomal gender plus her features profile constitute her qualifications for the job. According to NRT, the full-fledged version of the GL is found primarily in the Center/Perimeter SOC, but may also occur in pair-bonds and 50:50 groups.

The role of **Loyal-Helper (LH)** refers to the job of providing mutual assistance to all members of a group, no matter their age or gender. LH is not about leadership, but support – those who fulfill this role are loyal to the group as a whole, and particularly to the Grandmother-Leader, whom they acknowledge as the source of group wisdom, and unquestioningly follow her guidance. The role can be filled by males as well as females, but all LH candidates have versions of the same features profile, again related to brain types, as we'll see. The LH role is found in three SOCs: pair-bonds, C/P, and 50:50.

Finally, the **Focal-Asocial (FA)** role is filled by individuals whose social life, *particularly regarding long-term, complex relationships with other adults,* is almost nonexistent. NRT considers this role to be the only one found in both solitaries and eusocial species, and that the neural characteristics of individuals in these SOCs fit them perfectly for fulfilling this role.

* * *

In the next section, we will describe each of the five SOC options in detail, with examples from the everyday life of animals living them, and how the three social roles are expressed (or not), and function, in each of the SOCs. We'll see that from time to time (depending on economics again), the 'boundaries' between the SOC options may appear to become less definite. For instance, some solitaries have a kind of 'hidden Center/Perimeter' organization that can only be seen if one looks closely; and other animals who live in a basically pair-bond way may be able to tap into the benefits of a small group, and have 'helpers' that assist with many aspects of child-rearing. And, to close the circle, one of the rules for the Center/Perimeter organization is that some of its members actually end up living most of their lives as solitaries.

And all of these SOC versions *depend on individuals with the requisite features filling the component roles*.

We will also see that (again, depending on economics) a set of individuals from a particular species may temporarily adjust to environmental changes by shifting to another lifestyle option (a different SOC) as long as the change in circumstance remains in place. These within-species shifts suggests that the five main modes of social organization are a type of 'strange attractor' set of alternatives (not 'hard-wired' as part of a species' 'social genome'). In this way, animal social organization can be seen from the point of view of nonlinear dynamics ('chaos'), as characterized by a systematic, *small set of possible modes* that animals can 'choose' among, 'shifting gears' from mode to mode, depending on environmental demands.

The entire set of relations shown in Fig. 4.1 can also be described as a 'tunable device' for fitting a species into its environment. 'Tunable' in this case means that a fundamental change at any level in the niche-and-adaptation ladder can be propagated up and down the ladder. For instance, a fundamental change at the top of the ladder, in the environment (something like a change in food sources, or ambient temperature) could affect the dosage of prenatal sex hormones, resulting in changes in the proportions of brain types (at the bottom) produced, leading in turn to a new social-roles profile (next level up), with consequences for the species' social organization (next level up) and thus its 'degree of fit' to the changed environment (back to the top). If the environmental change is 'masked' in some way so that the natural potential for adjustment implicit in the system is not allowed to be expressed, the 'gyroscope' of the whole structure can be deeply perturbed – 'thrown off-center' – with the potential for causing local as well as long-range disruption in the daily life of the species, including the threat of extinction, if the species' 'gyroscope' cannot be reset.

NRT posits a direct connection between social organization and violence. In the discussion of each of the five options, we will begin by talking about animals who live in a *peaceful* way according to that option (that is, with a minimal amount of within-group aggression). With regard to this, we will take it as a given that anything beyond a minimal amount of such aggression (note that this does NOT mean protective aggression directed against intruders, or the feeding behavior of carnivores) is a sign that the animal group is stressed. We make this assumption based on the fact that for all animals (as suggested in Chapter Three), within-group aggression is behaviorally and biochemically anathema to the successful conception, gestation, and rearing of children (i.e., QRS).

At the end of the discussion for each option, we will illustrate this point by giving examples of animals who may be living according to that type of organization, but in a way that does not seem to be 'natural' for them – signaled by a variety of signs of stress, including violence. Eventually we will discuss some of the origins of such stress, and show how one very important source might be a mis-match between the brain types represented in the group, and the option for social organization the group is either trying to or is being forced to adopt (e.g., by being confined in too small an area, such as a 'preserve' or a zoo). Thus we will see that thinking about the *degree of fit between neural types and social organization might help us understand within-species violence*, including the many instances of that type of pathology offered by our own species.

And finally we will bring in our descriptions of the three-brain-types/six-genders complex from Chapter Three to discuss how the categories of individuals outlined there provide a good fit to each of these different lifestyles, specifically, combinations of the three social roles that support the five SOCs. (For that discussion, we will mention animals from a number of groups, but most of the focus will be on mammals including humans.)

Social organization up close: Choices and examples

Life in solitude

Ethologists have noted that for most animals who live as solitaries, the economics of making a living are difficult – that is, a very large territory is required to support a single individual. This is not a function simply of the type of surround (jungle vs. open country vs. ocean), as much as it is the concentration of food items – the amount of food per unit of space, and how much food it takes to sustain an individual. Thus tigers are solitaries, with their food sources so easily hidden in jungles – but so are polar bears, who live in wide-open spaces, with personal territories as large as 100 square miles, to accommodate to the rarity of food items, particularly in winter. (Lions, as we'll see later, live in a very different way, since their food is much more abundant relative to a particular space.) The following figure (an enlarged panel from Fig. 4.2) shows the spatial layout of the Solitary SOC.

Figure 4.3

Social organization map of the distribution of individuals living in a Solitary arrangement. (Circles are females, triangles are males; smaller symbols are children; as in Fig. 4.2, space is not to scale: individual-adult territories can be very large.)

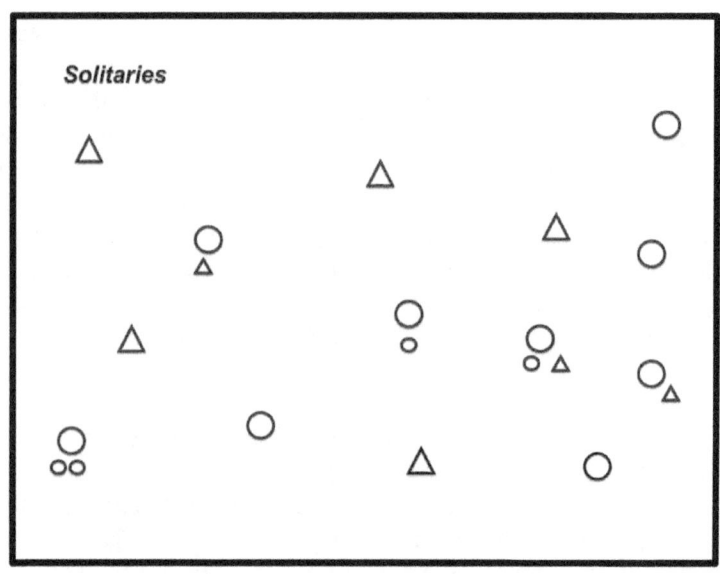

* * *

When a female living as a solitary wants to conceive, she finds a solitary male of her species to provide her with sperm, and then returns to living on her own. She gestates, delivers, and rears her children alone. The children of solitary mammals are typically able to care for themselves within 1-2 years of birth, at which time they go off on their own, and the mother looks again for a mate. The lack of complex daily relationships with other adults experienced by solitaries essentially defines the Focal-Asocial role, and the 'social' nature of interactions in those rare encounters with other individuals that do occur is extremely limited – either aggressive, for territorial defense; or reproductive, mating and (briefly) raising young.

As noted earlier, the job of 'finding a mate' may not always be as random as it might seem for animals who live far apart. Some solitaries (such as Komodo dragons – more below) seem to have a 'hidden pair-bond' arrangement, where a female and male who occupy neighboring territories exclusively mate with each other, and share in hunting and territorial defense; and still others (such as tigers) extend this to a 'hidden Center/Perimeter' format, in which a particular male's hunting territory overlaps with the

140

territories of several females – perhaps related to each other – and the group of females share his services as a mate.

One example of a reptile living according to a solitary pattern is the Komodo dragon, an imposing (10 feet long and 200 pounds) lizard living on several islands, including Komodo, in Indonesia. Among these lizards, individuals have fairly large but distinct territories within which they hunt and keep one or more burrows for sleeping. Getting food requires lengthy hunting forays, which may keep the lizard away from its home burrow for days at a time, and long hours of lying in wait along deer trails in the jungle. Hunting ranges of individuals may overlap to some extent, but each lizard is very protective of the places where they sleep.

For mating, Komodos show what we've called a hidden pair-bond pattern that may in fact be more common among solitaries than previously appreciated (as Paul MacLean has said – see chapter bibliography – Komodos are therapsids, or 'mammal-like' reptiles, which may be important for their behavior). The 'hidden pair-bond' in Komodos means that even though individuals live alone most of the year, they may have a favorite of the opposite sex whom they know well and with whom they prefer to mate. A female/male pair of Komodos will live in adjoining territories that have a large degree of overlap, much like a pair of people living in separate houses next door to each other. The members of these pairs are quite exclusive in mating with each other; the female of such a pair may even seriously injure other males who approach her, and can be seen entering into sexual relations with her favorite without the preliminaries of meeting and approaching that are *de rigueur* for strangers. Mating might occur when one of the pair 'calls' at the other's burrow, or if they happen to encounter each other at another place, such as near a site where some prey has been killed and is being eaten by several Komodos from the area. Part of the apparent enjoyment of these types of communal feasts is the lovemaking undertaken by bonded pairs.

It is notable that the behavior of solitaries, including lizards such as the Komodo, can be quite complex and exhibits many categories of behavior that we might think of as found only in mammals. This includes not only the details of day-to-day routines that are followed in and around the home burrows, and the evident planning and execution of hunting strategies, but also extends to patterns of interfacing with other individuals, whether strangers or acquaintances. For instance, when Komodo males meet, their aggressive displays (circling around each other, stretching up and out to appear as large as possible, bobbing and weaving as they close for fighting) are essentially identical to interactions among males of many species, including our own.

At the same time, descriptions of the ways that bonded pairs interact with each other, as they meet, greet, and caress each other during lovemaking (predictably using the same type of right-brain-activating 'support-communication' somatosensory receptors described in Chapter Two), are quite touching to read, and bear a striking resemblance to similar interactions in mammalian pairs such as wolves.

In fact, some scientists, such as Paul MacLean (see references in the chapter bibliography), suggest that many reptiles, especially therapsids, possess the entire behavioral repertoire of mammals – with the single exception the interactions associated with child care, and 'family life' in general, such as children playing together under the watchful eye of caring adults. Certainly Komodos do not show anything approaching parental care (though a few other reptiles can be attentive and caring parents). As soon as Komodo young hatch from their eggs, they seem to have a built-in drive to find a tree and climb it as quickly as possible. If any adult Komodo – including the female who laid the eggs – sees the babies, it will eat the children as prey. (Later we will see that this type of behavior which seems shockingly cannibalistic is not limited to 'primitive' reptiles – males of mammalian species also exhibit this type of 'conspecific predation' *where individuals living as solitaries* attack (and may also eat) children of their own species.)

Some animals living as solitaries at the present time may be doing this not in a 'natural way' but as a consequence of habitat degradation. Many signs indicate that the animals have not taken up the lifestyle out of 'choice' (that is, as a 'natural' adjustment response to changes in economics), but under coercion, as space constrictions literally reduce their range of choices. Symptoms of this type of coercion include marked conspecific violence and other signs of stress, such as explosive population growth and remarkable levels of disease, testifying to stress-related failures in immune function. Much of the stress may come from a radical shift from the 'expected' or 'natural' social roles for a species (e.g., C/P), to new role designations demanded by a new situation. For example, if a C/P female, who may be herself fitted to function as either a Grandmother-Leader or a Loyal-Helper, is forced into assuming the Focal-Asocial role by a new, solitary lifestyle, she may feel totally lost and as a result, suffer both psychologically and physically. If this happened to many individuals over a fairly short amount of time, the consequences could spell disaster for the species.

One example of animals forced to live in an 'unnatural' solitary way is provided by the terrible plight of whitetail deer in the Eastern U.S. These animals have undergone radical environmental restrictions over the past 100 years, losing access to meadows and open woodlands through human intrusions such as farms, urban developments, and roadways, which not only diminish the amounts of open country but also *island* the remaining areas from each other. Other American deer, such as the black deer of the plains or elk of the mountains, occupy much more open ranges, and as a result are able to continue living according to the more typically mammalian Center/Perimeter model. But whitetails in the Eastern U.S. live primarily as solitaries (a doe may be accompanied by her daughters from the previous year or two, but these young does will leave to live on their own when the mother conceives again).

Many observations in whitetails suggest that even though they are present in very high numbers (which only *appears* to be a sign of 'success'), they are actually doing this under conditions of chronic stress. For example, whitetail fawns are attacked by ticks to an extent that is seldom seem among other types of deer who have the freedom of larger spaces within which to choose places for birthing and rearing children. There are also known contrasts in stressed vs. non-stressed deer populations regarding adult incidence of parasite infestation, large disfiguring tumors, and bacterial skin infections.

The overpopulation among whitetail deer itself is a sign of stress, that the animals are being forced to live without appropriate access to feedback phenomena that would help them self-regulate their numbers. 'Feedback' does not only mean natural predators. For instance, as we will see, when animals are able to live in a Center/Perimeter model, this serves to limit population, since under this model very few males (sometimes as few as 10%) are reproductively active, and not all females in a particular group will give birth every year. On the other hand, for animals forced to live as solitaries through fragmentation of habitat, many more males will have a chance to breed, and thus more females will become pregnant, leading to explosive population growth – as has also happened with coyotes in this country.

In addition to sickness and overpopulation, stressed whitetails exhibit the same types of conspecific violence to be seen in other animals living under similarly unnatural conditions. If bucks and does are kept together in pens, bucks have been known to kill does during the rutting season, particularly if the bucks come into season ahead of the does. In the wild, the does could keep away, but when fenced in with a buck undergoing a 'testosterone storm,' they stand the risk of being gored. Violence among overcrowded deer even includes rape, as evidenced in one observed attack where nine bucks chased an isolated doe until she was exhausted, stabbed her with their antlers, knocked her down and joined in a gang rape.

Rape has also been seen in orangutans, who are themselves suffering a severe reduction in habitat quantity and quality. Orangs have definite sexual dimorphism (that is, females and males are quite different in size, shape, and body proportions) which should mark them as a species that in its recent past preferred the typical mammalian Center/Perimeter social style (we will talk more later about why sexual dimorphism and Center/Perimeter go together). Yet most observers report them now as living primarily alone, on the model of Komodo dragons or bears, where an adult female is accompanied only by her children, and the males roam on their own.

Orang females have been seen to be highly aggressive in defending what territory they have left, and some of the most horrendous tales of rape among animals come from observations of orangs. Interestingly enough, only one type of orang male ('the short ones') seems to commit these crimes, and later we will see that the details regarding the 'two types of males' which have been identified in orangs and many other animals provide strong support for the ideas in Chapter Two about physical and behavioral correlates of individual differences in brain type, and a tendency for conspecific violence.

Bonded pairs

Animals who utilize the pair-bond type of organization live in economic circumstances that make it moderately difficult for reproducing individuals to maintain themselves and support children at the same time. Thus animals living in this way have adapted to conditions in which the resources available in a given territory will support only two adults living together (the reproductive minimum) plus a few young children. The difficulties presented by the environment mean that individuals in such a species may not waste energy looking for a different mate from year to year – rather, once formed and stabilized, pairs will stay together for many years, even lifelong; they represent the iconic example of the Loyal-Helper social role. (We will see in a moment that some pair-bond animals, if the circumstances are right, may allow some of their children to stay with them for a few years after birth, as apprentice Loyal-Helpers, primarily to assist in caring for younger siblings, but even in these 'cooperative-breeder' groups, the 'breeding pair' remain a couple beyond a single season.)

The long-term commitment made by many bonded pairs suggests that another feature of the individuals forming these couples is that they find each other personally compatible. In the previous chapter we suggested that this might be based on 'matching' brain types that: 1) are not *exactly* the same, but 2) are within a 'sibling range' of each other. That combination should yield someone who is just different enough from you to be interesting, but who also feels comfortably familiar, as though you've 'known them all your life.'

The idea of a 'sibling range' might evoke visions of incest – would that mean actual genetic siblings should find each other sexually attractive and want to form pair-bonds? The answer is no – with the crucial qualification that avoiding this may depend on the way siblings *interact with each other* during childhood. We've said that postnatal as well as prenatal changes in brain connectivity have basic consequences for shaping individuals, and the array of physical, emotional, psychological, and social interactions shared by most animal siblings *as they grow up together* may be the way biology makes sure children from the same family will *not* find each other sexually attractive once puberty arrives.

144

Perhaps most important of these are *physical interactions*, involving many types of body and brain stimulations: olfactory, visual, auditory, somatosensory, and motor. Siblings that grow up in a nurturing environment where they play together, sleep together, and eat together, ideally with some caregiver adults (such as parents) sharing those same experiences at the same time, should grow up feeling supported and loved, confident in their own identities, comfortable and practiced in being with other people – but NOT sexually attracted to any of the individuals they knew so intimately during their formative years.

Wild animals, particularly mammals (horses, rabbits, elephants, etc.) 'take it for granted' this is the way to raise kids, as do many human societies, and the outcome testifies to how well it works. Sadly, some human groups (ranging from certain Apache tribes, to most of the upper-class families in 19th-century Europe – see the Fox reference in the chapter bibliography) have tried a different way of raising children – for instance, discouraging close contact between young opposite-sex siblings, or recommending parents distance themselves from children and assign a nurse or nanny to handle all close contact with the kids. (Interestingly, the societies who have imposed the most brutal penalties for incest are precisely the ones who virtually guarantee incestuous feelings by mis-managing children in this way.)

Some parents may have brain-types that make them treat their children in a similarly 'cold' manner, even if their society suggests otherwise – but the outcome will be the same: adult siblings with incestuous feelings for each other, even children attracted to an opposite-sex parent who may take on a mysterious, 'romantic' aura because they are seldom around, and on their rare visits, can afford to be overzealous in expressing love for the child, untested by the challenges of daily routine. (This last outcome may also be the origin of the 'Oedipus complex' as described by Freud, whose childhood may have included a seldom-seen mother who adored him, and a father who was jealous of their dyad.)

The idea of choosing life partners based on a 'sibling-range' of brain-types may account for the frequent observations, across a wide range of species, of same-sex individuals living in pairs (cf. Bagemihl reference in the bibliography). For instance, bonded pairs among geese may be made up of two males or two females who carry on from year to year without any attempt to reproduce. In other cases, female pairs may incubate eggs that one of them lays after mating with an outside male, and raise the goslings, cooperating in these tasks just the way a different-sex pair would. Male bonded pairs might take the opportunity of borrowing an egg from a nearby fertile nest and hatch it and care for the gosling. Again, many of these bonded pairs stay together for life.

Figure 4.4

Social organization map of the distribution of individuals living in a Pair-bond arrangement. (Circles are females, triangles are males; smaller symbols are children.)

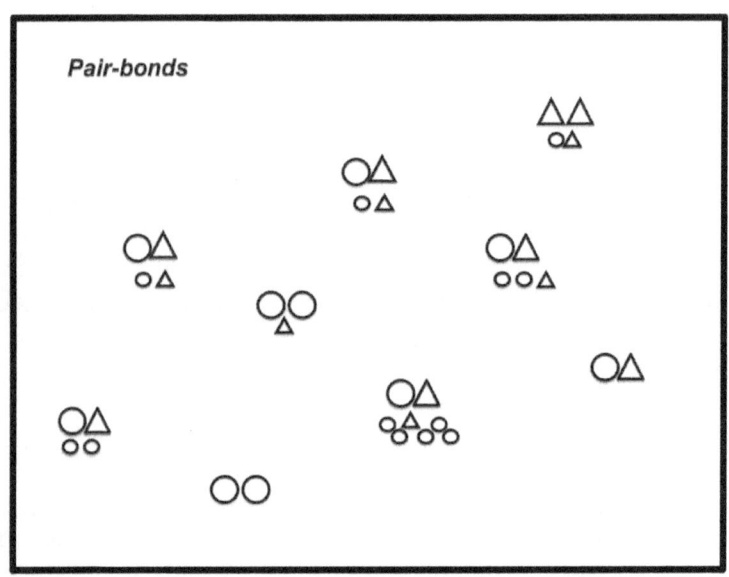

* * *

One of the outward signs that ethologists have come to recognize as a marker of adaptation to pair-bond life is the relative size of females vs. males. As a rule (with some exceptions), animals who live in pair bonds show very little sexual dimorphism, making it difficult for observers to use simple features such as body size to distinguish females vs. males. Thus in bonded-pair species such as crows, Canada geese, and gibbons, females and males look almost identical, although careful observation can usually reveal the subtle differences that are still there, such as the slightly more gracile head of a female Canada goose, or the finely formed hands of a female gibbon. (Animals who pair up only for the breeding season, such as songbirds, may be monomorphic in shape and size, but dimorphic in other ways such as coloration or singing.)

The behavior of members of a bonded pair is quite striking with regard to the degree of teamwork and cooperation regarding virtually all aspects of preparing for and caring for children. The mother is a 'perfect mother,' nurturing and skillful in her provision for every need of the children, and the father is a 'perfect father,' helping the mother out in whatever way he can, to prepare for children to be born (e.g., helping build a nest) and feeding them once they arrive. The two of them will fight side by side to defend their territory and children against predators and other intruders.

Where specialization of labor is called for, the two fulfill their roles in a remarkably coordinated way. For example, while the crow mother builds the nest, the male brings her sticks and other building materials; while the penguin mother looks for food, the penguin father patiently sits on the ice holding their egg nested warmly between his belly 'brood patch' and his feet. At other times, the members of the pair share the same roles. For example, both the mother and father gibbon take turns carrying babies and grooming them.

Mutual grooming among pair-bond adults and children is a regular feature of everyday life; it is an example of the right-brain-based 'support communication' via stimulation of deep-pressure skin receptors mentioned earlier, and as such it is a crucial part of the life of these animals, physiologically activating right-brain support for general health, and thus creating and expressing the bonds of affection that link the members of these small groups which depend so much on each other for survival.

It is very unusual if not impossible to find fish or reptiles living as pairs, and among mammals, the pair-bond lifestyle is also extremely rare (fewer than 3% of mammals live as pairs) – as we've said, the vast majority of mammals live according to the Center/Perimeter organization. (This makes the story of Noah's ark a curious fable, since the culture that produced it was certainly aware that very few classes of animals go 'two by two.' In actuality, the story was in fact not meant to be biologically accurate, but to make a sociopolitical point targeting humans, which we'll talk about later.)

By far the most pair-bond lifestyles are found among birds, very many of whom (more than 90%) use this mode, from songbirds to hawks and eagles – some only seasonally, others year-round, still others life-long. Certain carnivores such as crows, ravens, and wolves, have developed a modification of the basic pair-bond plan, in which a 'breeding pair' of a bonded female and male live year-round with a group of 'helpers,' three or four individuals who are children of the breeding pair from the two to four previous years. Occasionally a non-related individual obtains acceptance into the group, but for the most part members of these groups are related.

This lifestyle is called 'cooperative breeding,' and can be accommodated as long as a range has sufficient resources to support a group of this size, usually around seven to eight individuals. Within such groups, only the breeding pair are sexually active, even though at least some of the helpers are old enough to be sexually mature. Ethologists believe that this arrangement works to the advantage of propagating the genes shared by all members of the group, and at the same time, supports the considerable amount of social learning that takes place in the animals who live this way. Helpers earn their keep by assisting to gather food for the mother while she is attending to young, and teaming up with the breeding pair to make activities such as hunting more efficient.

Of course we know that canids such as wolves have highly complex behaviors, to such an extent that they appear very human-like in the ways that they interact with each other and with their cubs. This similarity must have been the basis for their early acceptance into human groups as companions. But these behaviors, complex and humanoid as they are, are not the exclusive domain of big-brained mammals such as wolves. Pair-bond birds such as crows and ravens have behaviors that are essentially identical. In fact, if one takes a description of crow behavior and changes the verbs appropriately (from 'preening' to 'licking,' from 'flying' to 'running,' etc.), it is virtually impossible to distinguish the behavior of crows from wolves. (Some references to books on crows and ravens are in the chapter bibliography.)

Crows live in cooperative-breeding groups of seven to eight individuals, with a single breeding pair and helpers who are their children from previous years. The breeding pair show great affection for each other, with frequent mutual grooming and 'baby talk' vocalizations as they court during mating season. The helpers assist with all aspects of group life, from bringing sticks for the mother to build a nest, to fetching food for the incubating mother and feeding the nestlings once they hatch. Parents and helpers also work together to keep the nest clean, carrying the chicks' droppings to discard them at a distance, and digging out parasites that hide in the nest materials.

Helpers also assist in coordinated group hunting like wolves. In crows, three or four individuals from the family group will shake the upper branches of a tree while the others stand on the ground below, looking up, ready to catch bugs and small animals that fall to the ground. Once the team members on the ground are fed, the two sets will trade places. Or one crow may bite at the tail of an otter who has just caught a fish while the others wait in a circle around him, and when the otter drops the fish to fend off the attacker, one of the waiting crows will grab the fish and all will fly off together to share the prize.

The highly social and affectionate nature of these types of birds has been observed many times by humans who have raised a crow or raven, such as chicks that had been injured in some way. The complexity and nature of their interaction is very similar to that of a dog, and demonstrates their natural abilities for recognizing individuals (including distinguishing among humans), mutual grooming, a large repertoire of vocalizations which they use in 'dialoguing' with their human 'family,' and protective aggression directed against others who are not perceived to be a member of the 'family,' such as strange humans or dogs.

The animals mentioned earlier who live as solitaries do not often gather into groups of any kind (except for cases of an attractive generous food source, as in the Komodos mentioned above, or the famous Kitchener polar bears).

However, pair-bond animals do occasionally come together for special events. For instance, migrating birds avoid travelling as isolated bonded pairs, which could be risky, and instead coalesce into flocks which are combinations of bonded pairs and unpaired adolescents. However, as soon as the destination is reached, the pairs often disperse again into separate territorial ranges.

Flocking may also occur during winter among birds who remain in colder regions, but some types of flocking seen during warmer months may actually signal habitat loss and stress. For example, in areas where habitat reduction is marked, not all animals may be able to find places to nest, and individuals that might otherwise form pair bonds and helper groups will gather into fairly large flocks which exhibit high levels of within-group aggression seldom seen in family groups, including stealing of food and fighting.

In our discussion of the solitary type of social organization, we mentioned two instances of species where obvious signs of stress indicated that living as solitaries is not a 'natural' way of life for them – whitetail deer, and orangutans. For example, among whitetails, we saw that symptoms of extreme stress included explosive population growth, dramatic signs of failure of immune function, and unusual acts of aggression, including males attacking females. All this sounds familiar to us, of course, and for good reason – many humans attempting to live as bonded pairs show similar signs of stress. We will return to this later and explain in detail that there is every reason to believe (including the telltale mark of sexual dimorphism) that humans in fact find the pair-bond model much less natural than the Center/Perimeter model. As a result, the high incidence of violence (including within-pair violence) in societies where the pair-bond model is imposed as the only allowed, 'legal' lifestyle, does not come as a surprise.

Center/Perimeter

The Center/Perimeter (C/P) type of social organization seems to be the one that almost all animals will adopt if given the chance. In the many instances where it occurs, from fish to reptiles to mammals, it is associated with 'the good life,' characterized by a 'cornucopia' of abundant resources combined with sufficient 'elbow-room' to accommodate this lifestyle, which we will see does demand a considerable amount of physical space.

Figure 4.5 shows a diagrammatic layout of the C/P organization, in this case: 1) two neighboring Center groups, each containing several adult and younger females (larger and smaller circles) along with one adult and several younger males (one large and several smaller triangles), and 2) the perimeter space between the Center groups, occupied only by post-pubertal males (triangles). The dimensions in the diagram are not to scale, as the space separating Center groups, where Perimeter males roam, may be fairly large.

Figure 4.5

Social organization map of the distribution of individuals living in a C/P arrangement (two Center groups are represented, plus a sample of that part of the Perimeter immediately between them; again, space is not to scale – for instance, too many Perimeter males are represented within this small space, and they would all be situated much further from the groups). (Circles are females, triangles are males; smaller symbols are children.)

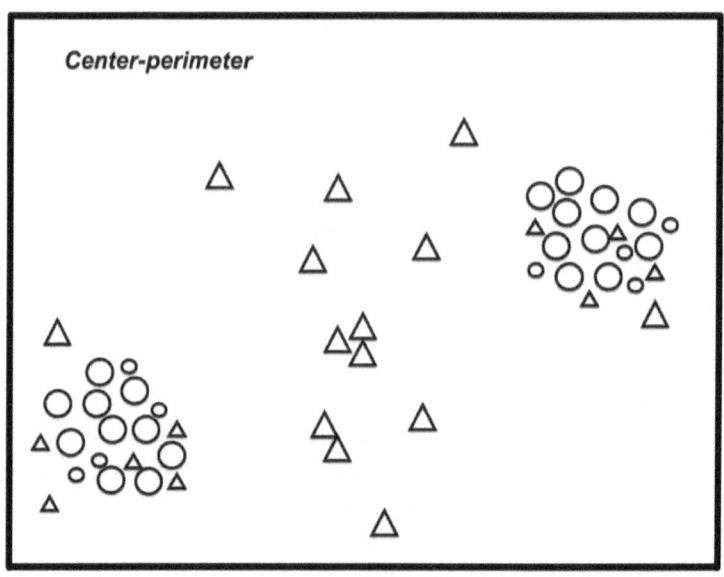

* * *

Many animals (including the vast majority of mammals) seem to be 'born' to Center/Perimeter, but the fact that economics is important is illustrated by cases where a species which typically lives in other ways can shift to a Center/Perimeter organization if resources permit it. For example, iguanas typically live as solitaries (like the Komodo dragon described earlier). But Paul McLean's 1990 book (see bibliography) reports on a group of iguanas living along a rock wall bordering a corn field in Mexico, who had taken the opportunity of the abundant, concentrated food supply to adopt a reptilian version of a Center/Perimeter lifestyle – complete with one adult 'alpha' male, a number of females with whom only he mated, and a number of 'outcast' males ranged around the perimeter of the group. (We'll talk more about these roles below.)

For those readers familiar with descriptions of animal ethology, this is the type of lifestyle that others have called 'harem.' For a variety of reasons, most of which should be obvious by now, we will not use that term. 'Center/Perimeter' is much more descriptive of the way this lifestyle is *arrayed in physical space*, an aspect of everyday life that we'll see is crucial for every species of animal. And as Darwin himself suspected, the male does not 'own' the females in these groups – it is the females who do the 'choosing' (the technical term is 'mate selection'). That is, those males who are (temporarily) accepted as mates undergo an 'audition' process to show that they possess qualities that can contribute to the genetic 'mission' of the females – i.e., achieving the QRS principle mentioned earlier. [It is remarkable, though perhaps understandable, to observe the difficulties some male authors have when they try to consider whether females play any active role at all in choosing a mate.]

In the Center/Perimeter plan, a group of adult females forms the 'Center,' where they live with their pre-pubertal children of both chromosomal genders, sexually-mature daughters and grand-daughters, and friends. Perhaps half of Center females are candidate Grandmother-Leaders – the current GL plus others like her, of different ages – and half are Loyal-Helpers. The Center male is also a Loyal-Helper, as are some of the pre-pubertal boys. Center groups typically consist of five to 20 individuals who represent a small number of matrilines which have proven compatible over time, perhaps over many generations. This proven compatibility means that the groups are generally friendly and cooperative, and tend to be both genetically and geographically stable, depending on a known group territory which may abut on territories where female relatives live in other Center groups – thus there may be regional communities that can peacefully band together for large-number movements such as seasonal migrations.

Ethologists often have problems analyzing relationships in these primarily-female groups, if they look only for the signs of rank-and-status characteristic of male groups such as within-group competitions involving (sometimes extreme) interindividual aggression and submissive displays. The stable nature of Center groups (at least, those not stressed by negative changes in habitat), deriving from their multigenerational history selecting for compatibility, means that relationships within the group are based on features of multidimensional personal profiles far more complex than 'who can beat up who.'

Mutual grooming among children and adults is as much a part of C/P life as in pair-bonds, discussed earlier. As a form of 'support communication,' it reassures individual group members – both the groomer and the groomed – each is valued and supported. As we've said before, the right-brain activation involved in this type of somatosensory stimulation provides not only a psychological sense of belonging, but also a 'brain treatment' ensuring that the right brain will be present and working for that individual in every way possible.

Depending on the species, each individual in the Center of a C/P arrangement is self-sustaining with regard to resources, and is also available to assist in the care of all, from very young to very old. Among mammals, co-lactation is standard – lionesses nurse one another's cubs, and female elephants who have not given birth in a particular season will begin lactating and suckle babies, if several are born into the group at one time; even females beyond child-bearing age provide milk when needed. C/P Center groups are the 'village' that supports all children.

The women of each group entertain 'auditions' by males to become their 'Center male,' a single male (with the personal features that make him a candidate Loyal-Helper – more later), to live with them and be their source of sperm for making babies, and assist the females with protection against intruders, including certain other males of their species – he is 'hired' to 'serve and protect.' Contrasted with the group females, these Center males are only 'penciled-in' – a given individual may be resident only for a single breeding season (e.g., two-three weeks), or remain with a group year-round, but no one male stays with a group very long, a strategy that over time, provides the females the benefit of genetic diversity for their children.

Sometimes Center groups will tolerate an older male and a younger one at the same time, a sort of king and prince, who may or may not be related, but who must get along well with each other – the males are not allowed to endanger either the females or young – their role as 'soldiers' must always be directed against strangers, never against group members. Examples of this type of 'silverback/ blackback' pair has been seen in many species, including gorillas, from which the term comes. The type of male who can function as a Center male must have a very special combination of skills. He must have good social skills, be loving and gentle, 'good with the kids,' and show good personal and sexual compatibility for interacting with the women – when invited by them, he must be interested in sex and have enough testosterone to perform. He must also be healthy enough to provide viable sperm to all females who are receptive, and to aid in group defense, if he is a long-term candidate.

As noted before, early descriptions of such groups described the male as 'owning' and controlling the women, on the model of the autocratic male owners of human harems (hence the old name). Subsequent observers, however, have shown that this is essentially upside down – that the women choose the male, not the other way around, and that the women manage the society, including making the decisions and teaching the male what to do (we'll review two anecdotes illustrating this in a moment). If there is any 'overseer' or 'boss' in these highly cooperative groups, it is the most experienced women, the Grandmother-Leaders, who draw on a long life of interactions with many children and many adults and in fact many Center males, to guide the group in maintaining peaceful relations and making decisions.

Paul MacLean has emphasized the crucial importance of the female-based management in these groups: "The female has been central to mammalian evolution for over 180 million years." He extends this to humans in a way which NRT predicts also applies to all C/P animals: "In regard to human evolution [a sharpened sense of empathy and altruism] has depended on the greater balance of function of the woman's brain." (For both quotes see MacLean 1996 in the chapter bibliography.)

Two instances observed in Center/Perimeter animals will illustrate the relations between the 'older-wiser' females and the younger male who is trying to fit in. One involved a lion and lioness kept in the same cage in a zoo (note the betrayal of the natural lifestyle, where the lioness would expect to live with several of her sisters and children around her, and the male would be one they would have themselves chosen as a group – it's not at all certain that the poor fellow in this case was really qualified for the job – and he was probably chosen by the zoo personnel, and may not have been at all compatible with the lioness caged with him).

In the incident observed, their two cubs began playing with the male's tail – chasing and catching it and sometimes biting it so hard that the male visibly jumped. Finally he had had enough – he stood up and growled menacingly at one of the cubs, who shrank away. Immediately the lioness sprang at the male and cuffed him hard across the face. The look on his face was amazing to see – he stood for a moment then turned around and walked as far as he could away from the cubs (that limited space again!), lay down pressing his back against a chain link fence, and pointedly pushed his tail under the fence, out of the range of the cubs' sharp teeth.

The second was a scenario observed in a Center group of wild mustangs, which included a fairly young stallion who had recently replaced a predecessor as Center male. The group of mares and yearlings was quietly grazing on a hilltop, and the 'grandmother-leader' mare lay down in the grass and fell asleep. As the group moved slowly in their grazing, they eventually moved out of sight over the edge of the hill from where the grandmother was sleeping. Eventually the older mare woke up – to find everyone disappeared. She got to her feet and began to whinny, walking in circles, looking for her family. The others heard her and came running, the stallion bringing up the rear. As they approached her, she trotted to the stallion and swinging around, gave him a sharp solid kick in the side with both rear hooves. The message was clear: "Why didn't you wake me up – you'd better learn that part of your job is to make sure we all stay together!"

So the Center male must be cooperative, too, and willing to take instructions from the women with whom he lives, with no hint of objection. At the same time, he must be willing to be aggressive even to the death against intruders – *but always and only against outsiders*. The Center male is one type of 'alpha male' – the top (usually only) male of the Center group. (Outside the Center group is a second category of 'alpha male' with a very different behavioral profile – more of this in a moment.) No group of women will on their own accept anyone into the role of Center male who gives even the slightest sign of being in any way aggressive toward either women or children. The group has enough to fear from outsiders – to ensure its survival, it cannot afford to harbor such a danger within its circle.

Thus the Center male, just as we saw was true for a good pair-bonded male, looks like what we would call the 'perfect father' (even though he often does not stay around for long) – loving toward women and children, but aggressive to the death against anyone who would threaten them with harm. Of course, this is just the male version of the perfect mother – every woman feels within herself the possibility of unqualified love for her children, combined with the capability for what is called the 'mother-bear response' where she would lay down her life for her children, 'throw herself at the dogs' or 'run into the guns' as a mother bear would to protect her cubs. The Center male is asked to take on this 'perfect parent' role in spades, and in return he receives continuing social companionship, the joys of sex with a variety of females, and the implicit advantage of having his genes continued into the future.

Thus the C/P Center group is the true Center, the 'civilization' of any species that is fortunate enough to be able to live this way. It is the heart of the species' life, where children are conceived and carried to term, where they are cared for and reared in the way of the species. We might say that its values revolve around the care and nurturance of the young, and seeking to ensure quality of life to all members in the implicit knowledge that what is good for each is good for all. This is a brief list of what we might call 'Center values.'

In human societies, this arrangement of cooperative, woman-guided group management is referred to as 'matristic' to distinguish it from the 'patriarchal' type of social organization which has sadly become all too familiar in very recent human history. In patriarchy (patri-archy = 'father-overlords'), the males take the upper hand, enforce hierarchical rankings of everybody down to the youngest children, and rule by intimidation including physical violence. There are vanishingly few instances of patriarchies among animals other than humans. Probably the best-known is hamadryas baboons, who have become famous for their X-treme male-on-male competition and the constant 'wife-battering' visited on the hapless females, whom the ranking males do indeed act like they 'own.' This pattern of battering violence suggests environmental stresses related to habitat encroachment or some other negative change that put these animals at risk. It is expected that females exposed to such treatment will have high-stress pregnancies, perhaps resulting in a majority of left-brain children, which may not bode well for the species' future. But this is the exception to the C/P standard – for the most part, Center groups are remarkable for their peacefully cooperative, woman-managed organization.

The behavior of males in the rare patriarchal groups such as hamadryas in fact leads us to look at the other component of C/P organization – the 'Perimeter.' This is the place away from the Center groups where all young males go when they reach puberty. This is the reason that ethologists often refer to males living outside Center groups as 'juvenile' males – some of them will live all their lives unattached to a Center group, so their identity within the species is fixed by the status they took at puberty, that is, when they were juveniles.

The boys leave at puberty because this is the time when their rising hormones make them naturally restless, and also because the resident Center male perceives their blooming sexual maturity as a threat, and will encourage them to leave. The boys physically disperse into the surrounding territory – what we've called the Perimeter. Human boys reaching puberty feel the same sort of restlessness, of course – this natural dispersal of males in early adolescence is the same phenomenon that Mark Twain was referring to when he said that Tom Sawyer, tiring of his childhood pranks with Huckleberry Finn, talked about "lighting out for the territories." (In some species, females rather than males may leave at puberty, but the norm is for the stable woman-centered groups to stay together. In fact, some cases of 'female dispersal' may be associated with a number of troubling features, which we will discuss later.)

Of course in any given region a species may be represented by several Center groups, and thus the space we've called the Perimeter refers to the spaces between the various Center groups, the 'no man's land' where, as it turns out, no one but men go. Thus for the Center/Perimeter organization to work, there must be enough space to absorb the young males as they leave their home groups. If there is not sufficient space for this, such that these ejected males are forced into contact with Center groups, serious trouble may ensue.

We will see in a later chapter that one of the problems many human societies face is that there are no more physical territories to 'light out to,' no more geographic Perimeter for our boys to escape to and distance themselves in this natural, healthy way. As we will see, the implications of this may have had devastating consequences for our species over the past several thousand years.

The lack of sufficient space for a functional Perimeter may also be the source of obvious social problems observed in other large primates such as gorillas, who are still clinging to a reduced version of a Center/Perimeter way of life. Common chimpanzees (not bonobos – more about them later), who are sexually dimorphic, though not to the extent of gorillas, may also be showing the effects of this type of spatial coercion. As their preserves become ever more threatened by encroaching humans, they have been forced into a lifestyle that is extremely different from the Center/Perimeter model their dimorphism marks them as preferring. (Observers have seen a single chimpanzee female go off temporarily with her children and a favorite male, to get away from the crowding and violence – thus as we've said, individuals living under stressed conditions may be able to 'shift gears' into a different lifestyle – in this case, a pair-bond arrangement – for some relief.) We should not be at all surprised that chimpanzee groups with their habitats under siege exhibit all the signs of an imposed lifestyle (in this case, a form of 50:50 – more in a moment) that in the case of common chimps seems to be stressful and unnatural, approaching social pathology, including murderous wars on neighboring groups, infanticide, and rape.

It may help us understand how things can take these disastrous turns, if we look again more closely at the males who roam the Perimeter. They are predictably of two types – one which is large, with the psychosociological profile needed for Center males described above; and a second type of male which is short and aggressive, not at all the kind that women of the Center groups would want to have around.

In fact, ethologists have observed that the phenomenon of 'two types of males' is widespread among animal species – these have been described in several species of fish, rodents such as mice and rats, mammals including pigs, orangutans, gorillas, bighorn sheep – and, as we'll discuss later, in humans. The two types of males (sometimes distinguished as showing 'two types of aggression') differ in: 1) *size*: the more aggressive ones, sometimes called 'sneaker males,' are smaller – in fact, the same size as the species' females; 2) *body proportions* (the shorter, more aggressive males have much larger genitals); and 3) *autonomic function* (in the more aggressive ones, the sympathetic nervous system dominates over parasympathetic – they have the high heart rate and hypertension of Type A personalities).

As suggested by these types of differences, we will also see that there are predictable correlations between the two types of males and the brain types described earlier – we'll return to this later in this chapter. The fact that the two types of males appear in so many species suggest that this is actually the norm among animals who use sexual reproduction, and is abandoned only in cases where environmental restrictions require that a species adopt either a solitary lifestyle or a pair-bond organization – in which case only those brain types appropriate to those lifestyles should appear.

The larger, highly-social males, the 'gentle giants' in the mix of males found in the Perimeter, thus form a pool of potential Center males. While they wait for a group to join (to do this, they will challenge incumbents from time to time, in audition battles which test which of two combatants can be the better protector), they wander in small, unstable all-male groups, having little if any interaction with any individual from a Center group. These males may not have to actually join a group to be able to contribute to the gene pool – their continuing mutual attraction to women may be the origin of the 'boy in the bushes' phenomenon noted in many Center/Perimeter species. This is where a female from the Center goes off with an outside male for a short time, conceives a child, and returns to her home group to have the baby. These 'nights on the town' might thus be another way of gaining additional genetic variety for such groups. (Even so, it is estimated that in most Center/Perimeter species, fewer than 10% of males ever get to contribute genes to the next generation.)

The shorter, more generally aggressive males are even less likely to join a Center group, due to their very different physique and psychology (their size may be similar to females, but their psychology is at the opposite, asocial extreme). These males will also wander the Perimeter either in small all-male groups, organized in rigid, pecking-order hierarchies, or as solitaries. (The 'top dog' in these hierarchical groups is the second kind of 'alpha male' – a 'Perimeter alpha:' short, hyperviolent, completely unfitted for life in a Center group.) These lifelong-perimeter males will not be attracted to joining Center groups – they may even be asexual (in spite of the large sex parts they usually have), and the women would not let them in, in any case. (In fish, the female-sized 'sneaker' males are apparently less violent than they are opportunistic. They use the 'disguise' of their female size and coloration to get 'under the radar' of a larger, 'territorial' male, to make rapid, almost comic dashes to fertilize a nest of eggs belonging to one of the Center females, attempting to get in and out before the territorial male notices.)

In mammals, the chances that the shorter, true-Perimeter type of male will ever contribute to the species gene pool are vanishingly small. It is curious that biology goes on producing this type of male, since we are taught that the goal of every organism is to produce offspring. But given the description in Chapter Two of the graded nature of prenatal testosterone, it is possible that this type of male is made only as a side effect of the need to make the gentle giants (who are the product of neither too much nor too little testosterone), and that sometimes the prenatal chemical processes simply get out of hand (due to genetic tendency of a particular woman, effects of stress, etc.) resulting in the second, truly 'surplus' type of male.

Thus the production of multiple 'surplus males' (that is, individuals who do not make a genetic contribution to a species' future) may be just another instance of biology's notorious casualness about 'wasting' the products of reproduction (an 'r-strategy' attitude – more later). As one of many examples, consider the astronomical number of acorns routinely produced by oaks, that never become trees; given sufficient resources, a single tree can go on doing this indefinitely without threatening its own survival. In the same way, the supportive environment that makes the C/P arrangement possible in the first place apparently allows the females to afford what has been called the 'cost of males' (that is, investing time, energy, and resources in individuals who will, like most of the acorns, 'not be used'). Of course, a radical reduction in environmental resources may invoke different rules, leading to differences in the types of individuals produced, as we'll see in the next section; but the standard is that many more males are made by C/P Center groups than will ever be needed.

Regarding the two types of males found in the C/P Perimeter, the nature of the second version of male, the '*long-term* Perimeter' ('Perimeters' for short) suggests that the greatest threat to the women and children of a C/P species is not from predators of other species, but from this second kind of male. Thus the displays of protective Center males would seem to be perfectly designed to intimidate would-be *conspecific predators*, who are known to attack and even eat children from the Center groups. There are horrific films of male lions killing and eating cubs, and the same type of conspecific infanticide has been observed in other, non-carnivorous, species such as gorillas and chimpanzees (NRT considers chimpanzee 'hunting' as yet another sign of environmental stress, not a 'natural' behavior). The aggressive, child-killing Perimeter males may in fact be the originals of the 'wolf in sheep's clothing' – that is, individuals who 'look just like us,' but are actually bent on killing. They may seem much more threatening than any other species of predator, precisely because of this chilling type of 'body-snatcher' masquerade.

Some ethologists have suggested that males who kill same-species babies and then rape their mothers is an expression of the 'selfish gene,' under the assumption that each and every individual seeks to propagate his or her genes at all costs – a genetic zero-sum game. However, this does not account for the fact that not all individuals do this – females don't tend to do so, and we might predict that Center males don't. If only short males are the ones who kill babies and rape, we might see that this is less an 'evolved male mechanism' as some ethologists have called (praised?) it, than a type of 'devolved' anti-social *pathology* that comes naturally to the type of individual who is 'made' (by high prenatal T) to live alone. We will see later that the brain type predicted by NRT for true-perimeter males is very much in keeping with such primitive, destructive, and sociologically-selfish behavior.

Note that in our description of the two types of males, we've referred to what are essentially *two types of violence*. First, there is the defensive, 'mother-bear' defensive fighting engaged in by the members of the Center group when they protect themselves and their children against predators, including conspecific predators, the short, aggressive Perimeter males. Second, there is the violence of the Perimeter males – not only visited on themselves within their rigidly hierarchical all-male groups, but even more dreadfully, directed against the people of the Center, including the cannibalizing of children.

These two types of violence and the individuals involved are often confounded by ethologists who talk about the 'big dangerous males.' As we've seen, it may be crucial to distinguish between *'good violence'* – the defensive aggression undertaken by Center females and males, which works to protect the members of the Center, and is 'dangerous' only to would-be predators, but to no woman or child – vs. *'bad violence'* – attacks on women and children, even extending to cannibalism, that true Perimeters commit, posing a potential threat to a species' very future. We will return to these ideas about violence when we talk about human societies, and consider the possibility that distinguishing between 'good' and 'bad' violence may help us to a deeper understanding of the nature of human violence and its origins.

All the species who live in C/P organizations abide by these same rules – women and children live in stable groups year after year, most of the males do not live in Center groups, and all of the males belong to one of the two classes we've described. There are, however, slight differences among C/P species, according to whether the Center males live with the women and children year-round, or only during the seasons when conception occurs.

In the first case, the Center male remains with the group year-round – examples of species which do this are gorillas, lions, and horses. In the second category, males live with the groups of females only during a brief, once-a-year (or more infrequent) mating season – examples are elk, elephants, and gazelles. In these species, for most of the year, the Center-group women and children form a society that may range within a particular territory, or join into larger, widely dispersed herds, gaining safety in numbers to defend against predators, or for migrating if they live in a climate zone where dramatic seasonal changes force them to accommodate to changes in food availability. During the same time, all males live in small, male-only groups that tend to stay away from the women. When mating hormones begin to rise, the Center-male candidates will seek out and 'ask' to join a group of females; when hormones fall as the season passes, the temporary Center male and the females separate to take up their segregated lifestyles once again.

In some species (such as some species of fish, quail, and deer) who follow this second type of Center/Perimeter plan, when mating season comes,

Center-type males do not individually seek out groups of women, but use a different approach. Those males who wish to breed take up temporary residence, each in a relatively small area, distributing themselves evenly over whatever space is available. Then the males simply wait for a female to visit and make her selection for mating, or they may make preparations that females will find attractive – fish may clear out a nesting area in the sand of the ocean bottom; birds may build a nest (European house wren males may make as many as 12 nests before they find a female who likes one). Perhaps the best-known example of this is the bowerbird, where males build elaborate 'houses' as ground-nests, and the females carefully inspect different houses; if one decides she likes a male's handiwork (actually, beak-and-foot-work), she will pick up a piece of building material such as a twig or leaf, and take it inside the little house, indicating her readiness to move in.

In talking about those males who wait for females, we used the phrase 'whatever space is available' – it is amazing to see small gazelle males spacing themselves out in a zoo-habitat setting, where each one may have only a ten by ten foot 'territory,' compared to what might have been an acre or more in the wild (the arrangement is called a 'lek'). While these males defend the boundaries of their small kingdoms with aggressive displays against other males, the females wander through the region without regard for any such boundaries. They choose males to mate with, and then gather into their all-women groups again, to gestate and deliver their babies. As the mating season passes, and the males' hormones fall, the males themselves begin crossing their own boundaries, as though their 'lines in the sand' evaporate with the hormones, and gather again into small all-male groups or resume their wandering as solitaries.

Are there any instances of animals living in Center/Perimeter groups who show signs of stress, indicating some type of recent coercion into that lifestyle? Because of our interpretation that Center/Perimeter is the 'ideal' lifestyle for many types of animals, the answer would probably be no. (As we've said, orangutans have actually been forced out of their preferred C/P lifestyle, and reverted to a solitary mode.) However, there are definitely animals still living in a C/P style, who show signs that external forces are making it harder and harder to maintain the way of life to which they are adapted.

The most obvious example is animals who are clearly trying to maintain a Center/Perimeter lifestyle in the face of extreme disruptive pressures, such as mountain gorillas. When they were first described in detail by Dian Fossey over two decades (1966-85), their Center/Perimeter arrangement appeared to be much like that seen in many other animals – a cooperative group of highly interactive females and children, living peacefully with a large silverback male, often with a younger blackback. These groups enjoyed a variety of social interactions among themselves, and were seldom if ever threatened by the Perimeter males who had plenty of room to occupy them, safely away from the Center groups, in the vast 'playground' of the jungle surround. (Fossey's unique and crucial work was ended abruptly when she herself was threatened by Perimeter males – from her own species: she was murdered in 1985, presumably by locals involved in the lucrative poaching trade.)

In recent years, with pressure increasing from destruction of habitat, and the escalation of poaching for trophies and 'bush meat,' gorilla Center groups are undergoing disturbing internal changes. They are being assaulted by their own kind – attacks by Perimeter males (forced into more and more contact with the groups as space for a Perimeter shrinks) are on the increase, with fatal consequences to females and children. As a result, the females, instead of enjoying their former life of a rich diversity of friendships with each other, spend much of their time anxiously fixated on their guardian, the silverback. The reduction in the variety and quality of life for all is disturbing, and would be of supreme concern were it not overshadowed by the even more ominous threat of complete extinction.

Finally, there are a few species, such as some types of baboons, who live in a strange type of Center/Perimeter mode that seems to have suffered an internal revolution, so that males rather than females have come to dominate. Such groups definitely merit the pejorative application of the term 'harem' – the males are overbearing and hyperviolent, quick to anger and strike out, not only against rival males (who are often encountered through overcrowding) but also against females and children within their own group.

(This violence against women and children is seen primarily in adult males – young males may develop friendships with a group of even younger, unrelated females, playing with them and gradually 'courting' them as future mates, and eventually leave with them to form a Center of their own. But once established, these 'kindly uncles' turn into autocratic patriarchs like their fathers, and lord it over their captive wives.)

A potentially important signature feature of such groups is that the dispersal pattern at puberty is reversed compared to the C/P norm – that is, it is the adolescent males who get to stay home with their mothers, while the young females are driven off, forced into exile. This clearly subverts the female-centered stability of the life in the Center, and also puts the isolated females at severe risk as they have to 'depend on the kindness of strangers' (which is seldom forthcoming among such animals) if they ever hope to join a group where they can have babies. In this as in some other features, baboon groups may offer an object lesson in how *not* to manage a mammalian society, with direct and disturbing implications for human social organization.

"Eusocial"

This SOC category refers to collections of very large numbers of individuals living in extremely close proximity to each other, where individual members are 'interdependent' in a way that goes far beyond what we've seen for the other social modes. (When compared with the other three SOCs described so far, this arrangement does not look 'social' at all, if that word is used to refer to the personality-based, mutual-assistance relationships among individual adults of a group; thus I use quotation marks around 'eusocial' [the word in Greek means 'beautifully social'] – clearly a term of approval that must have been coined by entomologists, not students of *mammalian* behavior including humans.)

Figure 4.6

Social organization map of the distribution of individuals living in a Eusocial arrangement. (Circles are females [largest is queen], triangles are males; smaller symbols are children.)

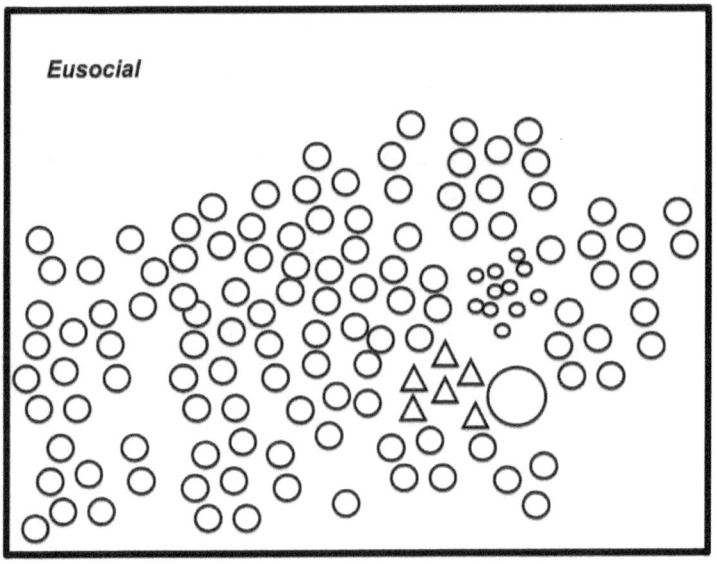

* * *

Examples of eusocial animals are insects such as termites, ants and bees. Of course not all insects live this way, so it is again not a case of genetic determination as much as the relevant economics – something about the nature of the preferred food supply predisposes a species to organizing in this way. (Note that there is one mammal which uses a eusocial organization, the naked mole rat from East Africa – it lives in massed groups of up to 100, who spend all their life underground, eating the underground portions of plants such as tubers and roots. For more details, see the Sherman et al. reference in the chapter bibliography.)

The eusocial SOC's way of meeting its food-gathering needs is based on: 1) the nature of the species' food and its distribution, *including its capacity for being stored for future use*; and 2) the ability of the animals to *construct some type of shelter* that can house all the members of the group along with their stored food, to protect them against weather events as well as predators. Richard Alexander and colleagues (see Sherman and Alexander references in the chapter bibliography) have outlined the ways that the eusocial SOC meets these needs: 1) prolongation of development of the young (i.e., delay of sexual activity of most members – similar to the 'cooperative breeder' version of pair-bonds discussed earlier) – this provides a large (non-breeding) worker base for managing the massive job of constructing and maintaining the all-important shelters; 2) 'extensive' parental care (a feature shared with some other SOCs); and 3) methods for designing and making the shelters – the signature feature of this SOC.

Eusocial shelters are impressive by any measure. Some consist of above-ground nests made of materials produced by the animals themselves, such as beeswax excreted from glands on the abdomens of young bees, or 'paper' made by wasps chewing woody materials to mix them with saliva. Termites make a similar material – a mixture of saliva, dung, and soil – and use it to create the above-ground mounds (some more than 20 feet high, with intricate internal structures) that are used to ventilate the complex tunnel systems of their below-ground nests. The work of construction and maintenance is on-going, and the result guarantees not only the immediate safety of the group and ready access to stored food (some nests even include extensive 'foraging tunnels,' protected means for accessing new food sources further from the nest, and returning the food safely to storage areas) but also long-term protection serving a series of successive colonies – some termite mounds have been dated as hundreds if not thousands of years old. We'll see later that the eusocial strategy of constructing shelters both for housing individuals and storing food is similar to methods employed by some human societies (though none with the longevity achieved by termites) and we'll also discuss why the human versions of eusociality often have problems.

As portrayed in Fig. 4.6, perhaps the most striking contrast between the eusocial way of life vs. other SOCs, is what appears to be an incredible degree of *crowding*. The other societies we've discussed seem always to involve substantial degrees of open space – even when individuals in small groups gather with others such as in migrations, they keep lots of elbow room around them. How then, do the eusocial animals manage their societies, accommodating to conditions which for other types of species would be unbearably crowded?

As we'll see later in the chapter, the secret may be that the vast majority of individuals in these large groups are not sexually active. While at first glance this may seem indeed like a radical departure – and it *is* predictably the difference that makes all the difference – it is still only a proportional change compared to the other societies we've reviewed. At the same time, as discussed later, an analysis in terms of social roles may provide more insight into how eusocial organizations work.

50:50

We have left this social style till last, because it is so extremely rare among animals of any class, order, genus or species. Yet it needs to be included, because as we'll see later, it is definitely related to brain types, and may also give us important clues about ourselves.

This is an organization where each group has equal numbers of sexually-active females and males – roughly fifty percent females and fifty percent males. Hopefully by this time in our survey of animal societies, such proportions seem preposterous, almost monstrous – 'too many males, for sure' – 'don't most of the members have to be sexless?' (etc.) Any farmer would tell you immediately that a 50:50 mix is impossible, and would precipitate a crisis – a pasture with as many bulls as cows, as many stallions as mares? – ridiculous – you've got to be kidding – it would be a war – animals injured, babies killed, fences smashed – the farmer would go bankrupt.

Figure 4.7

Social organization map of the distribution of individuals living in a 50:50 arrangement. (Circles are females, triangles are males; smaller symbols are children.)

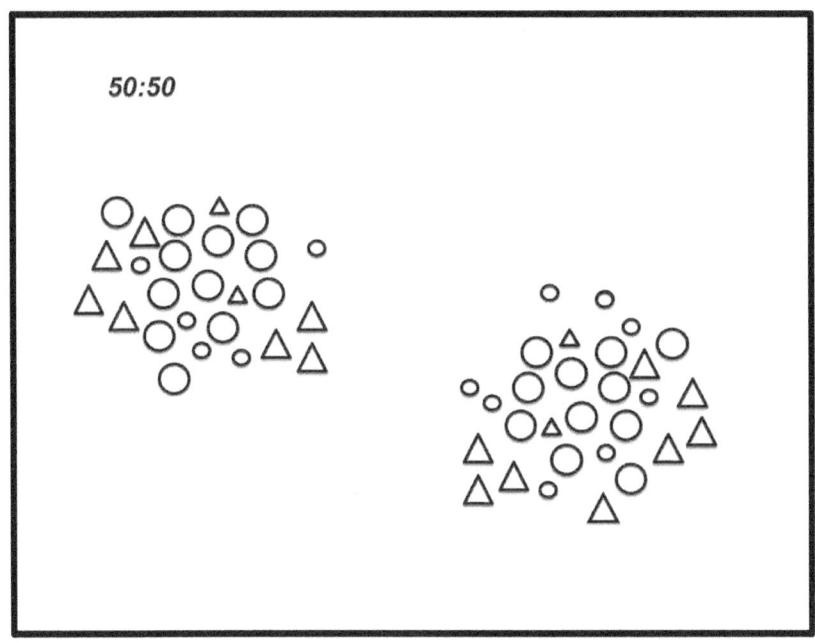

* * *

Neural Rainbow Theory suggests that this fundamental difficulty – all coming down to the presence of *'too many males'* – means that wherever and whenever 50:50 occurs, it is **not** the 'natural' (stable) state of a social group, but is most often the sign of a **transitional state** caused by some relatively recent (predictably within only a few generations) crisis, a degradation of the surrounding environment – e.g., dramatically increased predation (often at the hands of invasive-species humans), a reduction in the geographical range of local food or water sources, or some other disruption – that results in a *critical shrinkage of living space, particularly the space required for maintaining the C/P perimeter*.

Specifically, the prediction is that: 1) previously the group in question lived in a C/P arrangement; 2) the critical environmental change led to a 'collapse' of the Perimeter onto the Center, such that the excess males previously 'absorbed' by the Perimeter are 'suddenly' pushed inside the Center, bringing their inter-male competition and violence – their 'Perimeter values'

– into intimate contact with the cooperative, mutually nurturing daily life of the Center women and children; 3) this crisis, an attempt to mix 'oil and water'– just as the farmers would have predicted – *is* explosive: it brings the constant threat that the males will begin including women and children in their competitive 'wars.' [Of course, human women have experienced this, and worry: Will the men pick up automatic weapons, walk into schoolrooms, and shoot children in the face? Will members of armies rape and kill civilian women and children as part of their everyday, privileged activity as 'the meanest m*f*rs in the valley'? Will non-soldiers rape and kill women and children just because they can – no reason given? ..... For women living in the Perimeter war-zone, these are all rhetorical questions.]

It would be helpful if ethologists could conduct a survey of the few 50:50 species around the world (including species sub-groups that may have suffered a *local* habitat loss) to discover which groups now living in this way can be documented as having suffered a 'recent' history of loss of space for a Perimeter. (My sense is that what some ethologists refer to as the 'multi-male groups' – many of them distinguished for their level of marked intra-group violence – of species such as macaque monkeys and spotted hyenas *might* be examples of 50:50, though it is difficult in reading field descriptions to tell exactly what is going on; the terminology used to describe gender behaviors is often more obfuscating than explanatory or clarifying.)

Whether or not there is documentation about history, one could at least observe details of physical features (e.g., degree of sexual dimorphism such as body size and size of canine teeth) and behavioral patterns (e.g., do males rule the group by violence and threat, or females manage it via nurturance and cooperation?) in order to estimate *how far back in time* the possible perturbation might have occurred. The logic for making such estimates is derived from: 1) the original prediction, namely, that any group now living as 50:50 began as female-managed C/P; and 2) the further back the operative change occurred, the more time the group might have had to 'adjust' to the perturbation in order to survive. (The eco-evolutionary association of 'male' and 'crisis' is a pairing which goes well beyond questions of social organization, and is discussed further in my essay *First Things* included in the Volume Three Appendix.)

The nature of the required 'adjustments' might differ depending on a number of factors that together determine how much the Center-group females are able to manage the situation in order to control it, to keep group life on an even keel, with Center values firmly in place. The important factors include: 1) the health of the Center group (whether stable, or challenged by the same environmental change responsible for the loss of space); 2) food and water supply (whether abundant or scarce) and other details of environmental support; 3) the nature of the males themselves (their brain types – whether mostly middles vs. mostly left-brains; 4) whether the males are familiar to the females, or strangers from afar); etc. How quickly the change happened should also be crucial: was the process a slow, peaceful transition (allowing time for the females to develop protective strategies), or more like a blitzkrieg invasion?

Based on all these contextual factors, the females would have had either more or less freedom in finding solutions to the problem. If the change was sudden, resources scarce, and the males all left-brains prone to violence, the females may have had no options at all, no degrees of freedom for moderating the effects of the change. As a result the outcome might have been quick and unpleasant: a 'hostile takeover' by the males. The new masters would have dominated by force, with universal violence as their only 'social language,' replacing the cooperative nurturing Center values of the original group with zero-sum-game Perimeter values that stressed a rigid social hierarchy with a single top-dog male at the top, a coterie of sycophants below that, and women and children at the bottom – in particular, the Grandmother-Leaders demoted from their original honored place to the very lowest social level.

If we think of a peaceful Center group such as elk moving slowly through a forest, with one or more Grandmother-Leaders leading the way, the other women following with their young ones, and a lone male bringing up the rear in his role as lookout – and suddenly *switching the positions* of the grandmother at the front vs. the male at the rear, that is what the new 50:50 group after such a hostile male takeover would look like: a 180-degree flip in the 'poles' of its fundamental social structure: males now up front calling the shots, grandmothers relegated to the back of the bus.

(This may be what happened with common chimpanzees, thus making them an excellent example of a 'failed' attempt at an adaptive (sustainable) 50:50 arrangement. Perhaps for them, the change in environment came so quickly, and under such negative circumstances, that the females did not have enough time to develop strategies for maintaining the peace, and their Center values were overwhelmed and replaced by the invaders' Perimeter values. The same type of scenario may also look very familiar to those of us humans who know all too well what can happen when zero-sum males are put in charge, whether of single families, workplaces, or nation-states. Later in this book we will talk much more about the dire consequences of a 180-degree flip in the 'social compass' of a species, and how such an event has indeed deeply affected the past, present, and possible future history of humans on this planet.)

On the other hand, for another group, if the change was slower, and conditions more favorable for the females being able to maintain their position as group managers to keep Center values in place, the outcome might be very different. So, let's say in this case, that at the outset (at the point when the loss of space occurred), 1) all involved individuals (whether members of the Center group or the small sub-group of males seeking a new home) were healthy; 2) environmental conditions (such as food and water supply) within the Center's home range continued supportive; and 3) the males seeking entry were mostly socially-capable, nonviolent, and known to the females.

In such a situation (which may actually be more sanguine than many instances of the situation we're discussing), it might have been possible for the group females to make some simple behavioral changes sufficient to keep the peace; 'civilize' the males for living together with 'extra males' and women and children year-round; and even 'educate' each other in behaviors that would help keep the males happy yet would in no way undermine the essence of their Center way of life.

There are a number of human 50:50 groups who have been able to achieve this end, and we'll talk more about them later in the book. However, of non-human examples, perhaps the most famous are bonobo chimpanzees, the lemurs of Madagascar, and the muriqui monkeys (also called woolly spider monkeys) of Brazil. All of these groups have suffered increasingly radical habitat loss over the past 100 years, and have taken somewhat different paths to solving the problem of surplus males, but the basic results are the same: maintaining female group leadership, while at the same time developing ways to keep the peace, even with 'too many males.' In looking at these different solutions, it is notable that in all cases, the changes that occur involve a certain degree of *masculinization of the females*, both in behavior and at times, in anatomy (both of which suggest a possible underlying shift in the brain types produced, perhaps leading to a larger proportion of middle-brain females).

At first one might predict this is the result of an *overall* increase in prenatal testosterone exposure – but this should *not* be the case, given that the pivotal problem for these groups is the loss of a Perimeter needed to absorb left-brains, especially males, so the groups should want to go in the opposite direction, and *reduce* prenatal testosterone, in order to make fewer Focal-Asocial/left-brains than before.

There is a second, alternative hormonal adjustment that could yield *both* results, that is, the same one we've posited happens as a matter of course in all pair-bond animals – aiming for *moderate-T exposure in all pregnancies*, regardless of fetal gender. The outcome would be: females that are more male-like (in a good way), and males that are more female-like – both strategically effective changes for meeting the challenge of habitat (Perimeter) loss faced by these groups.

Several behavioral changes have been observed in more-or-less peaceful 50:50 groups that could be interpreted as 'females becoming more male-like.' These include: 1) an increase (relative to typical C/P groups) in the *overall amount of sexual activity*, especially outside of the breeding season, and a *mix of gender pairings* (both of these represent instances of separating sexual activity from reproduction) – in fact, these changes may go hand-in-hand with an increase in mutual grooming in general, as though stimulation of primary and secondary sexual parts is just a form of 'super-grooming' (cf. Bagemihl reference in the bibliography), yielding the same right-brain-based (thus female-associated) beneficial effects on body and mind we've discussed earlier; 2) *females' tolerance of multiple male sexual partners*; and 3) *females exhibiting male-type physical displays*, such as crotch-thrusting displays used to challenge outsiders or establish rank within the group.

One example of an anatomical 'masculinization of females' in these groups is the enlargement of the clitoris (the result referred to as a *'pseudopenis'*) that has been seen in elephants, lemurs, bonobos, and spider monkeys, among others – though none of the primate examples even approaches what spotted hyenas have experienced – more on that later. The enlarged clitoris makes it easier for males to see, and as a result, useful not only in greeting displays (which look more familiar – and thus more comprehensible – to males) but also for sexual signaling (via increased tumescence during breeding season), to inform the males whether or not a female is receptive.

Neural Rainbow Theory also draws on the model of pair-bonds to suggest that a 50:50 group with the best chance of surviving in a peaceful way will drift over time toward: 1) a *lack* of sexual dimorphism (females and males roughly equal in size, male canines roughly the same size as those of females, etc.); 2) equality across chromosomal genders regarding functions such as group defense as well as help with child care (no matter who the biological parents are); 3) a predominance of 'Center values' that is, a lack of intra-group competition (either female-female, male-male, or female-male); 4) minimal competition with neighboring groups (perhaps accomplished by building a female-based network of relatives to establish cooperation-based 'blood ties' to several groups in a region); 5) a 'horizontal' sharing of resources; and 6) an implicit recognition that it is the grandmother-type females (from the right-brain side of the 'moderate-T' spectrum) who are the acknowledged wise counselors and leaders. Regarding this last goal, NRT predicts that in general, any behaviors which *physiologically favor the right brain*, such as the 'pleasurable mutual grooming' described above, should help maintain the female focus of the *psychological* 'center of gravity' of the group, and in that way keep its personal and social compass pointing toward a universal acceptance of female leadership and female-centered values.

Thus one could compare 50:50 groups on all of these factors, to conclude which ones are being most 'successful' in adapting to the problem of 'too many males,' ranging from more successful (with the characteristics listed in the previous paragraph) to more unsuccessful (with the hallmark of frequent, often fatal violence against women and children, extending to include women and children of neighboring species, etc.) – predictably a maladaptive feature, since it targets the very individuals who represent the direct link to the next generation – those who *make* it out of their own bodies (the women), and those who *are* it, the children.

The interest in the history of 50:50 groups mentioned above originates in the NRT view of this SOC as a *transitional form* – beginning in C/P, moving toward 50:50 as a result of some habitat shrinkage that drove the invasion of Center groups by Perimeter males, and reaching a present state which may be more or less successful at reducing the stress associated with 'too many males.' It is important to recognize that even what appears *currently* to be a 'peaceful' state must still be seen as marginal – at best, there's only a 50:50 chance whether such groups will remain peaceful or become violent – *until* the condition of 'too many males' is resolved. Given what testosterone does to brains, as summarized in Chapters Two and Three, 50:50 is *not sustainable* in the long term because it is inherently *not stable* – individuals in the bottom row of the Trimodal periodic chart [Figure 3.2 of Chapter Three] are not and cannot be the same as individuals in the top row.)

Brain types, social roles, and social organization

To close this chapter, let's revisit the description of brain types from Chapter Three, and see how our current discussion about the different modes of social organization might help us understand 'why' the neural rainbow is made in the first place.

As we said, biology is all about persistence – making another generation, keeping the species going in a sustainable way. And thus as we suggested, it makes sense that animal societies will be organized around roles related to gender issues – the requirements of sexual reproduction mean that biology classifies individuals according to the way that they do (or do not) contribute to species persistence.

Chapter Three described the neural rainbow and the concept of the three-brain-types/six-genders complex as found in humans. But we also suggested there that this approach to classifying and grouping individuals might extend beyond humans, to apply to other types of animals. The specific mechanism invoked in Chapter Three for creating the rainbow was prenatal exposure to testosterone, and in fact Neural Rainbow Theory predicts that precisely the same mechanism is active in all mammals, with analogous versions in non-mammals, creating the same spectrum of brain and body types as described in humans.

The theory also predicts that mammalian brains are built according to essentially the same model across species, with the same basic patterns of functional asymmetries as described above for humans. These include the 'polypotent' nature of the right brain, important for overseeing social skills, general health, and right-left coordination – on which all animals depend – as compared with left-side specializations involving more limited skills which may not be as well developed or important for many animals. (There is evidence of functional asymmetries in non-human animals, and as research continues, more may be discovered. For example, if an animal's survival depends on being able to discriminate fine acoustic details such as those the EPIC model assigns to the left side of the brain, then functional asymmetries for such skills should not only be demonstrable in that animal, but the asymmetries will also predictably favor the left brain; for examples, see references to my articles on the EPIC model included in the Chapter Two bibliography.)

An important caveat for our discussion is that for animals such as birds, reptiles, and fish, which develop inside eggs instead of a uterus, the details of brain organization as well as the actual mechanism for creating the 'rainbow' may be somewhat different. But something equivalent must be at work, since as we've seen, these animals exhibit the same few types of social organization – revolving around the same few social roles – that characterize mammals including humans.

To see how this works, let's briefly review each of the types of social organization in turn, and see how the three brain types we've described *can be combined in different ways* to form a 'fit' to each of the different modes. For simplicity's sake in this discussion, we'll focus on the three brain types described in Chapter Three rather than the somewhat more abstract six 'genders' discussed there. We'll see that the three brain types provide a direct connection to the three social roles, which we've already seen can be filled (with the single exception of Grandmother-Leader) by versions of both chromosomal genders; thus the three brain types can be used to represent all six genders, since the brain types occur in both XX and Xy individuals.

Note that all of the matches we'll describe between brain types and social roles are in the form of predictions – Neural Rainbow Theory has only recently been proposed for humans, and this book represents the first tentative application of the theory to other types of animals. Thus all these predictions are hypotheses that remain to be tested. Also note that it will be easier if this first review is cast in terms that apply to mammals – as more is learned about the mechanisms that function in non-mammals, the same types of descriptions should be applicable to them as well.

The basic proposal, then, is that there is a biological mechanism (or set of mechanisms) which creates a continuum of individuals shaped to achieve certain social roles related to species persistence. The corollary is that the default 'setting' for this mechanism is 'free-running,' that is, in the absence of any type of adjustment (as might be needed, for example, to fit individuals for living within a particular mode of social organization), the mechanism will produce: 1) the entire continuum, shaped by 2) three concentrations of brain/body types, named earlier as 'polytropic' (right-brain/whole-brain), 'middle' (intermediate type), and 'focal' (left-brain favoring); with 3) versions in both chromosomal genders, giving rise to six 'genders,' all produced by dynamic individually-based variations in testosterone exposure.

Life in solitude

By definition, animals who live as solitaries must be willing to endure long periods of being alone. Coming fresh from our descriptions of peaceful Center groups with mothers and daughters playing with their children, we can recognize that the life of a solitary might be a psychologically difficult way to live – but only if an individual had the wrong kind of brain.

Thus Neural Rainbow Theory predicts that most animals who live as solitaries will be blessed with a brain type that prepares them for solitude, makes them actually prefer it, so that it is in fact not a burden at all. For solitary life, the left-favoring brain type should be ideal, since it is the one with relatively reduced access to right-brain skills (such as 'social intelligence'), by definition leading to a greater tolerance for a lack of social interaction.

Thus in solitary species, the rainbow mechanism will not be 'free-running,' but should rather *select for left-favoring brains* by ensuring that relatively *high levels of testosterone* are provided in virtually every pregnancy. (There is no reason to think that such a selective 'hormone setting' for making left-brains could not be possible – it is clearly at work in spotted hyenas, for example, who may represent a very extreme form, creating a species where even the females have 'penises' that are more than 'pseudo' – a greatly enlarged clitoris/urethra/birth canal combination, through which mothers must give painful birth – the organ rips open during birth, leading to a high mortality rate among first-time mothers; and the babies, many of whom suffocate while navigating the difficult birth canal, are born with their eyes open, and sharp teeth, and literally have to kill each other to survive.)

An impressionistic test of our predictions for solitaries would be to consider whether animals that typically live alone tend to be harder to domesticate. On a first consideration this would seem to be borne out, since trainers who work with large carnivores have reported that lions (C/Ps) are easier to manage than (solitary) tigers; and both tigers and bears, females as well as males, tend to remain quite 'feral' even when they are hand-raised with great nurturance and care.

Figure 4.8 is a graphic depiction of the match between brain types and social roles in the Solitary SOC. This diagram may appear to be identical to the 'SOC map' for solitaries presented earlier (Fig. 4.3), but only because the symbol code we use for both the Focal-Asocial social role, *and* the left-favoring brain type, is simply a shape with *no fill*. Later diagrams illustrating social-role/brain-type matches in the other SOCs will look different.

Figure 4.8

Solitary-SOC map with social-roles/brain-types indicated for females (circles) and males (triangles). (All symbols in this diagram are unfilled, indicating that all individuals have left-favoring brains supporting their Focal-Asocial role; as explained in the text, the other two roles and brain types are predicted not to be adaptive for a solitary lifestyle.)

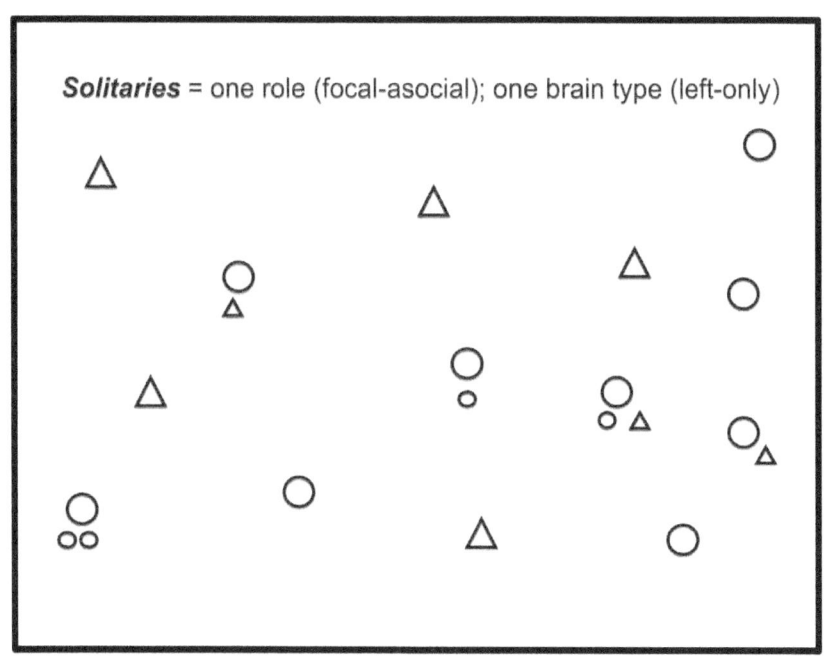

* * *

Bonded pairs

If we recall the characteristics of pair-bond life, where both female and male fill the Loyal-Helper social role, that is, required to do many of the same tasks, including the demanding combination of both caring for and aggressively defending children, we might predict that pair-bond species would be primarily made up of individuals with the *middle brain type*, produced via *moderate amounts of prenatal testosterone* (for mammals, at least).

Thus pregnancy for pair-bond mammals should be characterized as typically involving moderate testosterone exposure for every child. The result would be to complement a male's 'natural' abilities for defense, by adding 'middle-brain' tendencies for sociability and nurturing. At the same time, moderate levels of testosterone would complement the females' nurturing skills with a sufficient amount of aggressiveness to make them good defenders. Moderate testosterone creating middle-brains for both females and males could also account for female/male similarity in size – the lack of sexual dimorphism – which characterizes many pair-bond animals (excepting features such as coloration or vocalization patterns found in some same-size animals), as well as for the common occurrence of same-sex pairs in these species. Middle-brain features would also be consistent with some pair-bonds' high levels of sociability in interactions both with their own kind (for example, in extended family groups, as in cooperative breeders) and with humans.

Again, an impressionistic test would be to recall the long history of very successful domestication of animals which in the wild live as pair-bonds – obvious examples are canids and geese – along with the many descriptions of the strikingly 'human' behavior of large pair-bond birds from cooperative-breeding species, such as crows and ravens. For instance, we've noted before how observers remark on the way a pet crow or raven will readily 'adopt' a human family, enthusiastically grooming and vocalizing with adults as well as children, and defending the family vigorously against other humans (or animals such as dogs) who are seen as outsiders. These certainly sound like gregarious, Loyal-Helper, 'middle-brain' types.

Figure 4.9

Pair-bond-SOC map with social-roles/brain-types indicated for both females (circles) and males (triangles). (Gray symbols = Loyal-Helper/middle-brain; as explained in the text, the other two roles and brain types may not pertain in these species.)

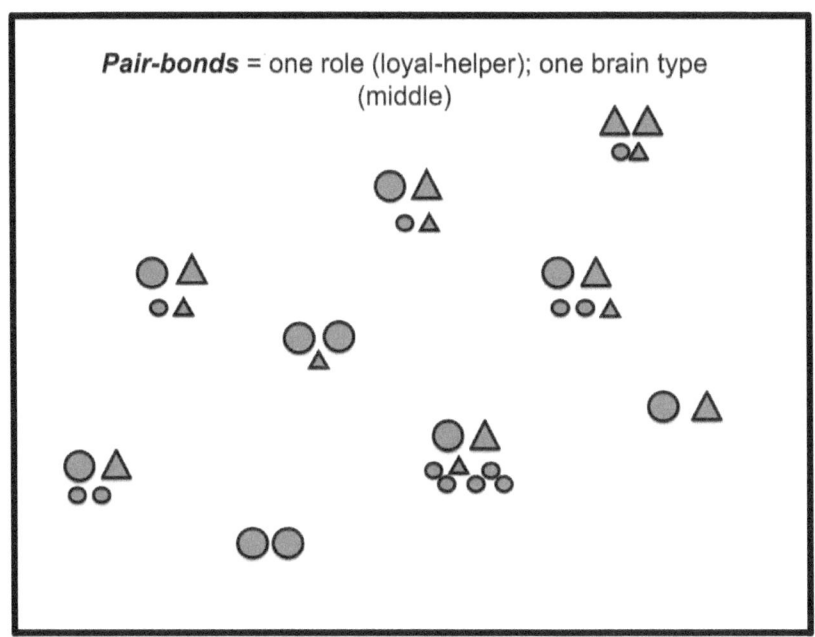

* * *

Center/Perimeter

What we've called the 'rainbow' mechanism seems to be custom-made for preparing animals to live in a Center/Perimeter style. Thus it is extremely interesting that, as we've seen, Center/Perimeter is the most common mode of social organization in the world, found in animals of virtually all classes, from fish to reptiles and mammals – and that animals living in other ways (like those typically-solitary iguanas in Mexico) may 'shift gears' into Center/Perimeter when conditions permit.

For Center/Perimeter species, the mechanism will function in its broadest, free-running mode, creating the full rainbow of individual differences, and all three brain types in essentially equal proportions, graphically represented in Figure 4.10, and described in detail in the text following the figure.

Figure 4.10

Center/Perimeter-SOC map with social-roles/brain-types indicated for females (circles) and males (triangles). (Black symbols = Grandmother-Leader/polytropic-brain; gray = Loyal-Helper/middle-brain; unfilled = Focal-Asocial/left-brain.)

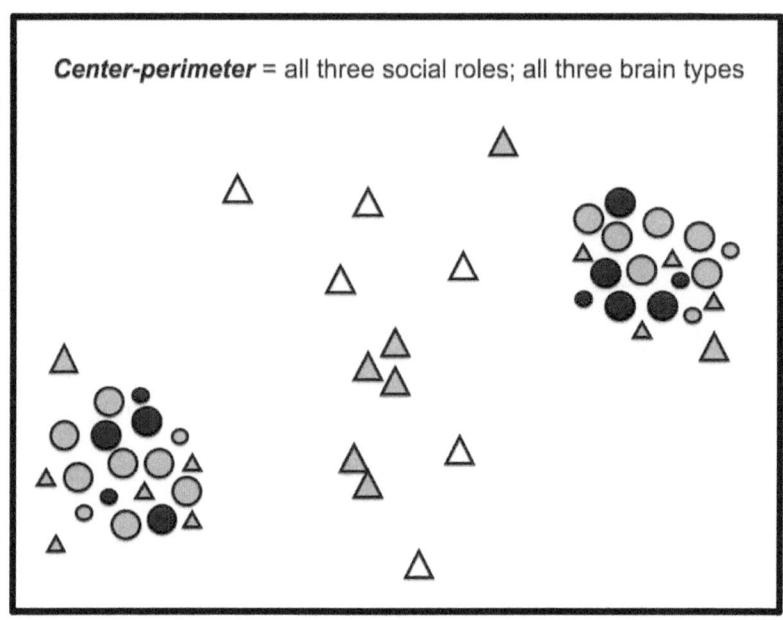

Center-perimeter = all three social roles; all three brain types

* * *

The *polytropic brain type*, made under conditions of *very low prenatal testosterone*, is ideal for the Grandmother-Leader women who constitute perhaps half the females of the Center group, and provide the multivariate management skills for dealing with the role's demands for high sociability, supreme social and emotional intelligence for judging the emotional state of individuals of all ages and genders, and great patience for dealing with babies, growing children, and the occasional Center male. This brain type will also endow a love of physical life including fondness for body-on-body contact, healthy sexuality, good instincts about what is nutritious to eat, exceptional general health physically and mentally to ensure successful pregnancies and a continuity of loving care for all group children, and good decision-making skills plus the ability to creatively draw on experience, providing a 'group memory' to ensure group accuracy and flexibility for responding to changes in environmental conditions.

176

The *female version of the middle-brain type,* created by moderate-T exposure, is ideal for the other women who live in the Center – not the grandmother type, but Loyal-Helpers: good with children, faithful followers of the Grandmother-Leaders, and friendly toward the Center males vetted via guidance from the grandmothers. The *male version of middle-brain* is *the* definition of the Center male – kind and loving to women and children, plus vigorously aggressive in defending the Center against intruders. As we said before, these 'big males' are 'dangerous' only to would-be predators, conspecific or otherwise – never to the people of the group. The moderate testosterone which produces a middle-brain will also make him tall and mesomorphic, an impressively imposing figure for showing off his full size to fend off intruders, and the advanced right/left coordination endowed by the middle-brain configuration will give him physical skills for the 'dance' of display, approaching and physically intimidating anyone who would threaten the group.

At the same time, middle-brain versions of social skills will also make him a Loyal-Helper, a willing 'servant' of his group – extremely loyal, emotionally bonded to them, and finding his interactions with them, both for nurturance and as their trusted 'defender,' deeply rewarding. Middle-brain females and males of the Center join with the polytropic grandmothers to 'serve and protect' group members from anyone or anything which threatens them.

The left-brain type, especially in males, created under conditions of *high testosterone exposure,* is perfect for Focal-Asocial life in the Perimeter – at least for those males who are not candidates for becoming a Center male (for one thing, the 'lifelong' perimeter males are too short, since high prenatal testosterone in the latter leads to early puberty which shuts down growth). (NRT predicts that very few focal-brain females are made in non-human mammalian centers. We'll talk later about why many human groups at present may be making more.) The lack of interpersonal social skills in the left-brain males (which also blocks them from being accepted into the Center) is not a problem for Perimeter life, since Perimeter 'society,' whether the individuals live as solitaries and or in 'pecking-order' competitive groups, is primitive at best.

The reduced nature of left-favoring brains, especially the general lack of connectedness, also fits the Perimeter males for a very empty life – what would be deathly boring to anyone with a polytropic or middle type of brain. Ethologists have described how young male monkeys on the verge of leaving their home Center group, may 'spend increasingly long periods of time doing absolutely nothing,' and another observer admitted that having to sit all day and watch an isolated (Perimeter) male gorilla for eight hours straight was extremely difficult, 'because he does so little.'

The dark side of the left-brain type, of course, lies in its generally challenged qualities with regard to mental and physical health. The sympathetic nervous system dominance of left-favoring brains means that they are prone to violence, which may become hyperviolence, of a particularly conspecific sort, directed either against other Perimeters or the members of the Center groups.

One expression of such violence may be the bizarre *'hunting'* behavior recently observed in some common chimpanzees, which has two features that suggest it is an outgrowth of the *infanticidal tendencies of Perimeter males*. First, this hunting tends to be directed to monkeys (who are a good approximation to chimpanzee babies). Second, it involves active sympathetic arousal instead of the very non-sympathetic 'cold-blooded' nature of hunting undertaken by 'natural' predators such as snakes and lions. In order to commence a 'hunt,' the participating chimpanzees (maybe only the short ones?) leap around and scream and work themselves into a rage-like frenzy before they launch into the frightening chase and harassment of monkeys. These are fearful tornados of activity which end by the gang of chimpanzees cornering and killing the hapless baby-like monkeys by literally tearing them apart.

Given these terrible propensities, it might be of some solace to remember that focal brains are also prone to a variety of problems threatening their own lives, such as an attraction to risk-taking behavior and generally poor physical health. Thus along with a tolerance for solitude and 'doing nothing,' these brains may also have built-in ways to assist them in 'shuffling off their mortal coil,' through being hyperactive around predators, or refusing to back down to a Perimeter alpha male who is just too strong, or simply dying of a heart attack during a self-induced rage.

"Eusocial"

It is hard to see how Neural Rainbow Theory can be applied in these same terms to eusocial animals, where the colony rather than the individual seems to be the real unit of organization – a 'superorganism,' as some have described them, where the individuals are more like specialized chemically-controlled cells inside a body than independent actors. Interestingly, insects are the only class of animals for whom this type of social organization has been a very common choice – as we said, no other set of non-human animals has adopted it, with the curious lone exception of the naked mole rat.

Figure 4.11

Eusocial-SOC map with social-roles/brain-types indicated for females (circles) and males (triangles). (As with solitaries, the unfilled symbols represent both the Focal-Asocial role predicted for all these individuals, as well as their left-favoring brains. Although a neural characterization may not be an appropriate terminology for insects, it is definitely accurate for describing the 'high-T' aggressive behavior of naked mole rats, especially the females.)

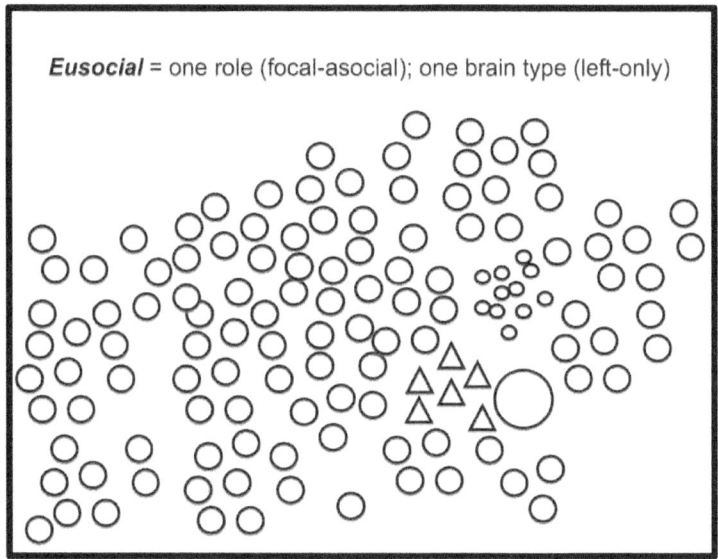

Eusocial = one role (focal-asocial); one brain type (left-only)

* * *

Certainly our concept of 'social roles' seems stretched a bit to apply to 'social' insects – for meeting the demands of everyday life, there is very little interaction between individuals (other than relaying chemical signals), and 'sex' in these giant colonies seems to exist in only a technical way, almost at the chromosomal level. The vast majority of eusocial individuals don't have social roles such as leadership, assisting others, or loyalty, as much as they occupy functional 'slots' or 'locations,' similar to interchangeable parts in a large machine, or cells within a greater organ. Examples are the 'castes' of ant colonies, where virtually all the animals are genetically female (though only one – the queen – is reproductive). In ant colonies, the queen may annually or semiannually produce a very few males for mating with new queens (to found new colonies), but even so, each colony's queen needs only a single mating to last her entire life (which may be 25 years or so, depending on the species).

She stores the sperm from this one mating within her own body, and draws on them over the years to produce eggs as needed.

However, because of the striking similarity of eusocial insect colonies to human cities, it might be helpful to consider whether the 'behavior' of such societies can be described according to the same typology we've used for the others – emphasizing in this case not brain type as much as behavioral style. This approach has proved useful for discussing the other social modes – for instance, animals living as solitaries do seem to be a good match to the Focal-Asocial role matching the 'social style' of a focal brain; pair-bonds have many of the middle-brain features we've described for Loyal-Helpers; and we've considered many details supporting the idea that the Center/Perimeter type of social organization is based on a mix of all three social roles and brain types.

How does the fact that most individuals in a eusocial group are 'not sexually active' fit into the way we've been talking about social organization so far? To understand that we need to return to the point made earlier, that the one thing all SOCs have in common is that *the* basic principle of their organization is the identity of each individual with regard to group persistence – not simply 'reproducing,' i.e., only making babies, but making sure the babies grow up so they can themselves produce the next generation. All the individuals of a SOC together form a matrix that generates persistence, and the matrix is shaped according to the three social roles we've been describing – Grandmother-Leader, Loyal-Helper, Focal-Asocial – and fundamental to all of these is how each contributes to group (thus species) persistence.

The 'social roles' we've discussed are based on three and only three 'reproductive roles'– breeding female, breeding male, and individuals who do *not* reproduce (though this is sometimes only temporary). Examples of the last category include: those solitaries who never find (or even look for) a mate; the crow and wolf 'helpers' who delay reproduction while in their home group to assist with caring for younger siblings; and the 80-90% of the males in C/P societies who for one reason or another (whether true-Perimeter males not fitted for group life, or Center-male types who never manage to join a group) do not pass on their genes. Thus we can see from even this brief review that an important difference between social styles, that is, the means by which they can provide alternatives for adjusting to different economic conditions, may be related to *different proportions* of the three reproductive functions.

In eusocial animals (bees, ants, termites, naked mole rats), no matter the number of individuals in the colony, there is only one breeding female (the queen). There is only a small handful of fertile males to provide the queen (or new queens for establishing new colonies) with sperm. The rest of the group – perhaps tens of thousands of individuals as in a termite hill – remain permanently neuter. They do not reproduce, but rather *work all their lives to support the children of the one breeding female and her consorts*. This is the

180

model of the crow 'helpers' carried to an extreme – but one which apparently best serves the food-gathering needs of the animals exhibiting this type of organization.

Many things about the eusocial SOC may make it seem so distinct from the other SOCs, that it appears to be a difference in kind, not degree, and yet the organization's dynamics can still be analyzed in terms of the same three social roles we've identified. The queen can be seen as a version of the Grandmother-Leader (she is literally the mother of everyone in the nest/hive, and her chemistry forms an integral part of the group's communication system, particularly regarding reproductive matters). The myriad 'workers' and 'soldiers' – depending on the species, sometimes numbering in the thousands – are definitely performing a Loyal-Helper role, trading their own reproductive function to instead work as support staff, to serve the reproductive success of the group as a whole. In addition, every member in its own way also fulfills the Focal-Asocial role, in this case, dedicated to doing a specific job where it is the combination of all the jobs that achieves group persistence, just as the cells of different organs of the same body are highly specialized for one thing only, and it is only through their combined effort that the body remains functional.

From this point of view, then, we might be correct in identifying the behavioral style, the principal social role, of eusocial colonies, as Focal-Asocial. Ants move about in response to external chemical signals; when the ants 'turn off' (if there are no current signals, there seems to be no other motivation to act), they just *stop* – 'ants don't play,' they don't gather with others to groom and relax.

The activities demanded of them as colony members seem very 'left-brain' as we've characterized that term – rapid, constant activity of individuals who are organized in rigidly defined ways to achieve tasks with ends that are beyond their individual scale, comprehensible only from a 'birds-eye view,' designed to accomplish the goals of the system as a whole. Success in a eusocial colony (whether it is an anthill or a large human city) demands left-brain attributes such as a tolerance for engaging in repetitive tasks, a disregard for personal danger, and self-denial regarding activities that in other animals are associated with reproduction – such as intimacy with a supportive partner, and children.

Thus we would not be surprised that in humans, it is the left-brains – not polytropics or middle-brains – who seem to get along best in big cities. Given the choice, polytropics and middle-brains may even decide not to live in big cities. If for some reason, circumstances force individuals with such brain types to stay in cities (and if we are right about their own behavioral styles), they will predictably exhibit signs of stress such as feelings of helplessness and social isolation, loss of individuality, lack of self-worth, a sense of being only a 'cog in a wheel,' nagging health problems due to challenged immune function, difficulty with sleeping, trouble with sexual function, and general feelings of being 'cut off' from themselves and their fellow human beings – *existential angst as the natural response to a mis-match between brain type and SOC*.

I would guess that if there were a way to ask an ant (or a naked mole rat) about how it felt about living in its home colony, it would not express such feelings. We might assume it is entirely adapted in every biological way possible to being there, the way a Perimeter male is happy with his solitary state which, from the point of view of people in the Center, looks like a sojourn in hell.

We've talked before about signs of stress among animals living under a different type of social organization than they are 'made' for (based on observations of sexual dimorphism, behavioral profiles, etc.), and we've suggested that these signs of difficulty are symptoms of the unnaturalness of that way of life for those animals. Thus we might ask whether there are any animals living in a 'forced' eusocial way, where the coercion shows in the signs of stress we've already mentioned – overpopulation, failures of immune response, intra-group violence particularly against women and children.

As suggested earlier, the answer is obvious – human cities. In almost every way possible, cities do not seem to be 'good for children or other living things' (borrowing a phrase from the antiwar protests of the 1960s, directed there not against cities but against war, though replacing the terms in this way makes my point). As we'll see in the next chapter, under very special conditions, humans do seem to be able to live peacefully in *somewhat* larger groups than the 5-20 of Center/Perimeter societies. But that 'somewhat' might still have its own limits. Even in large cities, people seem always to define a certain limited 'circle of social surround' for themselves, ranging from an inner ring of most intimate friends outward through several levels of relationships. One description of such a 'social surround' identifies the levels from innermost to outer as: a 'support clique' of five, a 'sympathy group' of 15, a 'close network' of 50, a 'personal network' of 150, and a circle of 'acquaintances' of 500.

If we consider the case of a typical C/P species living in Center groups of 5-20 individuals, one of these numbers, 150, could represent six to seven center groups living in a particular region – far enough apart not to encroach on each group's economic base, but still close enough to be personally known to each other (even perhaps related).

During the 1960s, the anthropologist Robin Dunbar, based on his studies comparing brain size and social groups in wild primates, suggested the 'Dunbar number' of around 150 individuals as the 'cognitive limit' of human acquaintances. Both his number and his general conclusions have met with criticism as well as acceptance, but several businesses have found that 150 is an effective upper limit for organizing workplaces (reports say that beyond 150, very different – and more implacable – personnel problems arise than in smaller groups). In addition, based on our descriptions of SOCs, we can see Dunbar's number might be of even wider significance, perhaps reflecting the nature of the *regional relations* maintained among members of a species living in a particular area – e.g., six to seven center groups of 20 individuals each seems like a comfortable – as well as a sufficiently entertaining and genetically diverse – social base to support a full and engaging daily life.

But even if humans living in cities do manage to create such personal support groups (and not everyone is successful at this), they are still impacted in many crucial aspects of their lives by social agendas designed to manage (and manipulate) much larger crowds of people, orders of magnitude beyond the tiny 'personal networks' of 150. The truth is, *no* animal, including humans, seems to have the capacity to live naturally (i.e., without violence, sickness, runaway population) in groups of thousands or millions – *unless* they follow the 'rule' embodied in the eusocial model, of assigning the majority of individuals to be sexless drones, 'slaves' to a tiny minority who are the only ones allowed to have children. This may sound like a science-fiction scenario, but it may also be a biological principle that no species dares ignore without suffering grave consequences.

50:50

I've already suggested that the biological mechanisms for shaping individuals according to the three social roles, if left 'free-running,' will generate the full continuum of individual differences, and that these will be grouped into roughly equal proportions of the three-brain-types/six-genders complex described in Chapter Three. I've also indicated that for some types of social organization – solitaries and pair-bonds – this system is *not* free-running, and that the C/P lifestyle is the only one that provides niches for all roles, brain types, and genders, such that all of them are 'adaptive' in one way or another.

If solitaries and eusocials are primarily Focal-Asocial/left-brain individuals (fitting them to tolerate living either alone or in impersonal crowds), pair-bonds are shaped to be Loyal-Helper/middle-brains, and the C/P style provides slots for all types, what should we predict for animals who are forced by environmental changes to live (at least for a while) in 50:50 groups? The first requirement is obvious – there *should* be *no* individuals with focal brains, because the crowded 50:50 arrangement definitely demands a high degree of social skills on the part of all concerned – which would rule out Focal-Asocial (grading to anti-social)/left-brain types.

Figure 4.12

*50:50-SOC map with social-roles/brain-types indicated for females (circles) and males (triangles). (Grandmother-Leader/polytropics are black circles, Loyal-Helper/middle-brains are grey. In **peaceful** 50:50 groups, shown here, there **are no Focal-Asocial/left-brains**, as they are too volatile for this crowded situation of 'too many males.')*

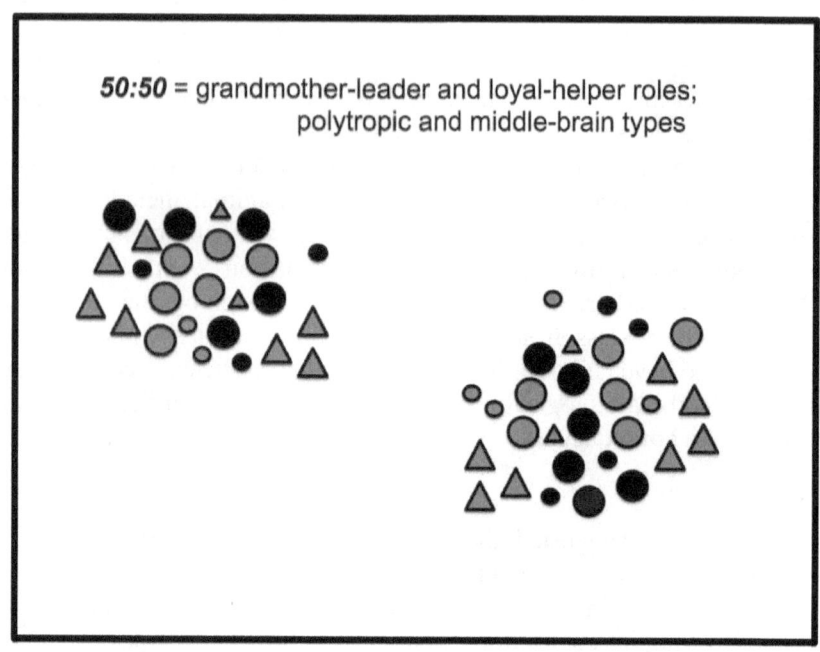

50:50 = grandmother-leader and loyal-helper roles; polytropic and middle-brain types

* * *

Thus we would predict that for a species to live in 'peaceful 50:50' groups successfully (that is, without any of the signs of stress we've listed), mothers would give birth to very few left-brain individuals. With everyone either a polytropic Grandmother-Leader or a middle-brain Loyal-Helper, universal good health and accomplished social skills should ensure a strong foundation for harmonious everyday life.

However, all by itself, this still might not be enough – remember that *space* is a crucial aspect of social organization – and we've seen that this essentially means the space separating reproductively active males. In 50:50 groups, the types of physical space we've seen are available to the middle-brain males participating in pair-bonds and C/P societies, are lacking. Thus there would probably have to be other, 'cultural' ways to manage all those males in such close proximity to each other – providing a *psychological equivalent of physical space*.

One very straightforward strategy might be simply to manipulate line of sight – for example, replace distance with walls, such as those used in human huts and houses. If reproductively-active males can be kept out of sight of one another – particularly with regard to their interactions with females – it might be possible to avoid triggering their naturally competitive response, and still allow them to live in relatively close proximity.

Another way might be to offer males experiences that mimic those provided in other social organizations, thereby defusing their sense of reproductive competition. Some of the primate 50:50 females we described earlier in the chapter do this by encouraging mutual grooming done for right-brain pleasure, not left-brain competition (that is, for displaying dominance or submission), and also by allowing all males in the group relatively free access to the sexual favors of more than one female – thus giving each male the experience of a Center male in a C/P society. For example, in muriqui monkeys, observers have seen a female have sex with one male, and when they are finished, go on to entertain several other males; this may be a good demonstration of how this can be done. Testifying to the effectiveness of this approach is the patient peacefulness with which the other males to be included sit together, waiting for their turn in line. With all females in the group behaving this way, there is no occasion for any one male to feel left out; each can enjoy the hormonal confidence of the C/P center male who knows that when any of his resident ladies is ready for sex, she will accept him as a lover.

Hopefully this sounds at least a little familiar from a human point of view. In fact, we will see in the next section that some 'peaceful 50:50' human societies have taken exactly this tack, that is, providing each male with a simulation of the experience of a Center male – which seems to go a long way towards keeping the peace. But we will also see that this type of management, clever as it is, may only be effective if it builds on the base of neural shaping in two ways: 1) all males in the society must be either right-brain or middle-brain types (under such explosive conditions, 'no left-brains need apply'); and 2) the entire scheme must be designed and managed under the oversight of right-brain/whole-brain, polytropic Grandmother-Leaders. If left-brain individuals are made, and are not sufficiently nurtured to develop their social skills as much as possible (the 'well-loved lefts' mentioned in Chapter Three), and/or the process is not overseen by the polytropic group members, any attempts at cultural management of sexual competition may be doomed to failure. In fact, NRT suggests that the different degrees of success at peaceful co-existence achieved by those animal and human societies using a 50:50 structure, may boil down to just three things: 1) exactly which brain-types/genders are produced; 2) whether or not a way has been found to ensure that every sexually active male has access to multiple females; and 3) whether the grandmothers are the ones in charge.

But no matter how momentarily 'successful' such management may in maintaining the peace (*no* intra-group violence, especially not against women and children), the most important thing to remember about the 50:50 arrangement is that, as suggested earlier, it does not ultimately 'have legs' – that is, given how sexual reproduction is managed by biology, just finding ways to *accommodate* the males does not have promise as a long-term solution to the short-term crisis of the Perimeter collapsing into ('invading') the Center.

That is because 'too many males' as a crisis is very different from problems such as temporary pollution of the local water supply or an insect infestation of a favored type of fruit tree – mainly because, unless it is female-controlled, *the presence of surplus males may drift the whole group toward the left* on the neural rainbow scale, resulting in behavioral and biochemical changes in *all* group members that can epigenetically propagate into the next generation, in ways that *undermine the sustainability of the group.* This undermining may begin with an immediate rise in *violence against fellow group members*, resulting at the very least in injury and death to crucially important, 'non-surplus' group members – women and children – and at the most, in stress-related neurological changes affecting all females, which can biochemically affect the health and brain types of subsequent generations.

If a condition of testosterone-based 'left-brain drift' is allowed to continue, the most devastating long-term change in group structure and viability may be losses regarding right-brain/whole-brain individuals – not only as a significant proportion of group members, but as the acknowledged leaders of the group, who are crucially necessary for guiding the group in making life-or-death decisions – such as how many males, whatever their brain type, can be supported at any one time, and for how long – a guidance absolutely central to group sustainability.

One might ask whether a condition of 'too many males' can be sustained at all for very long? The answer follows directly from what we said in Chapter Three about prenatal testosterone and its far-ranging effects on the brain – and is, simply, no. The NRT prediction is that biology's capabilities for adaptive changes DO NOT extend to handling a *testosterone-based crisis* as though it were any other kind – a disease outbreak, a drought, a change in food supply, etc. – because this kind of crisis, if not corrected, seems to quickly become permanent – *because the presence of the males themselves makes everyone in the group act more and more like males* – it's as though testosterone were added to the drinking water, and everyone ends up 'drinking the purple Kool-Aid' (a reference to the tragic 'Jonestown massacre' of 1978).

Only if a momentary situation of 'too many males' is reversed, and fairly quickly, *only* if the collapse of the Perimeter onto the Center is turned around, and the Perimeter males return to their roaming in the wide-open-spaces, can a *temporary* shift to 50:50 be managed. And in the real world, that qualification may itself be only theoretical – the observations available to date (in humans as in other animals betraying signs of such a change) suggest that *because of the way males are made, the reversal may never happen,* that once the males get in, they are there to stay, they never leave, and *their presence behaviorally and epigenetically masculinizes every other group member no matter the chromosomal gender* – with nothing but negative consequences for the long-term survival of the group.

QRS and the rules for reproduction: An acronym to live by

Earlier in this chapter, we briefly mentioned a set of general biological rules governing reproduction that apply to every organism on Earth – from single cells to multicellular creatures of all kinds – and we suggested that those rules are of basic evolutionary importance, and only those species which honor the rules can hope to persist.

As mentioned there, Neural Rainbow Theory uses the acronym QRS to summarize these rules. The acronym highlights the evolutionary importance of producing a next generation of *quality* individuals at *replacement* levels in a *sustainable* way.

For organisms in general, '*quality*' individuals are those whose nature makes it possible for them not only to persist and flourish themselves, but also serve their species as the producers and caretakers of a subsequent 'quality' generation. For animals, including humans, one component of 'quality' refers to the way an individual's brain type adaptively fits the social organization currently used by a species, and the extent of their flexibility for fitting into a different arrangement if environmental conditions require it. The catalog of individual features listed in Table 3.1 of Chapter Three provides a sample of some of the properties which allow individuals to accomplish these goals, including their 'wired-in' (brain-type-determined) social role in group life. If quality individuals are not made consistently by a group or species, this undermines the quality – the viability – of the group overall and can lead to extinction.

But making quality individuals is not enough by itself, if it is not done in a controlled way. The *replacement* rule refers to the need for population management, a basic requirement for all species. Even if all the babies a species makes are 'quality' individuals, having too many or too few – *based on the availability of resources* – can be fatal. Zero Population Growth (ZPG) is adaptive if the environment, including its provision of resources, remains stable over time. 'Replacement-level fertility' means reproducing at a rate that maintains zero population growth. Most simply, if two individuals have two children who survive to reproductive adulthood, the parents are said to 'replace' themselves.

Population management, even for achieving zero growth, is of course more complicated than this; under certain conditions, parental pairs may need to increase their birth rate, and in others, reduce it. For example, if one or both children of a pair do not survive to adulthood, the parents have not replaced themselves, and if this happens to too many parents, the size of the next generation may shrink, potentially threatening genetic diversity – thus to maintain replacement, parental pairs may need to produce more than the original two children.

On the other hand, if in addition to two children made with person A, one of the parents additionally has two children with person B, the three adults involved have exceeded their replacement limit (4 children instead of 3), and if too many individuals do this, the size of the next generation may expand, potentially exceeding its resources, which can either lead to a 'boom and bust' cycle as a crude way of regaining replacement levels, or to unchecked, runaway growth (with insufficient 'bust' drops in population) that can overload resources, also driving the species to extinction.

Depending on environmental conditions, zero growth may not always be the adaptive goal. Negative Population Growth (NPG) may be very useful as a group survival strategy if resources are rapidly dwindling (NPG was a goal often expressed in the population-control activism of the 1960s, when I was making my own decisions about reproduction). In contrast, if resources become more abundant and widespread, through climate change, etc., reproduction rates may rise to take advantage of the geographically-expanding niche, even leading to the formation of new groups, and beyond that, to dispersal, such that the increase in the number of new groups follows the geographical spread of resources.

For example, horses first appeared (as Eohippus) in North America, and when environmental changes occurred that encouraged population growth and dispersal, the changes 'led' the descendants northward, to eventually cross the Bering Strait and enter Asia. Humans followed a similar climate-based expansion of resources, spreading out of their original homeland in southern Africa, on a dispersal route that took them along a band of familiarly-moderate climate, from Africa into southern India and Japan, and finally, via the Bering Strait, to the Western Hemisphere. In such instances, it can be adaptive to increase growth rate, to exploit the new geographical niches.

But just making Quality individuals at Replacement levels is still not enough – it must be done in a *Sustainable* way. For instance, if a group goes on making healthy babies at the replacement rate in the face of declining resources, this is by definition unsustainable – *the only numbers that can be*

188

supported in the long term are those that are a match to the environmental niche in which the group is living.

As we said earlier, the infrastructure of social organization is a group-level adaptation to the niche of economics (the sum of the available resources, and access to them) – and in the same way, exactly *how* the next generation is produced (rated in terms of both quality and numbers) is an adaptation to the same niche. *In fact, social organization (and the brain-type means by which individuals support it) is the principal group-level strategy provided by biology for managing reproduction according to the QRS rules.*

Thus if a species is forced by some situation or event to change its social organization, its reproduction process may be undermined, leading either to a loss in the quality of individuals, and/or a lack of control over numbers (producing either too few or too many), and/or a state of unsustainability: a failure to maintain an accurate match to the environment, eventually resulting in extinction. [For more about QRS, see the end of Chapter Five.]

Again, as noted earlier, one or another of the QRS rules may be broken *as a short-term emergency measure* to help a species (or a local group) survive a temporary environmental crisis – but *continuing to break the rules even after the crisis has passed, particularly if the new version of reproductive management becomes permanent, by definition puts the species or group at risk.*

In the next chapter, we'll see more about whether and how this applies to humans – though the answer may already be obvious.

Chapter Four Summary: Taking stock

The science of ethology considers aspects of non-human animal behavior including *social organization*, for which we've suggested a more specific term *socioethology*. In this chapter we've made a brief survey of the modes of social organization found in animals, and we've suggested that there are only five principal ways to organize an animal society – solitary, bonded pairs, Center/Perimeter, eusocial, and 50:50 – and that each of the millions of animal species, no matter their other types of differences, lives according to one of these five.

We've also suggested that these types of organization take their origin in the basic requirement of sexual reproduction, that animals must in some way come together in order to mate. Thus all five types of animal societies can also be analyzed according to the inclusion and arrangement of the three basic reproductive functions common to them all, the 'basic elements' of social organization – the breeding female, the breeding male, and individuals who do not reproduce, either temporarily or permanently.

Finally, we have combined these observations with descriptions of the brain types from Chapter Three, to suggest some preliminary conclusions related to the science of *neuro-socioethology*, that is, how the organization of the nervous system is fitted to, reflects, and is reflected in, social organization. The result offers one way to understand 'why' animal social organizations have the form they do, and to explain how different individuals function more or less well within different types of societies, i.e., each SOC is a set of niches for social roles, and each role is a niche fit by a particular brain type. The same principles point to a possible new source of stress both for individuals and social groups, that arises if there is a basic *mis-match* between the brains of individuals, the social roles they are asked to fill, and the category of social organization they live in.

Table 4.1 summarizes these points, *by showing how each of the five SOCs depends on a particular set of brain types functioning in the social roles they were 'born for.'* The table also suggests specific possible sources of stress if brain types are required to undertake roles not natural to them – e.g., if middles or polytropics should have to live alone (top row), or if left-brains are 'forced' into a pair-bond (2nd row), etc. These simple correlations help us recognize the fundamental difference – with potentially disastrous impacts on health and happiness – between whether individuals are *allowed to express their brain type by fulfilling the role they are fitted for* – like a key in a lock, or a hand in a glove – vs. instead being *forced to assume a role that is not congenial* – 'a square peg in a round hole,' etc. The implications are clear, for *any* type of animal, including humans.

Table 4.1
Five social organization categories (SOCs)
with related social roles and brain types

SOC	roles*	principal brain types
solitary	1 = FA	1 = left
pair-bond	1 = LH, (GL)	1 = (polytropic), middle
Center/Perimeter	3 = GL, LH, FA	3 = polytropic, middle, left
50:50	2 = GL, LH	2 = polytropic, middle
eusocial	1 = FA	1 = left

GL = Grandmother-Leader, LH = Loyal-Helper, FA = Focal-Asocial

* * *

As noted earlier, this book considers humans to be just another of the multitudes of species on earth, governed by the same rules (such as QRS) that apply to all biological organisms. This point of view has naturally affected our choice of terminology, especially the avoidance of terms suggesting that the human version of a phenomenon (e.g., *woman, children, psychology, sociology*, etc.) is somehow different from (and thus implicitly privileged when compared with) the same phenomenon considered in other species (e.g. *female, young, ethology, social ethology*, etc.).

Based on this principle, we've suggested the term *neuro-socio-ethology* to refer to descriptions of how the *neurology* (understood in the widest sense, as described in the 'brain types' summaries of Chapter Three) of a species is related to the individual *psychology* of its members and their *social behavior*, including the *social organization* of the species. This chapter has for the most part focused on aspects of *neuro-socioethology* in non-human animals; in Volumes Two and Three of this book we will return to consider many issues related to neuro-socioethology in humans.

First, however, we need to take a larger look at human history, to see whether understanding more about human social organizations of the past and present – and how well they accommodate the different brain types – can give us a new perspective on the ways we live today. If so, then perhaps they can also offer guidelines for achieving a more human (and humane) future.

Chapter Four Bibliography

Ainslie T, B Ledbetter (1980) The body language of horses. NY: William Morrow & Co., Inc.

Alcock A (1973) The love of horses. London: Octopus Books Ltd.

Alderton D (2003) The complete book of birds. London: Hermes House.

Alexander RD, KM Noonan, BJ Crespi (1991) The evolution of eusociality. *In* PW Sherman, JUM Jarvis, RD Alexander. (Eds) The biology of the naked mole-rat. Princeton NJ: Princeton Univ. Press.

Altmann J (1980) Baboon mothers and infants. Cambridge MA: Harvard Univ. Press.

Attenborough D (1998) The life of birds. London: BBC Books.

Austin CR, RV Short (Eds) (1976) The evolution of reproduction. London: Cambridge Univ. Press.

Bagemihl B (1999) Biological exuberance; Animal homosexuality and natural diversity. London: Profile Books.

Barber C (1971) Animals at war. NY: Harper & Row, Pubs.

Barlow C (Ed) (1991) From Gaia to selfish gene; Selected writings in the life sciences. Cambridge MA: The MIT Press.

Barlow GW (2000) The cichlid fishes; Nature's grand experiment in evolution. Cambridge MA: Perseus Books.

Barlow N (Ed) (1958) The autobiography of Charles Darwin 1809 –1882; With original omissions restored, edited with appendix and notes by his granddaughter Nora Barlow. NY: Norton & Co, Inc.

Box HO (1984) Primate behavior and social ecology. London: Chapman and Hall.

Bright M (2000) Gorillas; The greatest apes. London: DK Publishing, Inc.

Browne J (2006) Darwin's Origin of Species; A biography. NY: Atlantic Monthly Press.

Budiansky S (1992) The covenant of the wild; Why animals chose domestication. NY: William Morrow & Co.

Burton R (1976) The mating game. NY: Crown Publishers, Inc.

Calef G (1995) Caribou and the barren-lands (original hardback 1981). Willowdale Ontario: Firefly Books.

Carroll SB (2005) Endless forms most beautiful; The new science of evo devo. NY: WW Norton & Co.

Colinvaux P (1978) Why big fierce animals are rare; An ecologist's perspective. Princeton NJ: Princeton Univ. Press.

Cunningham C, J Berger (1997) Horn of darkness; Rhinos on the edge. NY: Oxford Univ. Press.

Darwin C (2003) Origin of species [orig 1859; 2003 Intro by Sir Julian Huxley]. NY: Signet Classics.

de Boer SF, Buwalda B, Koolhaas JM (2016) Untangling the neurobiology of coping styles in rodents: towards neural mechanisms underlying individual differences in disease susceptibility. *Neuroscience and Biobehavioral Reviews*. PMID 27402554 DOI: 10.1016/J.Neubiorev.2016.07.008.

de Grahl W (1987) The grey parrot [translator W Charlton; German 1st edition 1976]. Neptune City NJ: TFH Pubs., Inc.

De Waal F (1982) Chimpanzee politics. Baltimore: The Johns Hopkins Univ. Press.

De Waal F (1989) Peacemaking among primates. Cambridge MA: Harvard Univ. Press.

De Waal F (1996) Good natured; The origins of right and wrong in humans and other animals. Cambridge MA: Harvard Univ. Press.

De Waal F, F Lanting (1997) Bonobo; The forgotten ape. Berkeley: Univ. of California Press.

De Waal F (2005) Our inner ape. NY: Penguin Books.

Discovery Books (2000) Mammals. NY: Discovery Books.

Dugatkin L (1999) Cheating monkeys and citizen bees; The nature of cooperation in animals and humans. NY: The Free Press.

Dunbar RIM (1988) Primate social systems. Ithaca NY: Comstock Publishing Assoc.

Edwards EH (1993) Horses. London: Dorling Kindersley.

Edwards EH (2003) Wild horses. NY: Hylas Publishing.

Eisley L (1958) Darwin's century; Evolution and the men who discovered it. NY: Doubleday & Co., Inc.

Eisley L (1979) Darwin and the mysterious Mr. X; New light on the evolutionists. NY: E.P. Dutton.

Eldredge N (2004) Why we do it; Rethinking sex and the selfish gene. NY: WW Norton & Co.

Elgin SH (1998) The grandmother principles. NY: Abbeville Press Pubs.

Elia I (1988) The female animal, 2nd ed. NY: Henry Holt & Co., Inc.

Fair J, L Rogers (1990) The great American bear. Minocqua WI: NorthWord Press, Inc.

Fedigan LM (1992) Primate paradigms; Sex roles and social bonds. Chicago: Univ. of Chicago Press.

Forshaw J (Ed) (1998) Encyclopedia of birds, 2nd ed. San Francisco: Fog City Press.

Forsythe A (1993) The natural history of sex; The ecology and evolution of mating behavior, 2nd ed. Shelburne VT: Chapters Publishing Ltd.

Fossey D (1983) Gorillas in the mist. Boston: Houghton-Mifflin Co.

Fox R (1980) The red lamp of incest. London: Hutchinson.

Freud S (1964 translation and notes by E Fritzen) Monarch Review notes & study guide: The ideas and writings of Freud [synopsis of Freud's 1909 Clark University lecture series]. NY: Thor Pubs. Inc.

Geist V (1991) Elk country. Minnetonka MN: NorthWord Press.

George M (1992) Mammals. North Mankato MN: The Child's World, Inc.

Gerardin L (1968) Bionics. NY: McGraw-Hill.

Ghiglieri MP (1999) The dark side of man; Tracing the origins of male violence. Reading MA: Perseus Books.

Giraldeau L-A, T Caraco (2000) Social foraging theory. Princeton NJ: Princeton Univ. Press.

Gould JL, CG Gould (1997) Sexual selection; Mate choice and courtship in nature, 2nd ed. NY: Scientific American Library.

Greenberg J (2006) Monkey portraits [portrait photography]. NY: Little, Brown & Co.

Gronefeld G (1965) Understanding animals [German original 1963; 1965 English translation by G Vevers, W Reade]. NY: Viking Press. Inc.

Haraway D (1989) Primate visions; Gender, race, and nature in the world of modern science. NY: Routledge, Chapman & Hall.

Heinrich B (1999) Mind of the raven; Investigations and adventures with wolf-birds. NY: HarperCollins.

Henry M (1967) All about horses. [1st edition 1962] NY: Random House.

Hinde RA (1970) Animal behavior; A synthesis of ethology and comparative psychology, 2nd ed. NY: McGraw-Hill.

Hird MJ (2009) The origins of sociable life; Evolution after science studies. Basingstoke, Hampshire, GBR: Palgrave Macmillan.

Hölldobler B, EO Wilson (1994) Journey to the ants; A story of scientific exploration. Cambridge MA: Harvard Univ. Press.

Hoyt E (1996) The earth dwellers; Adventures in the land of ants. NY: Simon & Schuster.

Huxley TH (1968) On the Origin of Species. [Introduction by Ashley Montagu]. Ann Arbor MI: Univ. of Michigan Press.

Jahme C (2000) Beauty and the beasts; Woman, apes, and evolution. NY: Soho Press, Inc.

Kaplan G, LJ Rogers (2000) The orangutans; Their evolution, behavior, and future. Cambridge MA: Perseus Publishing.

Kilham L (1989) The American Crow and the Common Raven. College Station TX:

Texas A&M Univ. Press.

Köhler W (1927) The mentality of apes [translator E Winter]. NY: Vintage Books.

Kowalski G (1991) The souls of animals. Walpole NH: Stillpoint Publishing.

Kummer H (1971) Primate societies; Group techniques of ecological adaptation. Chicago: Aldine-Atherton.

Lauter JL (1996) The Brain of Isis. Presented to Southwest Women's Conference, University of Oklahoma, Norman OK. [Unpublished; excerpt in Appendix]

Lauter JL (1999) The Center, the Perimeter, and the Neural Rainbow; The human brain and ways of being human – A neuroscientist suggests some new approaches to understanding individual differences, human types, social evolution, and the nature of good and evil. [Unpublished MS; limited circulation; excerpt in Appendix]

Lauter JL (2008) How is your brain like a zebra? A new human neurotypology. Bloomington IN: Xlibris. [Addendum section on social organization, titled "Other animals," was omitted from the 2008 edition, and is unpublished as of 2022; excerpt in Appendix]

Lauter JL (2011a) A new natural-selection approach to social organization in humans and other animals, based on the neurological effects of sex hormones. Part I: Propositions One and Two, linking economics, social-organization categories (SOCs), and social roles. Prepared for 86[6h] Research Conference of the SouthWest and Rocky Mountain (SWARM) regional division of the American Association for the Advancement of Science (AAAS), Wichita KS. [meeting cancelled] [Unpublished; excerpt in Appendix]

Lauter JL (2011b) A new natural-selection approach to social organization in humans and other animals, based on the neurological effects of sex hormones. Part II: Proposition Three, connecting social roles to hormone-mediated brain types. Prepared for 86[6h] Research Conference of the SouthWest and Rocky Mountain (SWARM) regional division of the American Association for the Advancement of Science (AAAS), Wichita KS. [meeting cancelled] [Unpublished; excerpt in Appendix]

Lauter JL (2012) SPINE: A new sociobiology for the 21st Century based on socio-psycho-immuno-neuro-endocrinology (SPINE), I. Prenatal hormones, six genders, and brain-based social roles. Plenary Lecture to 87th Research Conference of the SouthWest and Rocky Mountain (SWARM) division of the American Association for the Advancement of Science (AAAS), Tulsa OK. [Unpublished; excerpt in Appendix]

Lilly JC (1961) Man and dolphin. NY: Pyramid Pubs., Inc.

Lilly JC (1967) The mind of the dolphin; A nonhuman intelligence. NY: Avon Books.

Linden E (1992a) A curious kinship: Apes and humans. National Geographic 181(3): 2-45.

Linden E (1992b) Bonobos: Chimpanzees with a difference. National Geographic 181(3): 46-52.

Linzeh A (1995) Animal theology. Urbana: Univ. of Illinois Press.

Lorenz K (1952) King Solomon's ring; New light on animal ways. NY: Thomas Y Crowell Co.

Lorenz K (1979) The year of the greylag goose [translator R Martin; German 1st edition 1978]. NY: Harcourt Brace Jovanovich, Inc.

Loubach D, M Henckel (1987) Elk talk. Helena MT: Falcon Publishing, Inc.

Lyell C (1830, 1832, 1833) Principles of geology; being an attempt to explain the former changes of the earth's surface, by reference to causes now in operation. Vols I, II, III. London: John Murray.

Macdonald D (Ed) (1999) The encyclopedia of mammals. NY: Barnes & Noble, Inc.

MacLean PD (1973) A triune concept of the brain and behavior. Toronto: Univ. of Toronto Press.

MacLean PD (1990) The triune brain in evolution; Role in paleocerebral functions. NY: Plenum Press.

MacLean PD (1996) The limbic system and evolution of mammalian family-related behavior. AAAS Annual Meeting and Science Innovation Exposition 162: A62.

Marchand PJ (1996) Life in the cold; An introduction to winter ecology, 3rd ed. Hanover NH: University Press of New England.

Masson JM, S McCarthy (1996) When elephants weep; The emotional lives of animals. NY: Delta Books.

Masson JM (1999) The emperor's embrace; Reflections on animal families and fatherhood. NY: Pocket Books.

Masson JM (2003) The pig who sang to the moon; The emotional world of farm animals. NY: Ballantine Books.

McBane S (2001) Modern horse breeding; A guide for owners. Guilford CT: The Lyons Press.

McCarthy S (2004) Becoming a tiger; How baby animals learn to live in the wild. NY: HarperCollins.

Milne L, M Milne (1982) A time to be born; An almanac of animal courtship & parenting. San Francisco: Sierra Club Books.

Momatiuk Y (1997) Mustangs on the move. Smithsonian Nov 1997 28(8): 54-63.

Montagu A (1956) The biosocial nature of man. NY: Grove Press, Inc.

Montagu A (Ed) (1978) Learning non-aggression; The experience of non-literate societies. NY: Oxford Univ. Press.

Morris D (Ed) (1969) Primate ethology. NY: Anchor Books.

Morris D (1988) Horse watching. NY: Crown Pubs., Inc.

Napier P (1972) Monkeys and apes. NY: Bantam Books.

Perry N (1990) Symbiosis; Nature in partnership. London: Artillery House.

Petersen D (1988) Among the elk. Flagstaff AZ: Northland Pub. Co.

Portman A (1967) Animal forms and patterns; A study of the appearance of animals. NY: Schocken Books.

Richard UH, C Boesch (2003) Monogamy; Mating strategies and partnerships in birds, humans and other mammals. Cambridge UK: Cambridge Univ. Press.

Ritvo H (1987) The animal estate; The English and other creatures in the Victorian age. Cambridge MA: Harvard Univ. Press.

Rosenzweig ML (1996) Species diversity in space and time. Cambridge England: Cambridge Univ. Press.

Rue LL, III (1997) The deer of North America. NY: Lyons & Burford, Pubs.

Savage C (1995) Bird brains; The intelligence of crows, ravens, magpies, and jays.

San Francisco: Sierra Club Books.

Schaller GB (1976) The mountain gorilla; Ecology and behavior. Chicago: Univ. of Chicago Press.

Schmidt-Nielsen K (1972) How animals work. London: Cambridge Univ. Press.

Scientific American Books (1955) Twentieth-century bestiary. NY: Simon & Schuster, Inc.

Sherman PD, JUM Jarvis, R Alexander (Eds) (1991) The biology of the naked mole rat. Princeton NJ: Princeton Univ. Press.

Singer P (1975) Animal liberation. NY: Avon Books.

Skutch AF (1992) Origins of nature's beauty. Austin TX: Univ. of Texas Press.

Sleeper B (1997) Primates; The amazing world of lemurs, monkeys, and apes. San Francisco: Chronicle Books.

Smith A (1970) The seasons; Life and its rhythms. NY: Harcourt, Brace Jovanovich, Inc.

Southwick CH (Ed) (1963) Primate social behavior. Princeton NJ: D Van Nostrand Company, Inc.

Strier KB (1992) Faces in the forest; The endangered muriqui monkeys of Brazil. NY: Oxford Univ. Press.

Strum SC (1987) Almost human; A journey into the world of baboons. NY: Random House.

Thomas WD, D Kaufman (1990) Dolphin conferences, elephant midwives, and other astonishing facts about animals. Los Angeles: Jeremy P. Tarcher, Inc.

Turner JX (2000) The extended organism; The physiology of animal-built structures. Cambridge MA: Harvard Univ. Press.

van Baer KE (1828) Über Entwickelungsgeschichte der Thiere. Beobachtung und reflexion [On the developmental history of the animals. Observations and reflections]. Königsberg.

Van Lawick-Goodall J (1971) In the shadow of man. Boston: Houghton Mifflin.

Wallace AR (1859) On the tendency of varieties to depart indefinitely from the original type. J Proc Linnean Soc (Zoology) 3: 45–62.

Ward A (2007) Freshwater aquarium fishes. Neptune City NJ: TFH Pubs, Inc.

Waring GH (1983) Horse behavior; The behavioral traits and adaptations of domestic and wild horses, including ponies. Park Ridge NJ: Noyes Publications.

Watson L (2004) The whole hog; Exploring the extraordinary potential of pigs. Washington DC: Smithsonian Books.

Weber B, A Vedder (2001) In the kingdom of gorillas; Fragile species in a dangerous land. NY: Simon & Schuster.

Wilson EO (2000) Sociobiology; The new synthesis, 2nd ed. Cambridge MA: Harvard Univ. Press.

Wolkomir R (1997) From twigs to ravens, nothing escapes the notice of Bernd Heinrich. Smithsonian Nov 1997 28(8): 94-107.

Wrangham R, D Peterson (1996) Demonic males; Apes and the origins of human violence. Boston: Houghton Mifflin.

Zuckerman S (1981) The social life of monkeys and apes, 2nd ed. [orig 1932] London: Routledge & Kegan Paul Ltd.

* * *

Chapter Four Figures & Tables

◈ Chapter Five ◈

HUMAN HISTORY:
WHERE WE CAME FROM AND WHEN

In the last chapter we ventured into *socioethology*, describing the different types of social organizations used by animals. Toward the end, we extended this into *neuro-socioethology*, to discuss how different combinations of the rainbow of brains outlined in Chapter Three can be seen as providing biological support for the different types of animal societies.

In Chapter Four the discussion ranged from invertebrates to mammals, from ants to zebras, and was in fact the widest view we'll take in Volume One of this book [some items in the Volume Three Appendix will provide an even wider view]. We saw there that in spite of dramatic distinctions between animal species (in terms of body size, foods, preferred climate, etc.) the social organization of any species can be fit within a basic classification scheme usable for all animals: solitary, pair-bond, Center/Perimeter, eusocial, or 50:50.

From time to time in Chapter Four, we also suggested that human beings are no exception to this rule. (For the purposes of this discussion, 'human beings' will be understood as meaning 'Anatomically Modern Humans' or AMH, as identified by evolutionary biologists – the form of 'human' we are, that 'emerged' from the hominid lineage perhaps less than 200,000 years ago – abbreviated as '200 KYA.') Thus regardless of the variety of ways humans live now or have lived in the past, we can expect that all AMH lifestyles – simply because they are animal lifestyles – can be analyzed and categorized using the same five social forms. Human social organization may seem to differ dramatically from society to society, or change radically within the same society over time, but every type of human arrangement derives from those same five possibilities – ones that we share with all other animals on Earth.

In this chapter, we'll first talk more about *human socioethology* – the social choices that AMH humans have made during our history on earth. We will draw on a number of disciplines such as the study of human evolution, history, paleontology, and archeology. And as in Chapter Four, we'll then go on to take the next step, into human *neuro*-socioethology, to consider how the choices made by human groups regarding social organization either do or do not harmonize with the Neural Rainbow brain types.

By the end of the chapter, we will have surveyed all of AMH history (and be reminded how much time that really involves). We will also see how a neuro-socioethological analysis of the choices that humans have made, some of them long, long ago, can help explain why some societies have achieved peace and harmony, while others suffer from chronic, self-destructive strife and violence, no matter how hard at least some of their members try to move them onto a more sustainable path.

Human biology – older than our history

Just as the history of horses revolves around the fact that their digestive system fits them for eating grass instead of meat, and the history of seals depends on adaptations for living in cold water, so there are aspects of human biology that have been absolutely crucial in our own history.

I will approach this selective review as a catalog, noting how each feature places us within the context of other animals. Of course, we share basic aspects of biology with all animals, such as the chemical needs of respiration and digestion, and our dependence on a narrow range of temperature compatible with life. (Attempts to live outside our natural temperature range may have had disastrous consequences on human history, as we will discuss.) Humans also benefit from the sophisticated function of many body organs and systems, some of which are essentially unchanged from animals which evolved hundreds of millions years before us – such as sharks. Many other organs and systems are shared with virtually all air-breathing animals, from amphibians to mammals.

Size and temperature/humidity tolerance

The first way of comparing us with other animals is to say that we are moderate-sized mammals, somewhere between elephants and whales at one extreme, and tarsiers and field mice at the other. We are also relatively 'hairless' mammals – but not 'naked' as is sometimes said. We have as many individual body hairs as other primates, but most are so short they provide virtually no cover for the skin, significant for issues of temperature control, insect avoidance, and protection from solar ultraviolet radiation. The fact that our body hair is very short suggests that for extremely long periods of our history we lived in a warm, dry climate, where being able to sweat freely (and release the heat quickly through evaporation) was much more important than protection against cold. Our early warm homeland must have also provided sufficient shade to allow us to forego the other great advantage of longer hair – protection against solar ultraviolet radiation, for which humans substituted skin melanin to serve as a sun shield.

Child-bearing characteristics

There is a classification scheme used by biologists to sort organisms of all kinds – plants as well as animals – according to a cluster of characteristics having to do with reproduction. The basic distinction in this system is between 'r-strategists' vs. 'K-strategists.' The initials r and K are taken from technical terms used in equations expressing rules for population growth and maintenance, regarding the ways different organisms use reproduction to adjust to their environment. For our purposes, we can think of r as referring to reproductive rate, that is, how many babies are made per unit time, while K is a value related to the size of a stable adult population.

Organisms classified as r-strategists (such as most plants, fish, amphibians, and reptiles, along with mice, rabbits, and virtually all predatory land mammals) focus on making lots of babies – they typically have a relatively short gestation period, produce multiple babies per birth, and have a short time to sexual maturity. The r strategy is essentially, 'make as many babies as you can, as fast as you can, as often as you can.' The young of r-strategists typically experience high levels of mortality, but there are so many of them, at least some will survive long enough to start making babies of their own. This strategy is thought to be especially useful when the environment is *unstable* – a high rate of reproductive turnover lets the species cope with destructive or changing conditions.

In contrast, K-strategists such as giraffes, elephants, dolphins, whales, and large primates including humans, focus on ways to create a stable population of healthy adults. They have longer gestation periods (as long as two years, as in elephants), typically only one baby per birth, and the young live for years before sexual maturity. Thus the K strategy could be summarized as – 'invest heavily in each and every child.' This strategy allows an organism to flourish in a *stable* environment, because it allows them to create and maintain a population of a certain size, matching the conditions of that environment.

R-strategists tend to be smaller in size (though some carnivores break that rule) and K-strategists larger. All primates about the size of humans or larger are K-strategists (chimps, gorillas, orangs), as are most of the mammals larger than us (giraffes, elephants, cetaceans). R-strategists tend to have shorter lifespans (some not much longer than one year), while K-strategists tend to live longer (on the order of decades, some up to a century).

There is an intermediate case, one I will call the r/K strategy, seen for example in many grazer mammals such as elk, zebra, and white-tailed deer. This approach combines K characteristics for number of children per birth (one, sometimes two), and length of gestation (6-8 months), with r characteristics such as a short interval between births (typically only a year) plus a relatively short time to sexual maturity. The lifespans of r/K animals are also intermediate – one to two decades.

Humans are full-fledged K-strategists, since we: a) typically have only one child at a time (our two nipples mark us as a one-baby-per-gestation species), nurtured via a combination of b) a long gestation, and c) lengthy postnatal care including breast-feeding, that lasts much longer than gestation;

and d) our children take more than ten years to reach sexual maturity.

Women's monthly cycles, which make it possible to conceive year-round, resemble those of mammals who live near the equator, so our species may have spent a significant part of its history there, but humans living in more temperate zones also exhibit a statistical tendency to conceive in the fall, when reproductive hormones for both females and males are high, and deliver in the spring, when new plant growth promises a summer-long 'buffet,' so that a breast-feeding mother can replenish her milk.

Departing from the mammalian norm at any given latitude may introduce unnecessary handicaps, which have been suggested but not systematically studied. These might include: problematic conception, miscarriages (some occurring perhaps so early they aren't recognized, even by the mother), more difficult pregnancies, stressful deliveries, perinatal distress, higher incidence of learning difficulties, etc. As noted earlier in our brief discussion of 'season of birth,' conceiving off the normal seasonal/ hormonal cycle may result in less than ideal biochemical conditions during pregnancy and as a result, shift the baby's brain in an undesirable direction along the neural-rainbow continuum.

As suggested in the distinctions between r- vs. K-strategists, the relation between length of gestation and number of children per pregnancy is one of the most interesting aspects of animal classification, and may help us gain a better sense of 'who we are.' The human gestation time of nine months is similar to that of other moderate-sized animals who have single-child births, such as dolphins, zebras, and gorillas (all with gestations around nine months). Gestation times are shorter in single-birth animals who are smaller than we are – gazelles (three-five months), macaque monkeys and baboons (five-six months) – while pregnancies are longer than ours for animals who are larger than we are. For example, rhinos, giraffes, and sperm whales have sixteen-month gestations, and an elephant mother can expect to carry a fetus for a two full years.

Much shorter gestation times are found in those animals who give birth to three or more young at a time. This includes not only animals much smaller than humans, such as lemmings, who may give birth to as many eleven babies after only 20 days, and rabbits and prairie dogs, who produce litters of up to ten after a gestation of 45 days, but also carnivores who are about our size. Virtually all carnivorous land mammals, including lions, tigers, foxes and wolves, have more than three babies per delivery, and create these 'instant families' via gestations that seem more appropriate for rodents than for animals of this size – only 60 days for foxes and wolves, 90 for lions and cheetahs.

Most of our sister primates, from monkeys to gorillas, breast-feed, co-sleep, and body-on-body carry their children for three to four years. This period of nursing not only provides invaluable nutritional and psychological support for the growing child, but also suppresses ovulation in the mother, providing a natural contraception. Breast milk is crucial for child health. The very first breast fluid, called colostrum, 'jump-starts' the newborn's system regarding immunity, digestion, hormones, and growth in ways that may have lifelong benefits. In human newborns, there is no functional immune system at all until at least six months – antibodies in the mother's milk are the only protection the child has until then, and they continue to guide the development of the child's immune system into the fourth and fifth years.

During the second year in human babies, nutrients in breast milk may be particularly important for completing the connection between the two sides of the brain, ensuring harmonious, two-way communication between the hemispheres, to the extent that the functionality of that connection was not impaired by prenatal hormones. Because of this landmark event during year two, the general expression of the brain types described in Chapter Three may come into prominence at this time, as 'hidden' asymmetries are revealed when connections between the two sides develop; and other phenomena such as the 'terrible twos' and the 'appearance' of autistic symptoms may be signs that a pre-wired left-sided preference is already in place.

Many human societies have implicitly acknowledged the crucial importance to human health of the 'natural' length of breast-feeding, along with body-on-body carrying and close, nurturing contact between caretaker and child over the first four or five years of life. Other groups have not, but as we will discuss later, denying babies this type of postnatal care may have dire consequences for individual health and psychology, as well as disabling an important check on population growth, thus generating a host of problems that might be readily resolved by remembering we are *mammals* ('mammary-gland' animals), and for many reasons, need to act accordingly.

Nervous system

As seen in Chapter Two, the human central nervous system is more like those of other animals than it is different. The concept of the *triune brain* mentioned in that chapter, developed by MacLean and Papez, outlines how the 'snake' (fish/amphibians/reptiles) brain (spinal cord, brainstem, and parts of the limbic system) is present and functional not only in the brains of reptiles and birds, but also in mammals. As mammals evolved, they added on to this original foundation certain 'horse-brain' additions in both the limbic system and the cortex, followed by another step that created the 'monkey' brain of primates, expanding the extent and connectedness of neocortex not only across the surface of the brain, but also adding inclusive networks that integrated subcortical areas of the brain with the latest-developing neocortex, in the frontal lobes.

As a result, our nervous system is managed by a series of rules, some of them very old, tried and tested over millennia to effectively and efficiently support a variety of behaviors crucial to everyday existence including social interactions and successful reproduction.

Chapter Three also briefly referred to the autonomic nervous system, with centers within the brain, plus a network of neural pathways extending throughout the body. Here we examine some of its details, and see how its two parts (the parasympathetic and sympathetic systems) work together in complementary ways.

The parasympathetic nervous system provides crucial biological support for everyday life. It keeps the heart beating at a relaxed pace, oversees the regularity of calm, deep breathing, and handles all elements of digestion, from guiding us in judging what is good to eat, to activating digestive juices and controlling peristalsis (movements of the walls of the digestive tract), to allowing us to choose when and where to eliminate waste products.

The parasympathetic system is also very important in reproduction, not only to make sure heart and digestion are working well in the pregnant and nursing mother, but also for sex itself. All the 'right-brain' activities that we refer to as courting or foreplay, which can be observed in animals from Komodo dragons and crows, to wolves and humans, involve the parasympathetic system. Rhythmic, deep-pressure gestures such as stroking and licking, soft vocalizations, and the feelings of well-being and warmth as blood vessels near the skin surface relax and fill with blood – even the awareness that pleasures of this stage of sex resemble the pleasures of eating – all testify to the parasympathetic nature of foreplay.

In fact, the parasympathetic system continues to predominate throughout intercourse, right up to the point of climax. Orgasm, however, involves a sudden 'shift of gears,' transferring control to the sympathetic nervous system, which creates rapid physiological changes in both the female and male, including the ejaculation of sperm.

This contrast between the sexual involvement of the two parts of the autonomic nervous system may offer clues to many aspects of sexual experience. For example, those individuals who tend to be more parasympathetic in general (Type B personalities: high-PSNS polytropics and middle-brain types) may be almost more interested in the considerable and more varied pleasures of foreplay than in the ephemeral climax, and they therefore enjoy exploring ways to extend these whole-brain, whole-body, feelings throughout the experience.

On the other hand, individuals characterized by a high sympathetic tone (Type A personalities: high-SNS, left-dominant, 'high T,' or 'focal brains,' as we've called them) might be impatient with foreplay, prefer to 'get on with it,' and therefore appear cold, insensitive, and even violent as sex partners. As already noted, the psychological relation between sex and violence is supported by the close proximity of neural centers for aggression and sexual behavior deep in the limbic system, and high-T left-brain types might not have very good reciprocal relations between these very ancient parts of their brains that allows them to reliably distinguish between the gestures of physical love vs. attack.

The old observation that some people (mainly men, but some women) feel depressed after sex might also be explained by these autonomic complexities. For someone who tends to have high sympathetic tone, being 'forced' to spend much time in the parasympathetic stages of foreplay and arousal, might feel very unusual and even unnatural. Consequently, this type of person may suffer a kind of rebound or 'whiplash' reaction when climax restores their standard state of sympathetic dominance, resulting in feelings of disorientation, depression and loss of control. Thus people who feel this way (the "*post coitum omne animalium triste est*" response – Latin for 'after coitus, all animals are sad') might be thus identifying themselves as high-SNS left-brains, neither middles nor polytropics. (Interestingly enough, the original Latin quotation ended with – *praeter mulierem gallumque*, 'except women and roosters.' The reference to women here may be an unsolicited testimonial that most women are high-PSNS polytropics or middles themselves, while the 'rooster' presumably refers to a rooster's willingness to go on entertaining hens almost continuously, up to 30 times a day.)

The last thing we need to explore regarding the autonomic nervous system is a feature we will see later may have been of critical importance in human history – the relation between autonomic function and ambient temperature. When we are surrounded by the ideal air temperature for humans (around 20-25 degrees below body core – inherited from our geographical place of origin in southern Africa), the parasympathetic system is responsive and favored. After all, when you are comfortable – not too hot and not too cold – you usually have good digestion, your heart works in a relaxed way, you breathe slowly and evenly, and enjoy good circulation. Temperatures (or more specifically, the heat index – since humidity is crucial in body-heat regulation) which are higher or lower than the ideal can suppress parasympathetic functions, and actually lead to sympathetic activation. If you get too hot, digestion can be disturbed, and heart and respiration rate will increase as the body attempts to reduce body heat through heavier breathing, similar to a dog's panting. If the temperature falls too low, the sympathetic system is again called on, to shrink peripheral blood vessels (we turn pale not only with rage and fear, but also with cold), and to increase heart rate and respiration, thus keeping the heat-creating body core supplied with energy.

But as we all know, that's not all that happens when we get too hot or too cold. Sympathetic activation in these cases is much like the observation (which has been tested experimentally) that you can evoke emotions in yourself simply by mimicking the physical form of their expression – if you smile, you actually feel happy, and if you frown, you feel sad. These effects can be so strong, that some psychologists in the past went so far as to suggest that the origin of emotions was not in the brain but the body, that mental feelings follow changes in the body, instead of the other way around.

Thus if the heat index favors the parasympathetic system, so that you are warm but not too warm, cool breezes touch your skin, the air is dry enough for your skin to keep you cool so you can breathe slowly and evenly – you will *for physiological reasons* feel good, relaxed, happy, at peace with yourself and with the world. As we'll see shortly, this description of an environment that makes you feel happy also describes the conditions under which AMH humans originally developed – the cool, dry, breezy, tree-shaded savannahs of southern Africa. Little wonder then, that it sounds so comfortable – for us, that's home, that is 'Eden.'

In contrast, we've all experienced what happens if the heat index gets outside of the comfort zone. If it rises above this ideal range (too humid, too hot), you feel like you're choking, like your 'skin can't breathe,' respiration gets faster and more shallow, your heart starts beating faster, you feel out of sorts, and rapidly escalate into being edgy and irritable. Police departments know all too well such effects of a high heat index. Violent crimes skyrocket during heat waves, and this is particularly marked during 'Santa Ana' wind conditions, that occur (with different names) in various places around the world, where changes in the atmosphere involving ions related to brain chemistry combine with a rising heat index in a way that simply pushes people over the edge.

Emotional reactions to cold are not observed as commonly, since humans have developed a range of ways to protect themselves from cold – from fire to heavy clothing to climate-controlled shelters which maintain the 20-degrees-below-core ambient temperature that we find most comfortable. (Some students of human history like to brag that humans have adapted to many more climates than other animals – but putting on heavy coats and turning up the furnace are not true biological adaptations, only cultural adjustments – no more and no less than the towers termites build for controlling the internal temperature of their own living spaces – termite bodies, just like ours, also have their own preferred heat index. Deep inside our igloos and houses and layers of clothing, we are still the short-haired animals of 60,000 years ago, liking it best when the weather is comfortably warm and dry, just like the ambient air at 30° South.)

But our bodies do react dramatically to cold, by turning up the sympathetic nervous system. This not only redirects blood flow to the body core rather than the periphery (why cold skin gets very pale), and activates hair follicles to raise our hairs (though all we get are 'goose bumps' – our hairs are too short to provide an air-filled cover against cold, which animals with longer hairs achieve by the same action), but can also cause changes in emotional state, making many people feel more energetic, grading into more aggressive, in the cold. Experiencing emotional changes when the temperature changes, reactions that seem beyond our conscious control and make us feel almost 'possessed,' reveals the primacy of our biological nature, and the fact that (as MacLean and Papez have described at length) the involuntary, unconscious workings of the autonomic nervous system can have direct and sometimes very dramatic effects on behavior.

Digestive system

The design of the human digestive system, from tooth shape and salivary chemistry to the anatomy (and microbiome) of our stomach and intestines, provides another important point of comparison between us and other animals. Digestive details in humans make it clear that we are fitted to get our nutrition from 'energy-rich' foods, designed as *nutrient storage* devices for the *plants* that made them, such as tubers, fruits, leafy greens, nuts, and seeds. We do not have either the special type of digestive system needed to extract nutrients from woody grasses and leaves, or the digestive tools (from teeth to colon) to process raw meat. Even the length of our intestines (five to six times body length) is significant, falling somewhere between those designed to handle woody plant material (usually ten times body length, as in deer), and those designed to process animal muscle and fat (only three times body length, as in lions). As noted previously, the intestines of carnivores must be extremely short to minimize the time that the decaying flesh is kept inside the body.

The fact that our digestive system fits us for eating fruits and nuts (making us 'frugivores') rather than meat may be surprising to people who have been repeatedly told that 'animal protein' is essential to human life. I remember lessons in primary school claiming that meat and dairy products comprised one of the 'basic food groups' needed every day to stay healthy. In fact, the protein molecules in animal flesh cannot be used directly – they have to be broken down first, into the building blocks of amino acids, which are then used by the body to build up new proteins. This two-step process demands an energy investment to break down the proteins, and so is not the most efficient way to acquire amino acids. The most efficient way of getting amino acids is to take them directly from plants. We need to look at the plant amino-acid formula more closely, then, to understand more about the biology of human digestion.

The amino acids we're concerned with here are the eight 'essential amino acids,' which cannot be manufactured in the body (many other amino acids can be made internally), and so must be obtained in food. And again, contrary to what we are told in first grade – all eight of the essential amino acids are available in the plant foods which are an exact fit to the human digestive system, such as grains (we eat their 'seeds,' not the woody plant bodies), beans (representing the plant group known as legumes), and nuts. Grain-seeds have somewhat different proportions of the eight amino acids as compared with legumes and nuts, and so if every meal includes grains plus legumes/nuts, the body has all the amino acids it needs in order to synthesize proteins.

Many ethnic foods reflect an implicit knowledge of this, in the design of menu items such as a bean burrito, lentil dahl over rice, or even a peanut butter sandwich (if the bread is from whole-grain flour). The irony about the myth of the superiority of animal protein is that, as we have said, your body has to actually expend energy to break down animal protein, to free the amino acids for re-synthesis. This is like having to break down a brick wall that someone else has already made, then cleaning the bricks off one by one, to obtain the raw materials for building your own wall. Thus for any animal, even carnivores, eating meat is like a Catch-22 of financial investment – to make money you have to spend money. Meat-eating is a serious trade-off that biology has selected for some animals, but it comes with a high metabolic price, one which human digestive systems don't have to pay. We are designed to get our amino acids 'energy-free,' by taking them from plants, already 'pre-separated,' ready for use.

An additional feature of our digestive systems that shows they are shaped for plant-eating is the chemical content of saliva. There are special proteins in saliva that protect tooth enamel from the decay that might otherwise be caused by eating fruits and tubers and their 'stored energy' of carbohydrates, and is another of the many features we share with our fruit-loving primate relatives.

Sexual dimorphism

Finally, we need to consider this feature of human beings, to see how we compare with other animals. Chapter Four mentioned that ethologists believe the degree of physical sexual dimorphism exhibited by a species is a good indicator of the social organization preferred by that species. Thus, animals who lack sexual dimorphism, where females and males are almost identical in size, tend to live as pair-bonds, while animals who show marked sexual dimorphism most often use the Center/Perimeter social arrangement, where groups of women and children live with a single attendant male per group.

So – are humans sexually dimorphic or not? If we could determine this, it might give us some insight into what type of social organization is most natural for us. It's obvious that we don't have the very dramatic differences seen in some other animals, such as the color and form differences contrasting male and female peacocks, the striking distinctions in the size of canine teeth in chimpanzees, or the size doubling of silverback male gorillas compared with the Center-group females.

However, humans do have a certain degree of sexual dimorphism, involving a number of physical features. (It goes without saying that all of these should vary from person to person according to the Neural Rainbow model, resulting in large overlaps between 'female' vs. 'male' groups.) In general, the features most scientists agree as exhibiting sexual dimorphism in humans are: 1) body proportions (width of shoulders vs. waist and hips; size of vocal folds; size of lower jaw; etc.); 2) extent and amount of body hair; 3) muscle density and distribution; 4) fat distribution; and 5) height.

When ethologists discuss sexual dimorphism in humans compared with other animals, they usually describe us as being somewhere in the middle range. That is, although we don't seem to exhibit as large a size differential as animals like gorillas, at the same time, neither are human women and men virtually identical, as many true pair-bond animals, such as geese and gibbons, are. So humans are typically described as being 'mildly sexually dimorphic.' Ethologists then go on to point out that this is consistent with the fact that in virtually every human society known – even the ones that vehemently insist on pair-bond relationships – there is at least some degree of what is called 'polygyny,' that is, individual males having access to more than one female – *implying* (though seldom *admitting*) that we are biologically designed to live in Center/Perimeter groups, not as pair bonds.

I agree with all these observations, including the implication that humans are C/P animals. (In fact, we deny this at our peril, as we'll see in a moment.) However, the signs of our C/P nature may be even more definite than the mild degree of dimorphism usually reported. For instance, the typical way of reporting height measures of women and men, as *averages* for each gender, show only a fairly small difference – in one standard table, the average height for women between 30 and 39 years of age is given as 5 feet 5 inches, while men in the same age range average 5 feet 9 inches. By analyzing the data in detail, however, we can see that the statistical distribution for the women alone is almost a perfect bell curve (41% are shorter than 5'5", and 43% taller) while the distribution for males has an interesting skew toward higher values – only 28% of the men are shorter than 5'9" while 54% are taller. I would infer from this that if humans were indeed living in C/P groups, organized according to the choices of the women (and perhaps making fewer of the smaller, left-brain males than currently) ethologists would be less inclined to label our sexual dimorphism as 'mild.' Including the shorter 'focal' males in the same average with taller middle-brain males tends to mask the 'tallness' of human males compared with women. (At the same time, it may be true that in certain human cultures that have managed to accomplish a peaceful 50:50 SOC, women and men are even less dimorphic than in industrial societies, which as we'll see later, have a very unusual SOC signature.)

Chapter One briefly discussed the dangers of averaging across individuals – which can obscure or even erase crucial details. Using averages to report potentially dimorphic features such as height may also conceal another feature related to our C/P nature, the existence of two kinds of males in humans. As outlined in Chapter Three, Neural Rainbow Theory predicts that for all animals who live in a Center/Perimeter organization, two kinds of males will be created: the taller, middle-brain type and the shorter, left-brain type. Moreover, these differences in humans should parallel those found in other animals, such as the taller vs. shorter male orangutans, and the larger 'territorial males' vs. smaller 'sneaker males' described among fish such as bluegills (see Partridge et al. reference in Chapter Five bibliography) – that is, the smaller males approach the size of the typical female. In fact, the same statistical tables referred to above show that 28% of the human males fall exactly in the middle of the female range.

For the purposes of this book, then, we will assume that humans exhibit a more marked degree of sexual dimorphism than they are often credited with, and also that this occurs in the context of 'two kinds of males,' distinguishable according to all the features outlined in Chapter Three. This is not a trivial point, or mere statistical hairsplitting. In the rest of this chapter I will argue that differences in the proportions of brain types produced by any human society – particularly with regard to males – is of crucial importance. In fact, how well a society either controls the production of the 'two types of males,' or finds a way of accommodating the dramatic differences between them, has direct implications for the success of that society, measured in terms of signs of stress (cf. Chapter Four), including group survival.

* * *

To conclude this brief section on human biology, Figure 5.1 presents a summary of a few of the crucial biological features we've just discussed showing how we as humans compare with other animals. The summary is in the form of a 'Species Identity Card,' similar to other types of ID or business cards, that one might carry in a wallet. The front of the card (top panel) lists a few features each individual shares with the rest of their species, and the back of the card (lower panel) provides information about how each person's biological 'personal identity,' categorized in terms of the three major combinations of brain type and social role, shows how they fit into the social organization of their species, as described in the previous chapter. (If such cards were 'issued' to individuals, one of the three choices could come premarked for each person, to indicate which category they belonged to, or individuals could check the correct one for themselves.)

Since I designed this card in 2008, I've found it can have a strangely calming influence, as I gaze at it and realize that through the lens of this small list of a few simple facts, I can see myself as just another biological organism on Earth, someone who is a 'card-carrying' member of the world-wide community of creatures which biology has created on our planet since the beginning of life billions of years ago.

Figure 5.1
Species Identity Card (filled-in for humans)

SPECIES IDENTITY CARD

Name/Class Homo sapiens / Mammalia
Social Organization Center/Perimeter
Typical group size 10-25
Diet Frugivore
Reproduction K-strategist/ g = 9 mo. / single birth
Climate Preference Moderate temperature and humidity
Latitude Range 30 degrees S to 30 degrees N

PERSONAL

Brain-type / Social role

_____ Polytropic / Grandmother Leader
_____ Middle-brain / Loyal Helper
_____ Left-brain / Focal Asocial

Human history – Stage One, the making of
Anatomically Modern Humans (AMH)

Certainly we humans share our history with the earth itself, and all the other organisms of our world. After all, most of the atoms on earth, including those in our bodies and brains, had their origin in stars. But for now, let's just go back to what is generally considered the point where a biological arrow started to point more or less in our direction – about five million years ago (MYA). This was the point when our branch of the primate tree diverged from the two other closest branches, the ones that went on to create modern gorillas and chimpanzees.

Calculations based on DNA analysis show that already by this time, the developmental lines leading to all the other types of primates had long since gone their own way. New World monkeys split off more than 40 MYA and Old World monkeys (baboons, macaques, etc.) about 20 MYA. The other members of our 'great apes' group also branched off long ago – gibbons around 15 MYA, and orangutans around 10 MYA.

Of course, not all the specific types of animals present at each of these branchings, or which developed later along each line, are still around today. (The typical lifespan of a mammalian species is about 1 million years, and many don't last even that long.) It's believed that at one time there were as many as 6,000 primate species, compared with only 185 still around today. The fossil record shows an amazing degree of fluctuation as groups come and go – they either fit into an environmental niche or they do not, they may find ways to change in order to 'track' a changing environment, or move to find better-suited conditions, or die out. All these kinds of evolutionary experiences have happened to many types of animals, including our primate ancestors. Being able to change to adapt to different environments is at the very heart of the concept of evolution.

But successful biological existence does not always mean change. The same mechanisms that allow for change also make it possible for those animals fortunate enough to find a supportive, stable environment, to live harmoniously within that environment for millennia. Sometimes evolutionary scientists refer to this as a 'sluggish' or 'static' condition, whereas NRT holds that this is clearly what every animal group dreams of finding – the Right Answer.

The goal of adaptation after all, is not change for the sake of change (the means becoming the end), but rather to fit in, to match, like a key in a lock, to achieve a state of 'dynamic equilibrium' with the environment. *Stability can be as adaptive as change.* Many if not most descriptions of evolution, however, seem to forget this, stressing the points of change – the historical high-speed car chases and shoot-outs – at the expense of all the long millennia when things were quiet and life went on as usual.

This distinction is vital as we turn our attention to human history. We need to remind ourselves that the word 'interesting' in the saying (attributed to the Chinese, though the source remains elusive) "May you live in interesting times" is sarcastic – intended as a curse, not a blessing. And we might want to entertain the notion that there is nothing wrong with being 'static,' if it means that everything is working as it should – *stable* might be a more accurate word. When viewed from the perspective of long-term survival, the 'sluggish' stability of early human life will seem like a very good thing, when we approach the end of our story and find that many if not most of the recent changes for humans have in fact been changes for the worse.

It will also help to remember that when an animal group embarks on changes in response to some shift in conditions, this usually happens incredibly slowly, perhaps over eons, at the patient pace of 'natural selection.' Natural selection typically works over countless generations, waiting while some individuals fail to reproduce and others have more success, gradually molding a new profile for the group as a whole.

If the environmental change is too sudden to allow time for a group to adapt in this way (for example, if a large asteroid collides with the earth, or human hunters kill everything in an area), genocide *can* occur, and entire animal groups can be wiped out very quickly. If a few individuals survive a catastrophic change, even if the survivors have features that fit them for life in the new situation, the group still has to have a critical mass of individuals to ensure healthy hybridization – and this is precisely the grave problem facing millions of plant and animal species today, as they suffer radical habitat loss because of what humans are doing, leading to rapidly shrinking numbers.

So the wheels of biological change grind slowly – our line diverged from the one going to chimpanzees more than 5 MYA, and modern chimps represent as much change from that time as we do – but even so, we still share more than 99% of our genetic makeup with them, and only slightly less with gorillas. So although modern chimps might have changed somewhat compared with their progenitors of 5 MYA – as humans have, too – the differences that still exist between our lines are vanishingly small, giving support to the classification of humans as the 'third chimpanzee.'

The slight differences that do exist between humans and chimps are mostly morphological – we have shorter body hair, smaller canines, we can't use our big toes to help pick up things, our skeleton (including hips – making giving birth a heck of a lot harder, though delivery in many big primates is clearly painful) and muscles have changed somewhat to let us walk upright on our hind legs most of the time, and we have a little more neocortex. Upright walking (or bipedalism) is not unique to us, but the skeletal signs of it are important features used to follow changes in the fossil record that reveal the growing bipedalism of our departure from the chimp line (though it is notable that bonobo chimps seem to be more comfortable walking upright than common chimps).

Fossils discovered in Africa suggest that 5 MYA, on the cool, dry, wooded savannahs of the east and south, a series of animals appeared who were fairly bipedal, with skeletons that were different enough from those of other primates of the time to mark them as a genus of great ape that was neither a proto-gorilla or a proto-chimp. Because their bones were first found in the south, these animals have been given the genus name Australopithecus, meaning "southern ape." (A north-south geographical barrier, Africa's Great Rift Valley, separates the drier portions in the east – including the famous Olduvai Gorge region, the site of so many fossils – where our early development occurred, from the wetter areas in western Africa where chimps and gorillas now live.)

Several species of australopithecines have been described (the famous "Lucy" was a member of the australopithecine species *afarensis*) and we will not linger looking at them, except to note that they were successful enough to survive as a genus many times longer than we have, perhaps 4 million years. Fossils identified as Australopithecus have been dated as late as 1.7 MYA, well after the time that the line toward our genus of *Homo* had diverged from theirs.

It's been suggested that although Australopithecus was becoming more bipedal, the life of these creatures was not much different from that of their ancestors or other savannah mammals their size, ranging across a fairly large home territory, depending on a wide variety of plants for complete nutrition (modern chimpanzees utilize more than 300 plant species over the course of a year), and presumably living in a matristic, Center/Perimeter form of social organization (fossils indicate they were quite sexually dimorphic). Since they lived in open country rather than rainforest, their version of Center/Perimeter may have been less like gorillas and more like elk, revolving around multi-generational groups of females and children, with most males living on their own for the majority of the year.

The next hominid identified in the line toward AMH first appeared around 2.5 MYA, in the form of a creature known as *Homo habilis*, generally considered as a branch of one species of australopithecines. *Homo habilis* has been named as the first representative of our genus on the strength of its somewhat larger brain case, more rounded skull, and more human face than other hominids of the time. It is called *"habilis"* for its use of tools (stone tools are what this is based on, but of course, australopithecines could also have used 'organic' tools made from wood, bark, and reeds – these would just not have lasted long enough for us to find).

Tool use is not considered to have had much effect on the 'gatherer' diet of *habilis*, other than making it easier to dig for tubers and perhaps cut and mash different types of plant foods to make them easier to eat, which might have helped bring about the gradual changes in *habilis* teeth which appear over time in the fossil record.

Early conclusions identifying *habilis* as a hunter who killed and butchered animals, that led some authors to credit meat-eating as the basis for human evolution, may have been premature. The most famous instance of this type of archeological re-interpretation is a site where remains of *habilis* are found along with massive amounts of bones from other animals that show evidence of having been broken and 'butchered' in a crude, savage manner. One early analysis by a scientist (who himself enjoyed the occasional steak) suggested that this was an abattoir run by *Homo habilis*. However, later investigators have concluded that all the animals represented were probably killed by a family of leopards, and that *habilis* was among the eaten, not the eaters, as much a victim in this case as the gazelles, zebras, and wildebeests whose bones were also found in the pile.

This is an illuminating instance of fossil *interpretation*, which is after all, only that – interpretation, intuition, a guess about what fragments of stones and bones tell us about the animals whose lives they represent. As fossil remains of proto-humans are subjected to new techniques, including chemical analysis of teeth and bones, the 'hunter' part of the common designation of proto-humans as 'hunter-gatherers' is coming to be modified, to 'gatherer-hunters' or even simply 'gatherers,' acknowledging that like all hominids, biologically we were then and still are plant-eaters. Only in very rare instances have our human forebears turned to eating meat (usually only when they are caught outside their normal climatic range, where their favorite foods no longer grow). But those exceptions do not define us as we are now – AMH – and they do not change the fundamental facts of our biology – we still have fruit-eaters' teeth, saliva, and intestines. In the future, we can only hope that more objective interpretations of the evidence, free of the culturally biased POV of investigators who take their children to MacDonald's on a regular basis, will acknowledge that this is true.

So again, it is reasonable to see *habilis* continuing to live a matristic, C/P lifestyle, perhaps making shelters for their life in the open (as suggested by remains at Olduvai Gorge), and slowly perfecting their use of stone implements to shape even more advanced organic tools to exploit a widening variety of plant foods found on the African savannahs.

No evidence of *habilis* has been found outside of Africa. But the next-appearing member of *Homo* not only boasted a larger brain case than *habilis*, but was also the first to leave Africa. It has been named *Homo erectus*. Fossils classified as *erectus* have been found across a wide span, from Africa to Southeast Asia and China, and also into Europe, all dating between 1.7 MYA and 120 KYA.

The extent of world-wide migration exhibited by *erectus* is not unusual. Paleontologists find such wanderings in many species, as well as patterns of migration repeated over and over again throughout history. For example, as noted earlier, horses first developed in North America (the modern genus *equus* emerged at about the same time as *Homo habilis*), and from there spread around the world, crossing and re-crossing the land bridge called Beringia at the Bering Strait a number of times, as fluctuations in glaciation over the last two million years created an on-again-off-again dry-land connection between Asia and the Americas.

Remains associated with *erectus* offer evidence of advances in skills for making stone tools, and there are indications that these continued to be used for further improving organic tools (including bamboo in China) for working with plant food sources. In some cases, stone tools might have been employed to collect materials such as hides and bones from dead animals, and bones gathered in this way might have been used in turn as yet another type of tool.

Bones might also have been used as a substitute for firewood. Several sites suggest that *erectus* did have fire, which they might have used to clear areas so that favorite plant foods could grow more readily. Fire would also have assisted in helping them cope with cooler temperatures. In Europe as well as China there is also evidence that *erectus* lived in shelters such as huts and caves, another strategy for dealing with cold.

However, it is also clear, from evidence such as the distribution of fossils over time, plus the lack of cold-adapted skeletal features, that *erectus* for the most part followed warm temperatures. Their groups moved north in times of global warming, and back south again as the cold encroached from the north. Thus there is no reason to suppose they would change their warm-adapted lifestyle of matristic, C/P living.

The changes in weather during these times could certainly be quite dramatic, as indicated by fossil finds of animals associated with radically different climates. For example, excavations in London have uncovered skeletons of hippos, lions, and elephants, deposited in times when the climate in Britain was quite African (thus attracting such animals to migrate north just as *erectus* did), while bones of mammoths and reindeer in other layers of British excavations signal periods when temperatures became much colder there.

During one of these long Ice-Age cold spells, *erectus* in some parts of Europe may have transformed into a form called *archaic Homo sapiens*, and either *erectus* or *archaic* may have been the predecessor to *Homo neanderthalensis*, whose remains start appearing around 150 KYA and persist for more than 100,000 years, until about 35,000 before the present (BP). In fact, Neanderthals may have overlapped AMH presence in the Middle East by about 5,000 years.

Neanderthals lived throughout Europe from Britain to Spain, in regions around present-day Israel, and as far east as the Caspian Sea. They are associated with many of the same features as *erectus* – fire, cave-living, and advances in stone technology, but took each of these much further. For instance, more powerful stone tools were developed for working with larger pieces of wood, perhaps for building shelters and fires for warmth. Neanderthals definitely lived for a very long time in very cold conditions; their skull dimensions and the proportional lengths of upper vs. lower limbs show striking signs of cold-adaptation, matching patterns (similar to those in present-day Eskimos) which require thousands of years of exposure to such conditions in order to develop.

The glacial climates typical of most regions where Neanderthal remains are found indicate that they might also have been the first proto-humans forced to undertake a radical change in diet. For many long dark months of these cold years there would have been no plant foods available at all, and there are clear signs in the fossil record that Neanderthals responded to this by becoming aggressive hunters. Many tools found in their sites are clearly made for killing, and imposing piles of bones from animals of all sorts and sizes indicate a skill for butchery. They did not shrink from taking on even the largest and most dangerous prey, such as woolly mammoths.

Other stone tools found at Neanderthal sites are very similar to leather-working tools employed today (now made of metal), which may have been used in preparing at least some of the skins taken from all those animals, to serve as shelter roofs, bed covers, and clothing. One cave site on the Mediterranean in the south of France included remains of a hut shelter which had been built against one inner wall, with clues suggesting that wooden posts were arranged to hold up a hide roof, accompanied by hearths and areas for sleeping which may have included seaweed bedding, judging from scatterings of tiny seashells.

We've already noted that cold created anatomical changes in Neanderthals, namely, skeletal adjustments in body proportions (which helped conserve heat). But the combination of exposure to cold plus a growing dependence on meat as the only food source might have brought about drastic physiological changes as well. For example, the sympathetic nervous system would be activated by the extreme cold, resulting in a general state of 'fight or flight' arousal, in everybody, all the time. For the women, this would increase testosterone levels during pregnancy, leading to larger numbers of children with brain types toward the left on the Neural Rainbow continuum. In addition, eating nothing but meat for so many months of the year might have evoked an adaptive mutation in blood chemistry, similar to changes posited for the origins of the A and B versions of the ABO blood group family (the O subtype is the oldest, while A and B are known to have originated relatively recently, in colder latitudes).

The combination of metabolic changes related to digestion, plus chronic sympathetic arousal and increasing numbers of focal brains, would have certainly have been adaptive given the groups' needs for continuing and perhaps escalating aggression against other animals. But there would have been cultural fall-out from these changes, as well. In a state of constant sympathetic arousal and surrounded by more and more focal brains, the Center groups would have taken on more and more of the features of Perimeter groups. This awesome (and awful) transformation, the 'perimeterization' of the hominid Center, might have been augmented by the addition of actual unattached, roaming Perimeter males, recruited by the Center male to help with hunting. Certainly the evidence that Neanderthals hunted and killed very large, dangerous animals such as woolly mammoths says that cooperative hunting was involved, with a high premium on risk-taking behavior.

Some scientists suggest that Neanderthals lived in gender-segregated groups that came together only seasonally for mating, as elk do; but it might be that their life in the Ice-Age cold forced Neanderthals to take a much more radical step, and depart from the hominid C/P norm to adopt a 50:50 group arrangement. This would accomplish three important things, none of which is needed in C/P gathering groups: 1) keeping the men close together to plan and conduct hunts (they would find this very congenial given their propensity for 'men in groups'); 2) assuring that women and children shared the meat; and 3) allowing all the men who shared the dangers of the hunt to also share other rewards, including the pleasures (and reproductive advantages) of sex.

It's doubtful that this re-organization would proceed according to Center rules, that is, be managed by the women. Rather, this perimeterization process would naturally produce new groups structured along Perimeter lines, with an emphasis on rule by force and hierarchical rankings based on strength and hunting prowess. It would have been extremely difficult for the women to withstand such a change in the center-of-gravity of their societies. The Perimeter males would have had a rapidly- growing sense of solidarity, as their aggression and primitive (focal-brain) social skills became more and more indispensable in the harsher, colder environment, and this would surely have led to the general intimidation of women by the males' greater physical strength. The women's situation would have been even more compromised, because of the fact that they also were also being transformed biochemically by the cold – in terms of digestive metabolism, sympathetic arousal, and elevated adrenal testosterone. Finally, and perhaps the most sinister of all, the women must have had a pronounced psychological reaction to their new and unprecedented state of economic dependence.

In warmer places, where each woman in a Center group could gather sufficient food for herself and her children, all group members were essentially equal from an economic standpoint. That is, no one got exclusive credit as the breadwinner, because everyone could find their own food. But when getting food came to depend primarily on male attributes such as physical strength and propensity for violence, it must have been hard for the females as well as the males to continue seeing males only as adjuncts to a woman-centered group, as 'guests' of the women, as *servants* of the mothers and children. If male violence put the meat on the table – and that was the only way to keep from starving – male violence and male rules would not only have to be tolerated, if only for the sake of the kids – but also, eventually, perhaps considered as signs of superiority.

Under such severe climatic and psychological conditions, how could the original matristic C/P society survive? From the women's point of view, becoming dependent on males' predatory violence for food would have deep implications not only for the logistics of everyday life, but also for the culture of these groups. The old Center values emphasizing democratic cooperation and interpersonal support so important for child-bearing and rearing must have been superseded by 'Perimeter values' glorifying muscle strength, risk-taking behaviors, hierarchical relationships and violence.

Thus in the case of Neanderthals, hominid society may have suffered a radical transformation – the 180° flip in the social compass mentioned earlier – what Riane Eisler refers to in later cultures as the change from a 'partnership' to a 'dominator' model. It is hard to overstate how drastic a change this was. Caught in cold northern lands where no primate should live, forced to survive 'by the sword,' having no food for their children except the dead flesh of other mammals, the women in essence experienced a 'hostile take-over' of their nurturing Centers by Perimeter brains and attitudes.

Clearly, the new social ethos was far more oriented to death than to life – and it is extremely interesting that Neanderthals are the first hominids known to bury their dead. Many Neanderthal sites include burials of children as well as adults. The bodies are buried in strangely contorted positions (described as 'crouching') and are often accompanied by items such as animal bones and stone tools. This attention to the body after death has long been taken by orthodox anthropologists and archeologists as a sign of 'advance' among these people – but there may be other, darker implications. As we will see, a variety of cold-adapted, 'dominator' cultures which appeared long after the Neanderthals were gone, also show evidence of preoccupation with death, such as: ritual burial; sacrifice, including various types of 'sati,' in which healthy individuals (humans and other species) are killed to 'accompany' a high-ranking person in death; the building of grandiose tombs; and increasingly elaborate attempts (such as embalming and the framing of immortality fantasies), to delay or even deny the biological fact of death. Indeed, such practices are so common in 'dominator' cultures (like most of those we know today) that they are recognized as a signature feature.

As mentioned, this focus on burial rituals and the dedication of large resources to building tombs, particularly for rulers, are frequently praised as signs of 'advanced' societies. However, such societies are also typically very violent, both internally (they are 'stratified,' that is, a few people command most of the resources) and externally (significant resources are drained off into war and aggressive expansionism, which again benefit only a privileged few). So we might suspect that 'advanced' is not really the right word. Rather, these societies might be better described as having a 'death fetish,' or practicing a 'death cult,' where death and making life miserable for most people take priority over birth and quality of life. (We'll see later that most of what are valorized as the 'great world religions' are unabashed death cults.)

Given all this, we can only feel relieved that Neanderthals are not believed to be our ancestors, that is, the forebears of AMH. When the last Neanderthals died out in about 35 KYA, they were the end of their line. Modern *Homo* had a different, more matristic set of grandparents, and to find them we must return again to the natal warmth of Africa. In fact, 'out of Africa' is the current theory of AMH origins, extending from our first hominid ancestors, the australopithecines, to modern humans.

Around 120 KYA, at about the same time as a long period of cool, dry weather was peaking over the lower half of Africa, signs appear both in central East Africa (Olduvai Gorge again) and in far South Africa, of a new animal with a completely human face – sometimes called *Homo sapiens sapiens*. Fossils found in several sites in these regions are essentially identical to us, and are often therefore referred to as *Anatomically Modern Humans* (AMH). They are generally assumed to have developed from an African form of *Homo erectus* which stayed in the south (while others migrated out) and in that supportive homeland changed gradually into us.

The most curious – and perhaps decisive – feature of early AMH is the fact that about 20,000 years after they appeared, something happened which reduced their numbers severely, finally reaching a minimum of only around 10,000 individuals. The causes for this so-called 'bottleneck' in the history of AMH are not certain, but it did occur during a time of dramatic climate changes associated with Ice-Age cycles – a perfect context for the appearance of a new disease vector, perhaps a novel pathogen such as those that are known to have decimated whole populations of animals around the world from time to time in the past, and continue to do so today.

In any case, molecular biologists have documented and dated the time of the bottleneck, revealing a frightening near-miss with extinction for our species. (So we've done that twice in our history – the second time was at the end of the Cold War, in the agreement to disarm ICBMs, with their thousandfold overkill capability. Of course, as we'll see later, we are not out of the woods yet – this and other threats of extinction looming on our current horizon may not be so easily avoided.)

There is scant information about these AMH people between the time of the bottleneck (around 100 KYA) and approximately 80 KYA, when their remains are first found in the Middle East. Perhaps during this interval, they were recovering, gradually increasing in numbers, and small groups were slowly migrating northward, following climate changes and/or favorite foods. Perhaps we do not find evidence of them because their numbers were so small that any remains they may have left are too few and far between. But after this time our human ancestors must have increased their numbers, because their fossils begin to appear like footprints leading out of Africa, taking a route north and then turning east, following a warm band of familiar climates from the east end of the Mediterranean across southern India, into Southeast Asia, and (somehow) across what must have been fairly daunting expanses of sea, to arrive in Australia around 50 KYA. (It's possible that the islands of the Malay Archipelago, stretching between the south-Asian mainland and Australia, like the islands of the Bering Strait, may have been available from time to time to serve as stepping-stones.)

As bands living all along this route became established, they in turn apparently began to migrate elsewhere on their own, arriving in Europe by 40 KYA (the 'Cro-Magnons'), other parts of India by 35 KYA, China by 30 KYA, and Japan around 17 KYA. Some groups in the Far East moved up the coast during a cool period around 30 KYA, taking the Beringia route earlier used by horses, and then travelled down into parts of North and South America by 25 KYA.

So somehow these people found a way not only to step back from the threshold of near-extinction, but then to increase their numbers sufficiently to support a slow but steady migratory spread. Just as with horses and many other species before and since, these migrations established within a relatively short time resulted in at least some presence of AMH on every habitable continent.

There are numerous theories as to how AMH accomplished such a dramatic turnaround. The standard idea is the 'man as hunter' story. Supposedly these early humans fought off extinction by changing their diet, as we've seen Neanderthals doing – taking up cooperative hunting and thus increasing their meat consumption. This seems implausible, since, as we've shown, eating meat was probably a desperation measure for living in extreme, year-round cold. If plants were available, there is no logical reason to assume such a radical dietary (and behavioral) change – any more, say, than a paleontologist suggesting that at some point, wild horses started chasing and eating ground squirrels and mice they found in the prairie grass.

Some scientists (who don't seem to know much about amino acids, in flesh or in plant foods) have even gone so far as to posit that there can be no advanced thought without meat ('meat is mental,' cited earlier), and that by increasing their intake of animal protein, these early humans were literally 'force-feeding their brains,' resulting in a dramatic expansion of the neocortex and associated advances in the capacity for abstract thought.

Given what we've said about the rich amino-acid mix available in plants, this seems nutritionally naive. From a comparative ethological standpoint, it is even less likely. After all, there are many full-fledged carnivores who have remained evolutionarily 'static' for hundreds of thousands of years, and despite a regular and exclusive diet of meat, give no signs of expanding their neocortex, speaking in inflected languages, or designing writing systems. At the same time, many animals which some have suggested are among the most intelligent on earth – such as elephants and some cetaceans – are thoroughgoing vegetarians. And of course, millions of humans today flourish and think quite well without ever consuming any meat whatsoever.

A second and more interesting possibility is that these early humans, faced with shrinking numbers (whatever the cause), actively decided to make *a basic change in their social organization, with the goal of 'rescuing' every individual they could.* If we think of their *erectus* forebears living according to a C/P plan, or even in gender-segregated groups, we can see that this becomes an evolutionarily wasteful lifestyle once disease or climatological disaster starts dramatically reducing the species' numbers.

So AMH women might very well have decided they couldn't afford to give up any of the children who survived to adolescence; they could no longer send anyone off to the Perimeter, and still survive as a species. As we'll see in the next section, they may have therefore taken a tremendous gamble, much like those few rare species who have responded to environmental stress by shifting to the 50:50 lifestyle, and in effect, erased the Perimeter, finding ways to keep more than one male inside the Center group.

Their goal is illustrated in Figure 5.2, using the same type of SOC maps employed in Chapter Four. The AMH women needed to transform the peaceful C/P arrangement (top panel) they shared with virtually all the other mammal species around them, which had worked well for millennia, into an equally peaceful 50:50 group style (lower panel). We still do not know whether that gamble, that throw of the dice, *abandoning C/P for 50:50,* will prove to be a winner or a loser for humans.

Figure 5.2

Recasting the peaceful C/P SOC originally employed by AMH into an equally peaceful 50:50 arrangement. Top panel = original C/P (as in Fig. 4.10); lower panel = the 50:50 result, the 'kindest SOC of all,' where no one is exiled to the Perimeter. Symbol codes as in Ch. 4: circles/triangles = women/men; black = polytropic Grandmother-Leaders, grey = middle-brain Loyal-Helpers, unfilled = left-brain Focal-Asocials.

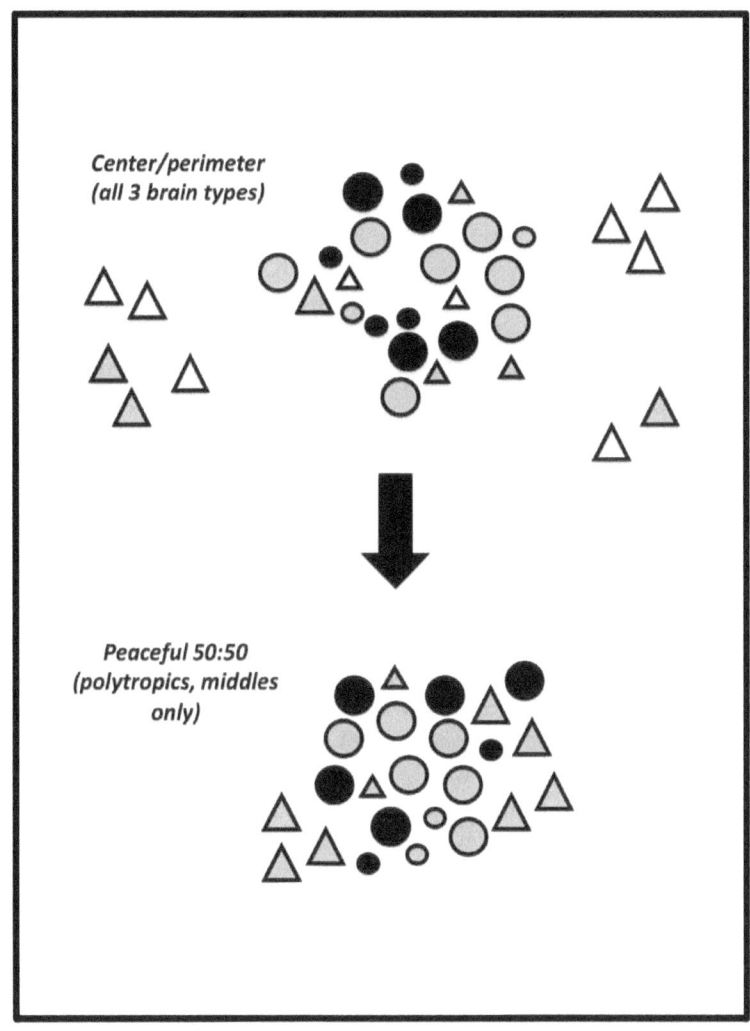

Human history – Stage Two, a new kind of Center

One of the fundamental features of C/P life is dispersal at puberty, which for virtually all mammalian species means that most males leave, departing to wander the Perimeter for the rest of their days. However, since for most C/P animals, there are two kinds of males, it's clear that quite a few of the ones who leave – maybe as many as half, or more – will actually be middle-brain types, making them very sociable fellows. It is this subset of the exiled males which is the candidate pool for recruiting new Center males (though few may be fortunate enough to actually return to a Center).

Now almost everyone who studies human evolution has a 'just-so' story about the mysterious early steps in human history ('just-so' stories are explanations – 'the giraffe has a long neck just so it can reach leaves growing high up,' etc.), and in particular, the puzzling and disturbing time of the AMH population bottleneck – and I am no exception.

My theory is that it was indeed a new disease that arose in South Africa in the climatically unsettled times around 100 KYA. Certainly diseases have had devastating effects at other times in human history, as documented in books such as *Rats, Lice and History*, *Plagues and Peoples*, and *Guns, Germs, and Steel* (all included in the Chapter Five bibliography). The course of history has been changed for many human societies when trading ships bring an old bug to a new country where immune defense has not been established, or when a change in climate triggers the mutation of an old bug into a new one against which people are not prepared.

The new pathogen in 100 KYA may have attacked other animals in addition to AMH, but in any case, the effect on us could not have been sudden, or there would have been no time at all for any kind of adjustment. A rapidly spreading, completely fatal disease might have left a few scattered survivors, but in such small and separated numbers that they would not have been able to coalesce again into a healthy reproductive base.

There was a definite, dramatic population drop, but luckily for us, it was not a completely devastating 'wildfire.' Perhaps the pathogen made it more difficult to conceive, or bring a baby to term, either through a direct effect, or indirectly, by changing a mother's immune system so that more embryos were rejected. Or it could have been a disease like polio that increased infant and child mortality, or selectively attacked young adults, as did tuberculosis in 19th-century Europe.

In any case, the early AMH women apparently had sufficient time to make a conscious decision to save themselves by finding a way to hang onto all the warm bodies they could, for help with gathering food and protecting against predators. The obvious pool of 'extra people' was the substantial group of individuals who typically went away at puberty – most of them males, who in better times this society could afford to 'throw away.' I believe these early women saved the human race by salvaging at least some of these erstwhile dispensable males as helping hands – not because they were males, but because they were humans.

Pondering such a decision, the women would have known it was not going to be easy. They knew (just as we know now) that in close proximity, adult males (even middle-brains) can be like tinder and matches to each other, that anything approaching a 50:50 arrangement would be almost impossible to manage without making some very basic reproductive adjustments, which we'll see was done in a very different way from Neanderthals. Chapter Four discussed the inherent difficulty of this change, most easily pictured by imagining what would happen on a ranch or farm if a group of stallions were suddenly released into a small pasture of mares and their foals, or if that same thing were done with bulls and cows. The chaos would be immediate and perhaps fatal for some individuals. The 50:50 mix is simply not natural for C/P mammals.

So our early mothers (perhaps like bonobos, or the muriqui monkeys also described in Chapter Four) would have started very slowly, one step at a time. Their goal was to create *peaceful* 50:50 groups configured as in Fig. 4.12 – relatively small, moving toward more or less equal numbers of adult females and males, living together year-round in woman-managed communities, according to Center values. The problem was: how to do it?

They could have taken some of the steps described in Chapter Four, that seem to be how peaceful 50:50 groups have been formed by some humans groups, as well as the few other species who live that way today.

If they were living in seasonal-breeding groups of women and children, perhaps they first invited one Center-type male to join them full-time; if they already had an attendant 'silverback,' perhaps they encouraged him to accept one or two younger 'blackback' candidates – perhaps his brothers from his home-group family, or some of their friends from yet other groups. Such additions, although modest, could offer a significant boost to group survival against disease, and add more hands for help with gathering and protection.

If this limited experiment worked, the women might then take the next step, inviting in boys from neighboring groups as they came of age, and sending their own in exchange, particularly if it was hard to predict who would prove more resistant to the pathogen. (They wouldn't keep their own young men – not good for genetic diversity.) In any case, whatever the numbers they started with, and however quickly they proceeded, the women also had to do something cultural to make it possible to manage so many males in such unnaturally close proximity. (Remember the stallions and bulls.)

The current examples of this discussed in Chapter Four – muriquis, bonobos, etc. – suggest how this might have been done. For those early groups of AMH, the process amounted to the first human experiment in *domestication* – in this case, of their own males. After all, males who disperse at puberty essentially become feral – they wander as solitaries, or in highly competitive all-male groups, far from the civilizing influences and interpersonal demands of Center groups. Once the women figured out the general strategy – that they needed to 'domesticate' the guys – ideas for implementation would have been obvious.

First, it was clear that the males could not be bullied into being nice – they had to be 'gentled.' The point was not to compel them but rather to 'kill them with kindness.' The women already had a model for that, in their own society and that of many other mammals – the trick was simply to make each male feel like a Center male, the apple of the ladies' eyes. This required two things: 1) lots of sexual access – in terms of both frequency and variety of partners; and 2) cultural props as constant reminders to the men of how lucky they were, and just who it was that was making all this possible. (Of course, the women could not ignore the importance of 'men in groups,' predictably as strong a 'drive' for males as their attraction to females. We'll talk about how this was managed in a moment.)

Sexual access to the women was not a problem. If early AMH women had not been warm-land primates, that is, if they were more like deer living at latitudes where mating hormones were active only during a short annual season, it might have been almost impossible for them to overcome this aspect of their biology and provide lots of sex more or less year-round for the extra males. But as Old-World primate females (sisters to chimps, gorillas and doubtless, the australopithecines, *Homo erectus* and *habilis*) these early women had menstrual cycles all year round. So they could honestly be receptive at almost any time (even when they themselves were not particularly interested, i.e., enjoying the mid-cycle hormone surge of ovulation). As it turns out, this is precisely the way that some non-human primate women today also manage their males.

Nor would it have been a problem to provide each male with a variety of partners – C/P groups had a clear precedent for that, in which all the non-lactating women in the group will accept the Center male as a lover. In the new social structure, with many extra males involved, the women would simply make it clear that all the males are welcome. These two innovations (providing the males with lots of sex, with lots of women) were, I believe, a major turning point in human evolution – one that is scarcely whispered about in orthodox texts. Such changes, incidentally, might have been new to AMH, but as we've seen, were not new to peaceful primates such as muriquis. Early human women, in dire straits for a future, simply invented the same wheel that bonobo and muriqui females have done – that is, all the ladies all the time, every guy's dream.

226

The new-found sexual access for all the males also led to important cultural innovations, designed as strategies for male management. There is overwhelming evidence from every part of the world where these people came to live, from Africa to the Americas, that in addition to giving (woman-managed) sexual freedom to multiple men within a group, the women also created a powerful, complete set of symbols and rules, customs and artifacts, practices and systems, which must have served as an effective means of acculturation, with the primary aim of *helping the men live together within a woman-centered culture*. This system has been given many names, based on the many names of its divinities worshipped by thousands of cultures around the world, from ancient to modern times – but in general, it was the religion of Woman, Gaia, The Great Cosmic Mother, the Goddess.

This culture in fact became a world culture as it was carried from continent to continent by the burgeoning AMH groups wherever they moved, from Europe to Australia, from China to the Americas. Its nature is revealed in the artifacts it produced, all of which celebrate the beauty and vigor of all animal mothers who give birth and support life – humans along with a multitude of other human-sized, non-predatory animals such as horses, bison, and deer, all of whom also live in woman-centered groups.

These artifacts have become well-known from numerous archeological finds over the past century. They include the tens of thousands of 'Venus' figurines found around the world, representing human women often shown as pregnant, round-figured and well-supplied with body fat, and therefore ready for child-bearing and sharing their stored food via breastfeeding. Many sites include varieties of beautifully stylized symbols representing female anatomy, as well as counting symbols referring to monthly cycles and the months of gestation. Other evidence of these cultures is found in the astounding cave paintings in Europe and China, some as old as 35 KYA, depicting herds of human-sized mammals such as horses and deer painted in vivid colors and realistic motion, as well as figures of pregnant women, men with erections, and other male animals with glorious horns.

Interestingly, archeologists sometimes refer to the artists who created such art as if they were males – "Stone Age Michelangelos," one text says. However, there is no reason to assume that it was not in fact women who sculpted the gracefully *enceinte* ('pregnant' in French) figurines from stone and clay and bone, or guided the charcoal pencils outlining the graceful body of a running horse or deer. When I look at such paintings, I can feel the pencil in my hand, and the muscles of my arm tracing the beautiful grazer heads and bodies across the cool stone walls. (As a girl I spent many hours drawing birds and trees and horses, and these women may have done the same.)

Another unmistakable fingerprint of this woman-centered world culture, also dating from the earliest finds, is the red clay pigment called red ochre (primarily hematite, iron oxide). (Red ochre has been associated with pre-AMH remains in Africa, and European Neanderthals in Europe, perhaps relating to its function as a sunscreen which may have dated to early hominid experience in Africa – see the 2015 paper by Rifkin and colleagues in the Chapter Five bibliography.)

Red ochre is found in virtually all sites connected with early AMH, from locations in Africa dated from 90KYA to 40 KYA, the European caves painted with horses and deer sometime after 40 KYA, sites in Australia dated to more than 50 KYA, and others throughout the Americas. Although some archeologists are puzzled as to what was being colored with red ochre in many of the earlier instances (perhaps answered by the Rifkin paper from 2015 cited above, suggesting it was widely used as a sunscreen), anthropologists do not find it confusing at all. They know that red ochre is a universal sign which has been used by women of many cultures, around the world and over many millennia, to represent the color of life: the red blood of birth and menstruation. That women use a red-clay pigment also connects their reproductive powers to the fecund earth herself, a relation articulated in many matristic religions by creation stories describing emergence of tribal ancestors from under the ground, and by underground ritual chambers such as the Hopi kivas, and the association of women with pot-making, makers of mud huts for sleeping and food storage, crafters of vessels (as metaphors for their own bodies) for holding and carrying water and food.

Girls on the Gold Coast of Africa, in Brazil, and among the Cheyenne, are painted with red ochre to celebrate their first menstruation. Women in many parts of the world have used red pigment to signal that they are either menstruating (Chinese women used to put a red mark on their forehead) or expecting (Kaffir women of Africa paint themselves with red ochre when they first become pregnant); brides in Nigeria get ready for their weddings by painting their bodies with red dye from the camwood tree. In other societies, women keep some type of red color on their bodies all the time they are breastfeeding, to signal that they are not available for sex. Australian indigenous groups say that deposits of red ochre at some sites familiar to them are actually menstrual blood from women of the ancient past.

So red ochre at an old site is a signal to archeologists that early AMH may have lived there, with their Culture of Woman, their celebration of life, and their matristic, 'partnership' mixes of men and women. After all, symbols to mark the onset of menstruation would not have been needed in a Center group. Women know about the reality of such blood; they do not need a symbol. Nor would they need paint to advertise that a woman is pregnant or breastfeeding in a Center group – she would simply not be receptive to the Center male at these times, and he would not approach her without invitation. And the other women would know all the signs, and accommodate to her condition without the help of artificial visual aids.

Only in groups where many men mingle with women, would such symbol systems be needed. These would have been important not only to keep the men informed of the status of the women, but also to educate the boys as well the girls in these cultures about the special power and centrality of women. Puberty celebrations may also have been instituted for early AMH girls using red ochre, as so many contemporary groups do, to emphasize yet again the mystery and importance of women, to help the men and boys, along with the women and their daughters, appreciate and celebrate the centrality of women: they are the ones who bleed without being wounded, who create the next generation from their own bodies – giving miraculous birth to tiny living replicas of themselves – the ones who guide the growing children, and nurture individuals of all genders and ages – who, in short, embody the past, present, and future of the group, and the wisdom of the tribe. Signs of the use of red ochre and other woman-centered artifacts from all these millennia and over vast geographical ranges are thus evidence suggesting that such cultures did in fact include males who had through this and other means been 'domesticated' to live under the guidance of 'partnership,' Center rules.

In her book *Male and Female*, Margaret Mead suggested that "The recurrent problem of civilization is to define the male role satisfactorily enough ... to have a solid sense of irreversible achievement." So along with symbols and practices designed to educate males regarding the nature of females and the primacy of Center values, another cultural strategy might have been to develop symbols for males to aspire to, specifically, the middle-brain type of male the women favored (and needed, if their new 50:50 groups were to stay peaceful).

This of course was the big 'gentle giant' who, although not always very bright (he did not need to be, the women knew what to do), was entirely trustworthy as a loving companion to the women, and great with the kids. To be most useful, such symbols for male aspirations would have been based on C/P mammals familiar to all, chosen to have features that clearly demarcated males from females, such as horns. This would explain the various forms of the 'horned god' in matristic cultures, one of which is the 'curly-headed bull,' whose image is found repeatedly in archeological sites of matristic groups around the Mediterranean. Being praised and pampered as big lovely bulls could have given the men a gratifying (and socially useful) self-image which, combining strength and gentleness, fertility and docility, graphically illustrated their role in these new human groups.

Finally, the 'men in groups' drive, the need men felt to spend lots of time with other men, as they used to do in the Perimeter (and as their brains still prepared them to do), would have been easy to arrange. In many non-industrial and industrial societies even today, when given the choice, men as well as women are attracted to spending time in same-sex groups – the men sitting around the cracker barrel in the general store, or in other types of 'bachelor houses' such as gyms or garages, or out in the open, talking and working together; and the women in their own common areas sharing the jobs of caring for kids, gathering food and gardening, sitting and talking together while they make pots and blankets and clothes. In some cultures, family units may spend nights together, and may mix with other families for eating or sitting together during ceremonies and dances, but for most of the time, the distribution of individuals is much as in the old C/P groups – a comfortable, gender-based segregation of women with women, men with men. The universality of this arrangement speaks to its biological primacy, its testimony to our nature as C/P mammals.

But the early AMH women would also have recognized the potential danger of encouraging their men to spend time with other men, the threat of a psychological drift away from Center values – perhaps you can take the boy out of the Perimeter, but can you take the Perimeter out of the boy – especially if he is still hanging out a lot with other boys? One important way the women may have countered such a threat was to develop storytelling, crafting tales about characters who acted out the lessons they wanted to impart to the men and boys in their new 50:50 groups.

One example of such a character is the Trickster, who appears again and again in stories from cultures around the world. Anthropologists have been fascinated by the trickster figure, and have come up with many ways to 'explain' him. But when we look at the central character in these tales – his personal characteristics, the way he behaves, and the terrible things that happen to him, we can see he may be a very old figure indeed, dating from these earliest times when the women were trying in every way to encourage Center behavior in their men – in many ways, the Trickster seems to be a parable of the Perimeter male.

Virtually all the stories not only present him as male, but one who is *small in stature*, certainly compared to most humans. In most of the tales, the part of the Trickster is played by a small non-human animal – almost always an omnivore which is *particularly fond of meat*, so much so that it is willing to be both a scavenger and a predator. Examples of such animals used as trickster figures are Coyote, Jackal, Raven or Crow, and Mink or Weasel. (Even when a trickster is a human character, he is again portrayed as a *small* (left-brain?) male – examples, as suggested in Ruth Finnegan's wonderful *Oral Literature in Africa* (1970), include the Lambas' Kantanga [described as "a little mischievous fellow"], and the Zulus' Uthlakanyana ["a deceitful and cunning little dwarf"].)

The Trickster is never shown as belonging to any one human group or even to a group of social animals – rather, he is always a loner who 'wanders aimlessly,' on the periphery (the Perimeter?), as noted by Lewis Hyde (*Trickster Makes this World*, 1998). He is often shown as hypersexual, but has no babies of his own. When a Trickster is confronted by the rules for living as expressed by people (or animals) who do live in groups, he consistently expresses his conviction that those rules don't apply to him – 'that's your way, that's not my way.' As summarized by Lewis Hyde, Tricksters are depicted as always hungry (mostly for meat), shameless in many ways that people living in social groups are not (the tales are highly scatological – one or more egregious events of urination and defecation can almost always be counted on to figure in the plots), and attracted to all kinds of dirt.

Sometimes Tricksters are shown as foolish and stupid, sometimes as clever, but their antics are almost always presented as dangerous either to themselves or to others. In fact, the 'tricks' they are so famous for are often designed to fool other animals into doing things that end up getting them killed – and eaten – by the Trickster. Sometimes the Trickster fools mothers so that he can eat their babies.

Trickster stories are definitely funny, though sometimes in a cruel and almost surreal way. The early AMH women knew (as we still know now) that guys are charmed by humor, and particularly by crude and physical humor – the more pratfalls and bad words and shit hitting the fan, the better. In trickster tales, humor is used as a way to convince the audience NOT to be tricked into behaving like this metaphorical version of the Perimeter male. The things Trickster does to fool other characters may at first seem funny (and it may sometimes seem as though he is actually going to win), but the outcome, when the Trickster himself is tricked and one way or another brought to justice, is even funnier – though the laughter may be macabre, often very black humor indeed.

Several anthropologists have noted that trickster tales end in only a few ways. In some, Trickster finds a way to escape the fix he's got himself into, and continues wandering, planning more mischief (the picaresque tale that appears in much of medieval European literature is one example). In others, he is domesticated, changed in basic ways so that he can be brought into a group – this is clearly the ideal outcome of these stories, underlining the importance of behaving like a Center-type male – "Desperado, come down from your fences, open the gate," sings Linda Ronstadt. But in others, his exasperated opponents simply force him to stop causing trouble – they might drive him far away, sometimes after gravely injuring him, or imprison him (locked inside a mountain, etc.) or actually kill him, often in a very violent way.

In all their variety, these tales are carefully crafted so that the audience is both entertained *and* educated. The message (to use the Trickster's own words) is simple – 'his way is not our way.' (If you're familiar with trickster tales, you may know some in which the cleverness of the small male is presented in a good light – he might be shown fooling people who have become too big for their britches, or his inventiveness might actually contribute in some basic way to the welfare of a group. However, I believe these are versions that were created much later, by human groups with very different social needs than the ones we're talking about now. We'll discuss those other groups in a moment.)

Another thing the early AMH women may have done not only to encourage the men to observe Center values but also to give them things to fill up their time, was to use a 'ju-jitsu' strategy, that is, exploit the strength of the 'men in groups' drive to accomplish a cultural goal of the women, namely, the furtherance of Center values. I believe the women gave the men the job of 'inventing' the paraphernalia of religion, what I've always called the 'totem-pole' aspect of religion. This refers to all the hours needed to design the ceremonies and craft the costumes and sacred objects, dream up the various taboos and the names of divinities, create and elaborate long, detailed stories filled with all sorts of fictional characters, etc. – but (an important *but*) all framed in terms of Center values. (Of course, many aspects of the religions we know most about now don't seem like Center values at all, but that change came much later, motivated, as we'll see, by agendas very unlike those of the early peace-keeping women.)

All this definitely gave the men something to do, that not only drew on their special abilities – physical strength, fondness for somewhat focal behaviors, displaying (performing) in front of admiring audiences – but also gave them that "solid sense of irreversible achievement" Mead identified – allowed to believe that only *they* could dig the kivas and build the special huts, only *they* got to spend hours and hours in deliciously-restricted, men-only-places planning and rehearsing ceremonies, making 'magical' costumes that supposedly endowed their human wearers with a divine presence, acting out the ceremonies in the presence of women and children who responded with gratifyingly realistic signs of wonder, awe, and admiration.

One interesting example of this busy-work encouraged for the men are the musical instruments made only-by-men and played only-by-men that are claimed to have magical properties, endowed with supernatural powers, and thus taboo for women to see or even know about. Many groups around the world have such things – they are often obviously phallic, such as the big tubes kept in men's houses away from the sight of women, and blown into by men where the women can't see: the *karoko* of the Amazonian rainforest, the *molimo* of the BaMbuti in Africa, the *didgeridoo* of Australia.

Anthropologists note that it's obvious the women of these groups know all about the 'big tubes' – where they come from, that they're the source of the strange noises that emanate from the forest (after all the men have disappeared there) or from behind the walls of the men's house – but they also know they're supposed to pretend that they don't, and clearly display how mystified and impressed they are by the obvious power of such sounds and the unseen entities that produce them.

Handing over the 'totem-pole' aspect of religion to men was a terrific strategy, which addressed many goals – the men had their 'men in groups' needs answered, everyone in the village got to enjoy the diversion of ceremonies and unusual get-ups and the 'games' of rituals and 'supernatural' identities walking around in the (costumes') flesh – and the message of Center values became ever more clear and part of the culture. (As we'll see, the early strategy of giving guys responsibility for the details of 'religion' may have seriously backfired, but not because of any inherent flaw in the logic – more of that later, too.)

And yet, our early mothers did even more – they did not stop at 'taming' the boys they kept in the group, by allowing them access to women, giving them time to themselves, finding ways they could contribute to the culture of Center values. The final triumph of these women in shaping matristic human society may have been the control they came to have over *which brain types they produced*. They could have recognized (as all of us can, once we see it) that there was no need to risk the huge investment of pregnancy on creating disruptive individuals, and they found ways to manage pregnancies so that few if any far-left brains were made. Thus they effectively *shut down the Perimeter* – simply by ceasing to make the kind of individuals who would have to be banished there, as we earlier suggested muriqui monkeys seem to have done. This was the final, crowning 'savings' accomplished by ancient AMH women – every child was a healthy, socially-capable child, every child a wanted child who could count on living with or near an extended family throughout her or his life. In the matristic groups created and managed by these women, the village raised every child, and nobody was banished to live all their lives in the dog-eat-dog world outside.

The hypothesis outlined here may sound too good to be true, like the tales of the 'golden age' which have been pooh-poohed by so many males in our own culture – one prominent writer even refers to the 'myth' of modern anthropology that humans have spent 99% of our history living in exactly the types of small, peaceful groups I've described here.

In fact, there is evidence, and lots of it, that hundreds if not thousands of such societies have existed. Moreover, they were managed by women, they cared for their members, and they were peaceful and prosperous for tens of thousands of years. (A persuasive, fictional picture of such cultures is provided by Ursula Le Guin in *Always Coming Home*. If you want to see what it might have been like to live in a matristic 50:50 society, find and read this book. After a number of years out of print, it is thankfully again available, in an expanded edition.)

Moreover, a few of these cultures are with us today (more later), and several fairly large ones survived until relatively recent times, and were extremely successful by every measure of human culture. History books in our schools do not describe these matristic, flourishing cultures. The omission is purely political, however, motivated by reasons which will be all too clear in a moment; and there is a growing consensus among archeologists and other students of human history that the women of these cultures were responsible for accomplishments which are typically considered to define 'human' achievement – agriculture, weaving, pottery, writing, business, law, accounting, and art.

A special group of woman-centered cultures which flourished most recently, bloomed in several places on the globe around 10 KYA, a period when world climate changes made it possible to conduct agriculture on a somewhat larger scale than previously. The best-studied of these so-called 'goddess cultures' were located in the Near and Middle East. Archeologists have gathered information about them for more than 100 years. Perhaps the most famous are two sites, one at a place in modern-day Iraq called Catal Huyuk, founded around 8500 BCE (Before Common Era – the new secular revision of Before Christ), and the second on the island of Crete.

The story of these sites and others has been surveyed in many excellent books over the last few decades, most notably *When God was a Woman* (1976), by Merlin Stone; *The Chalice and the Blade* (1987), by Riane Eisler; *The Once and Future* Goddess (1989), by Elinor Gadon; and *Evaluating the Myth of the Goddess: Evolution of an image* (1991), by Ann Baring and Jules Cashford – see the chapter bibliography for these and similar books, the basis for the descriptions that follow.

It is impossible to adequately represent in the space we have here the revolutionary, refreshing view of human culture offered in these works. I encourage everyone who wants to be assured that humans have been and can again be a peaceful, loving species, to read them. But I will briefly suggest what these cultures were like, and most importantly, how they accomplished the incredible task of including males within a woman-managed society. I also want to offer a sense of all that we have lost, before I go on to describe the third and tragic stage of human history, the catastrophe that took it all away, and therefore fully merits the metaphoric label of "The Fall."

Catal Huyuk was a full-fledged town, reaching its peak in the seventh millennium BCE, with as many as two thousand inhabitants. The city was laid out like the pueblos still used by the matristic Tewa people of the Southwest U.S., with flat-roofed adobe houses, each with an open courtyard in the middle. There is no evidence of any type of social stratification – that is, no larger, grander houses, mixed with smaller, meaner ones, no great plaza, no palace.

Each house had rooms clearly assigned to different aspects of living, with adobe 'built-in' furniture – kitchens with counters and ovens, open living spaces with benches fitted with rush cushions, bedrooms with sleeping platforms and woven bedding.

Rooms thought to be shrines were included in every house, and the rooms of some houses were all shrine, with paintings on the walls, and small sculptures of 'goddesses' and other sacred figures, including stone and clay figures of mammals. The shrine houses might have served people coming in from surrounding areas. One of them, containing a large room with special benches, carefully-laid limestone flooring, and raised flues for bringing in water, has been identified as a special place for giving birth; painted symbols adorning the walls recall those found in many caves and other sites associated with matristic cultures from preceding millennia – cream circles with red centers representing the cervix, a thick cream line for the umbilical cord, wavy lines and spirals representing water and amniotic fluid.

Other rooms were clearly meant for ceremonial events, with 'throne' chairs fitted with horns from bulls, and murals showing life-size figures of humans and animals. There are pictures of women dancing, their hair swirling out around them as they spin, and representations of the 'three ages of Woman:' the maid, mother, and crone (the Wise Older Woman – our 'Grandmother-Leader'). Throughout the shrines of the town there are pictures of bulls and other horned animals, personifying (and validating) that previously mentioned image of Center males as 'gentle giants.'

With regard to the cultural management of males, it is interesting that one mural at Catal Huyuk shows an older, bearded man riding a bull and a younger man riding a leopard. This might be a symbolic depiction of a silverback-blackback pair, a visual representation of the strategy used by women to incorporate men peacefully into the center. (Much later records from other cultures which moved into this same area note that an old custom among the matristic people was for a woman to have two husbands – perhaps an older and younger, a silverback and a blackback, chosen so that their difference in ages helped them get along.)

Yet another room seems to have been used in 'secondary burial' celebrations. Earlier we mentioned the burial practices of Neanderthals, in which whole bodies were placed in the ground in crouched positions, accompanied by tools. The people of Catal Huyuk followed a different practice, still used in many matristic cultures around the world, called 'excarnation.' First, the body is placed well away from living areas so that scavengers such as foxes, weasels, and vultures, 'nature's purifiers,' can clean away the flesh, re-cycling it for their own children. Only then is the skeleton retrieved and buried. The Plains Indians of North America used vultures to clean skeletons in this way, as some groups in Iran and India continue to do today.

This special, valued role of scavengers is acknowledged by celebratory sculptures and murals in the Catal Huyuk shrines. On the walls of one funeral room, large pictures of vultures are painted alongside much smaller, headless human figures. With the flesh cleaned away, the bones of a family member could be returned to become part of the physical foundation of a family's house, kept close instead of being banished to some remote 'city of the dead (like modern cemeteries). In Catal Huyuk, the bones of loved ones were actually buried under the family's sleeping platforms, and children's bones were placed near their mother's bed. In many cases, buried skeletons of women show that red ochre had been scattered on the bones.

Those who have studied Catal Huyuk emphasize the sense of joy and life-giving energy embodied in its art and iconography, the celebration of birth and the natural cycles of biology, and above all, the primacy of women. There are numerous sites in the Middle East that resemble Catal Huyuk, towns up and down the Tigris and Euphrates, a settlement at Jericho, and many others. Some have cobbled streets, at others pieces of metal jewelry have been found along with ceramic vases painted with goddess figures. And at site after site are the goddess figurines, some with serpents coiling over one shoulder, double axes (perhaps a butterfly symbol), the tree of life, and doves, all attributes of female divinity which continued even after what we'll call The Fall. (It is amusing to read standard archeological descriptions of these joyous, woman-centered places. For instance, the sculptures and paintings are taken as evidence of 'cults' – the goddess figurines represent a 'fertility cult,' bull figures indicate a 'bull cult,' and the wonderful pictures celebrating vultures preparing the dead are signs of a 'death cult.')

The most exciting aspect about these cultures is the evidence of the way they were managed – their government – which is in a direct line from the management strategies for peaceful 50:50 groups presented earlier. Much of this evidence comes not from the archeological sites themselves, but from observations recorded by later cultures who came into the area. In each matristic town or settlement, there was evidently a building known as the Temple, which was the core of the community (the shrine house at Catal Huyuk was perhaps an early form). The Temple was where certain groups of women, including older women, sometimes referred to as the Elder Women, or the *qadishtu*, lived and worked (*qadishtu* means 'those who stand apart,' and 'the pure').

The Temple was the heart and soul of the town. As an institution embodied in the *qadishtu*, the Temple owned the low-tech agricultural farm land around the town, and kept the records of births, deaths, and commerce. The *qadishtu* were responsible for all such aspects of town life, overseeing agricultural activities, planning and directing the building of new houses when needed, and guiding the citizens of the town and surrounding areas in everyday interactions. They served as judges to settle disputes, and were also responsible for the religious celebrations having to do with landmarks of life such as puberty, birth, and death. In addition to their many civic duties, the *qadishtu* also offered their sexual favors to men who came to the Temple to worship the goddess (a continuation of the strategy making every man feel like a Center male.) Their children were raised within the Temple, and when they grew up, they might take a house in the town, or if they were girls, choose to live in the Temple and carry on their mothers' and grandmothers' work as *qadishtu*.

The Temples and their customs persisted for many thousands of years. For instance, laws pertaining to the Temple oversight of inheritance, property rights, business, and legal relations between parents and children were recorded in systematic codes of other cultures in the area composed many generations later. When the temple of Yahweh was built in Jerusalem, it was sited next to a Temple of the Goddess where the *qadishtu* continued to carry on at least some of their governance, including its sexual aspects, and women from Jerusalem and the surrounding country went on attending this temple to worship the goddess for many years afterward.

Crete was even more amazing than Catal Huyuk, taking all of the same features to another level. Crete was founded around 7000 BCE by people who may have come from the area of Catal Huyuk. On the fertile slopes and plains of the island they created a peaceful, prosperous society which flourished in the Mediterranean for more than four thousand years. The women in the Temple designed and oversaw a far-flung trading network which connected many areas around the 'Goddess Lake' of the Mediterranean, and provided for exchange of goods of all kinds.

One of the most important and incredible facts about the cities on Crete is that they were not fortified – this was a peaceful culture, living (for a time) among peaceful cultures. The mural art of Crete is unsurpassed, and is always in praise of the power and vigor of biology and of women. The most famous are the 'bull-leaping' murals in which young women and men gymnasts do handsprings over the back of that 'curly-headed bull.' Others show flying-fish and dolphins, or a blue bird ready to fly from a high cliff.

Areas around the Mediterranean (Crete; Catal Huyuk and neighboring river valleys such as the Tigris and Euphrates; the upper Nile valley in Egypt) were not the only places where these burgeoning farming cultures began to appear. There were similar developments of accomplished matristic cultures around the world – along the Indus and Ganges Rivers in India; the Mekong in Southeast Asia; the Yellow and Yangtze Rivers in China; and in North America, including communities in central Mexico.

In a moment we will see that all this was to end. The end came, not because of an inherent flaw in design – as we've suggested, these represented the ideal human society, in harmony with brain types within and the world without – but (as I'll talk about in the next section of this chapter) because of invasions from another place, by people who had not stayed in the warm climates where hominids belong, but had lived for too long in cold (like the Neanderthals), and consequently had been changed away from the matristic human norm into something terrible and predatory.

But it is critical to stress at this point that the depredations of these new people, as murderous and misogynist as they have been, have not succeeded in totally erasing the legacy of the tens of thousands of years of matristic, truly human society. Long after the 'Ice People' as I will call them, descended and started making catastrophic changes, female divinities continued to be worshipped around the world, in cultures large and small, by people in tiny matristic tribes and in giant patriarchal cities.

Although the last Temple of the Goddess in Rome was destroyed in 500 CE (Common Era, the secular revision of *Anno Domini*), there has been no abatement of interest in the divine nature of the Human Woman, with all her Goddess features – sexual, maternal, all-powerful, all-wise, and infinitely nurturing. Even under the rule of the most patriarchal religions, the all-embracing love of the mother goddess is remembered and revered. She became Queen Isis in Egypt, Sarasvati in India, Mary in southern Europe – and many, many others. It is also no accident that even today, the life of a mammalian Center male is still the dream of virtually all men. Even under the worst manifestations of rule by puritanical Perimeter males (such as the virulently misogynist Taliban of Afghanistan), the best heavenly fate for men that can be imagined, the greatest and finest reward, is to be able to have sexual access to many women.

Human history – Stage Three, the descent of the Ice People

You already know about Stage Three – it is the only 'history' we are allowed to know about in school (beginning with Greece and Rome, for heaven's sake – which did not even come into existence for thousands of years *after* the women in Catal Huyuk were dancing with their hair floating out around them).

Stage Three is now. It is the stratified, war-mongering, genocidal horrors of the last 10,000 years, misogyny and sexism and racism and species-ism, a nightmare pretending to be a real society. But I want to reassure you that in spite of what the history books preach about 'progress' and 'civilization,' *the last 10,000 years is not human history, it is not Center history, it is not my history – it is Perimeter history.* Looked at objectively, it appears as though Neanderthals, with their strange, cold-adapted perimeterized society, rather than dying off 35,000 years ago, inherited the earth – instead of the matristic, warm-loving AMH.

To understand how the Perimeter has come to dominate these last few millennia, we need to learn where the change-over from Center to Perimeter came from, and how it happened. Even though this transformation is what I consider to be 'The Fall' for human beings (almost a literal loss of a Garden of Eden), I am certain that knowing how and why it happened is crucial – to show us the way to set things right. Knowing how and why will help us see that the worst horrors of the last 10,000 years are exceptions to the rule, *deviations from the main matristic line of human history.* This will give us some badly-needed perspective on our contemporary problems, change The Fall to a fall, allowing us to pick ourselves up, brush ourselves off, and get back on the matristic track.

As I've said, at about the same time in 10 KYA, weather patterns were changing all around the world – away from Ice-Age cold, to conditions that were warmer and wetter and much more conducive to horticulture. Farming on a scale that could support villages and small towns began to be practiced almost simultaneously in several locations within a band of about the same latitudes around the globe – in the Middle East (such as Catal Huyuk), Southeast Asia, southern China, and southern Mexico. The simultaneity of these meteorological developments is too perfect for advanced agricultural practices to have started at just one place and travelled. Rather, anthropologists think that the people in all these zones had carried along with them the methods for 'pre-agriculture' present in Africa during the earliest years of AMH (this might have included clearing space around favored plants, so they could spread; hand-planting certain plants to increase their number; small-scale burning of unwanted plants; or helping plants endure heat by using small-scale irrigation to bring them water). In 10 KYA, when the weather permitted, the women who lived in just the right places (with good soil and water) at just the right latitude, were ready – and evidently at the same time, all started slightly more advanced agriculture.

In these early agricultural societies around the world, women led the worship of various forms of the Goddess, and managed non-stratified, peaceful and nurturing societies for the good of all. And, left to their own devices, there is no reason why these cultures would not have become the norm for us today, ensuring a healthy, nurturing, sane human future. They were living the legacy of the matristic way of life 'invented' ten millennia before by the AMH women in Africa, an achievement that saved themselves and their kind from extinction. The new agricultural societies found new ways to build on all those eons of success, of woman-centered wisdom for harmonizing human society with the Neural Rainbow of brain types, including modifying the rainbow in a way so that everyone could stay in the Center, and live the good life.

Based on the progress they made in the time they had, these cultures clearly could have developed along a number of lines and accomplished just about anything they wanted. After all, the brain types represented within them – polytropics and middles – provided a great combination of skills, ranging from right-brain emotional intelligence to left-brain fine-motor skills for designing non-invasive, sustainable technologies; and from middle-brain abilities for sports and entertainment such as acting, singing and dance, to all-embracing polytropic 'judicial' guidance to keep the inevitable social friction that arises among any group of animals in proportion.

What I want to stress here is that the human condition for these cultures was *not* 'solitary, poor, nasty, brutish, and short,' as Thomas Hobbes described life for people around the world who had not yet 'benefited' from English colonialism. Hobbes himself lived in 17th-century London, where by 'civilized law' men were allowed to beat horses to death when they collapsed pulling heavy carts, and beat women to death when they objected to being treated like horses. Many sincere and good-hearted people even today who wrestle with issues of morality, of good and evil, still do not believe that human life can be any other way. They believe that cruelty is endemic to human beings, and war a human universal. Some serious students of human behavior have declared that 'we are all genociders.'

But the evidence suggests that things were not like that in the matristic cultures. The case was precisely the opposite – a good birth, a good childhood, a good adult life fulfilled by making a valued contribution to an integrated society of relations and friends, and finally, a good death, surrounded by that same supportive community. Of course there were accidents, and birth defects, and disease. People got sick and died. But as we know from studies of groups living in similar societies today, their medicine was very sophisticated, combining a diverse pharmacopeia of natural medicines, implicit knowledge of the right-brain context of immune response, the importance of treating the 'whole organism,' and perhaps most important, drawing on the very concrete connections between social support and physical health.

There were years when the rains didn't fall, the crops failed and times were hard. But like all K-strategist animals in harmony with their surroundings, these people lived where their bodies were at home, and knew more than one way to make a living. They were not an overspecialized key made for only one kind of lock, as most humans are today. (Think of it, all the gadgets that surround you – which ones could you make for yourself? Could you survive without them? If grocery stores disappeared, could you feed yourself and your children by gathering plants in nearby woods and fields, could you find clean water for drinking?) Nor were the matristic cultures set on a course, as we are, to destroy themselves and every other life form on the planet; rather, they were living as one species among many fellow species, fulfilled by life in the human Center.

But now we need to stop for a moment – freeze-frame, and fast-return back to about 40 KYA, a time when anatomically modern humans were living in the Middle East, southern China, Australia, and the Americas, long before the agricultural innovations came in that made Catal Huyuk possible. About this time, the warming trend mentioned earlier attracted some AMH groups to move *north* of the original band that formed the track of the main west-to-east migration. In fact, some of them must have gone as far north as the 55th parallel (which passes through Ireland and Moscow), because AMH sites with 'signatures' such as goddess figurines have been found at that latitude (but no further north), stretching from Britain into the lands south of the Baltic Sea (northern Germany and Poland), and out across the steppes of Russia, all the way to Lake Baikal in southern Siberia.

Apparently the groups of AMH (still based on that peaceful 50:50 profile of Fig. 4.12) who established themselves in all these locations, from far south to far north, from east to west, pretty much stayed in place – for the next thirty thousand years. Although there were major changes in global weather during this long period (several fluctuations of colder then warmer temperatures), the populations established by about 35 KYA were essentially non-migratory. For nearly thirty thousand years, AMH bands carried on their everyday lives in these new homelands, without much interaction with people from other regions. (Toward the end of this period, around 12,000 BCE, a small migration of AMH peoples crossed Beringia into the Americas, where they formed the Clovis cultures. Unlike their AMH predecessors, however, this group originated in northern Mongolia rather than further south – a crucial difference, as we will see.)

Over the enormously long time during which these populations remained within their environments, the process of 'genetic drift' slowly helped fit them for living in four major geographic regions. The regions were: 1) southern Africa; 2) a warm belt around the world extending from the equator north to about 40 degrees latitude (taking in lands around the Mediterranean, India, Southeast Asia, southern China, southern North America); 3) northeastern Europe (the western steppes around the Caspian Sea); and 4) Mongolia (the eastern steppes north of Tibet).

The adjustments made might be called 'chameleon' changes, that is, mostly affecting external appearance to match physical features of their environment. Today we refer to these as 'racial' differences, but they are more properly called geographic differences, because all the people were AMH and remained so. The changes were merely adjustments to the demands of living in different regions, whether the air temperature was warmer or colder (e.g, affecting the size and length of the nose), or there was more or less sunshine (thus more or less skin melanin), or one type of food was more plentiful than another (leading to differences in teeth and jaw).

The first set of changes is one previously mentioned in relation to Neanderthals – adjustments in body proportions for either maximizing or minimizing heat loss, the sort of changes often seen in other animals. In consistently warm climates, AMH populations were able to retain their original 'gracile' shapes, with slim, cylindrical bodies that helped them lose heat easily. In contrast, people who settled in areas (such as the steppes from northeastern Europe to Mongolia) which eventually underwent long periods of cold, gradually changed away from this standard pattern to have rounder bodies which helped conserve heat.

Another population characteristic related to geography is the distribution of body melanin. Melanin is important in two ways for managing the body's response to ultraviolet (UV) wavelengths of sunlight. There is good news and bad news for humans about UV radiation. The good news is that UV (in limited amounts) is important for human nutrition, because it changes a chemical in the skin (related to cholesterol) into Vitamin D, which is crucial for calcium metabolism and strong bones. Thus AMH groups living where there was abundant sunshine throughout the year ('natural' places for hominids to be) could make all the Vitamin D they needed, simply by letting the sun fall on their skin.

The bad news about UV radiation is that too much of it can cause burns, and even skin cancer. (These very short wavelengths can damage DNA.) However, melanin in the skin, hair, and eyes will break up the UV waves, and prevent this type of damage. Thus AMH peoples living in sunny places (Africa, and the warm belt around the world from Mediterranean to Mexico) retained their original dark (perhaps generally a cinnamon-brown) coloration, or became even darker (brown-black to black) as needed, to protect themselves from too much sun.

The case was very different for the populations which ventured into the far north, where sunlight falls much more obliquely, and is often blocked completely by clouds for long periods of time. The people there, seldom in danger of sunburn, needed all the sunlight they could get to make Vitamin D. In fact, they may have turned to fishing to make up the deficit, since the livers of northern-Atlantic fishes such as halibut and cod are high in Vitamin D.

As a result, over time the northern populations, particularly those in the western steppes (the western third of the Great Eurasian Steppe, that extends from Hungary to Chinia), underwent severe de-pigmentation, a genetic change leading to underproduction of melanin in skin, hair and eyes. As we discussed in Chapter Three, this reduced ability to make melanin may also have predisposed these people to biochemically-related disorders such as Parkinson's Disease. It has certainly caused fair-skinned races major problems as they move back into warmer areas in modern times – rates of skin cancer in white men living in Arizona and northern Australia are the highest in the world.

The third area of geographic adjustment relates to diet. In addition to using the sun to make Vitamin D in their own skins, the people living in sunny regions also enjoyed the benefit of year-round growing seasons, and so could continue their age-old dietary practices, depending on a rich and various cornucopia of plant foods providing complete protein and the other nutrients they needed. Thus nothing about their digestive systems would have to change, including aspects of blood chemistry related to food metabolism, such as the ABO family of blood types. The O subtype of the ABO group is believed to be the original human blood type, and its historical distribution in many ways matches the locations where the original warm-adapted AMH groups lived – throughout Africa, in India, Southeast Asia, southern China, and the Americas. (The ABO story is complicated somewhat by interaction with certain types of diseases, but the match between blood types and the geographical adjustments at issue here is too close to be coincidental.)

A vivid contrast is again presented by the people who moved into regions that were cooler than the AMH home-place and eventually became very much colder. As I've said, the lack of Vitamin D from sunlight (which may have given them a high incidence of rickets early on) could have been answered by turning to animals as food sources. Groups with access to the Atlantic might have gotten their Vitamin D from the livers of fish like halibut and cod, while those further inland might have been the first to domesticate animals for their milk, cheese, and eggs, which are also sources of Vitamin D (though fairly poor ones, affected by how much sunlight the animal itself receives).

For anyone older than weaning age to be able to digest dairy products (in fact, for them not to go blind as a result of lactose intolerance, which happened to many third-world children in the early years of the CARE program), these northern people would have had to retain lactase in their systems all their lives. (Lactase is the enzyme which metabolizes lactose, the sugar in breast milk; it disappears in mammalian children as soon as they are weaned, leading to the perfectly normal state which modern medicine deplores as 'lactose intolerance,' as though it's a failing.)

During the long periods of increasing cold in the north, the people may also have been cut off from their usual supply of plant foods for most if not all of the year, and like the Neanderthals, turned to predation as a source of food. Their first efforts at hunting might have targeted smaller-size, r-strategist animals that were adapted to the cold and dryness of the steppes, such as hamsters and gerbils (found in large numbers throughout Asia, and as far north as Siberia). The fact that these animals were r-strategists would have ensured a reliable annual new 'crop' of young adults that the starving humans could regularly 'harvest' for their needs. As the blossoming hunters became more proficient, they may have sought a higher return on their predatory effort by switching to r/K strategists as prey, such as the many species of 'goat antelopes' that are also found across Asia and into Siberia; again, the annual reproduction of these animals would have served the needs of the humans well.

Finally, a growing need for meat plus the possibility of exploiting dairy products as a Vitamin D source may have led the humans to start *domesticating* r- and r/K strategist mammals, in order to have more physical control over them and also to exploit their rapid reproduction as an efficient way to ensure a constant supply of meat-on-the-hoof. Thus these people eventually became 'pastoral nomads,' following their r/K herds as they tracked the seasonal variations in the sparse vegetation of the harsh and inhospitable steppes.

As time went on, the blood chemistry of these people may have changed to make use of non-plant sources of foods more efficiently, both to support the energy drain involved in breaking down animal protein, and to store food (as body fat) from animal sources characterized by extremely low levels of carbohydrates. It is believed that the blood-group subtype A arose on the steppes of western Asia/northeastern Europe between 25 KYA and 15 KYA, and that subtype B originated much further east, in the Mongolian steppes around 15 -10 KYA. My point is this: although individuals with A and B blood types may now be vulnerable to diseases of several types, these mutations away from the original type O were originally an adaptive response to the radically different diets forced on the people living in cold areas of the world.

Finally, these different environments proved to have dramatic cultural implications, as well. The cold-adapted Ice People would have undergone the same types of changes outlined earlier for Neanderthals: increased chronic sympathetic arousal, higher general aggression, the production of more left-brain babies (especially males), and the transformation of woman-managed groups by the invasive presence and attitudes of Perimeter males, resulting in the perimeterization of culture for people living in these areas.

This process would have radically transformed their social organization map, away from the peaceful 50:50 shown in Figs. 4.12 and 5.2, into something so different as to represent a difference in kind. The first change from the old to the new is illustrated in the top half of Figure 5.3, where the original peaceful 50:50 group format (panel A), consisting only of polytropics and middle-brains, an SOC which they had actively created out of their original C/P, and which had served them so well for so long, *became infiltrated by left-brains*, whose nature was anything but peaceful (panel B)

This quickly led to the next and most fateful change (panel C), the 180° 'flip' in the 'social compass' of these groups mentioned earlier, in which group leadership (thus power) was taken away from the polytropic women and appropriated by left-brain men. As illustrated in the panel, this change was accompanied by a radical rearrangement in terms of rank – which translated directly into resource allotment – from a 'horizontal' (cooperative/ sharing) organization to a hierarchical one (unequal distribution of rank and resources), with left-brain men at the top, middle-brain men in the middle, and women and children relegated to the lowest levels (a somewhat higher 'rank' might be recognized for certain women and children associated with the higher-up males, but ultimately, all prestige and privilege flowed from the men who held positions at the top of the newly 'pyramidal' society).

Figure 5.3

Forced conversion of peaceful 50:50 AMH groups (polytropics and middles only) (A) into aggressive groups combining all three brain types (B), soon re-organized as rigidly hierarchical societies (C) based on unequal resource distribution, privileging left-brain men over all others, men over women and children, and polytropic women banished to the lowest level. As in Ch. 4, circles/triangles = women/men; black = polytropic Grandmother-Leaders, grey = middle-brain Loyal-Helpers, unfilled = left-brain Focal-Asocials.

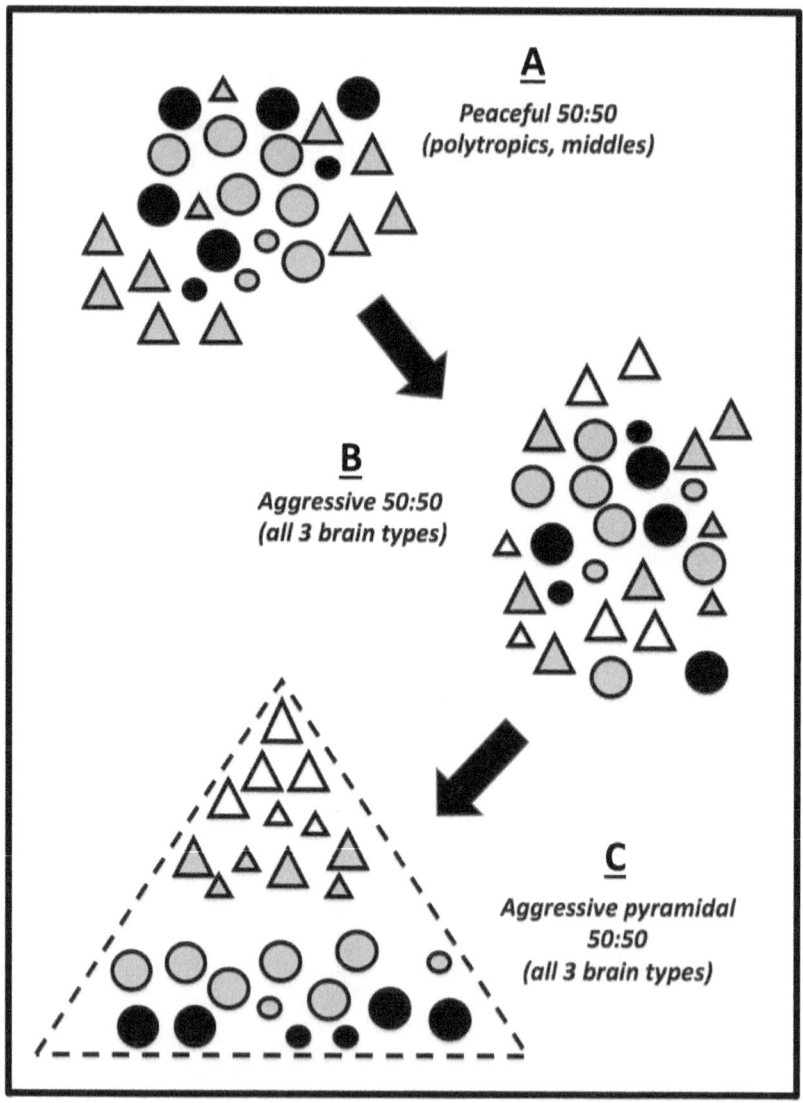

Thus, these perimeterized, 'dominator' societies of the steppes (as Riane Eisler calls them in *The Chalice and the Blade*) became rigidly hierarchical chiefdoms, with rank depending on (or signaled by) ownership and the unequal distribution of wealth. They might have extended their sense of ownership over domestic animals, to ownership over humans, as well – not only enslaving people kidnapped during wars with neighboring groups, but also insisting on dominance hierarchies within their own groups, such that women and children came to be seen as the property of males, and the men themselves were aligned in a pecking order, as strict as an army, from the chief at the top, down to the unlucky few at the bottom.

The nomads' experience with domesticating r/K animals such as goats may have led them to encourage their own 'domestic-animal' human women to shift their reproductive style in an r/K direction, and produce babies faster – one every year like domesticated goats instead of taking the normal 4-5 years between births like the large primates they were. (In many of the societies which have descended from these cultures, the best wish for a man is that he be blessed with all the signs of wealth and power – "many cattle and children.")

The features of hierarchy and dominance by males are clearly indicated in burials found from these cultures, showing the telltale signs of social stratification – a very few males buried with great riches (daggers and knives and rings of copper), while most others, including women and children, are left in poor graves. The Ice People were also fond of blood sacrifices, killing healthy animals from their herds as offerings to violent male gods who were distant, non-biological, and destructive – different types of 'sky gods,' gods of the blazing sun of arid lands (not the life-giving sun of the south), of thunder and lightning (not fertile rain), and maybe most significantly, volcano gods. Many of these cultures practiced a generalized kind of *sati* (a practice where a widow is routinely burned alive on the same pyre as her dead husband) – that is, murdering humans and domestic animals to 'accompany' high-ranking men into death. At one burial site in Russia just west of the Caspian Sea, the skeletons of 13 people and 22 horses were found arranged in systematic squares around the remains of the one man, apparently an important steppes chieftain, at the center of the grave. The whole crowd of corpses had been enclosed in a wooden chamber with a pyramidal roof, which was apparently set afire (volcano-like) and then buried under a mound of earth.

In these dominator cultures, where women and children are 'owned,' and the women are bred as the men bred their goats, the ancient wisdom of women for managing society would have been dismissed as worthless 'old wives' tales.' This is made abundantly clear in the writings and laws of societies that can trace their ancestry directly back to these early steppes people – for example, "Let the woman learn in silence and with all subjection. But I suffer not a woman to teach, nor to usurp authority over the man, but to be in silence" (I Timothy 2: 11-14).

As we've said, all these changes would have been gradual; but well before the time of the dramatic global warming around 10 KYA, the four geographic types were firmly established – warm-adapted, matristic blood-type-O people with very dark skins in Africa and Australia; warm-adapted, matristic type-O people with brown skins in the belt stretching from the Mediterranean to the Americas (though no humans were in Polynesia yet); cold-adapted, perimeterized type-A people with very pale skins in northeastern Europe and the western steppes; and cold-adapted, perimeterized type-B people with their own type of depigmentation (combined with epicanthal folds, etc.) in Mongolia.

In spite of the 'dark side' of the cold-adapted changes for the people up north, things still might have gone on in this way indefinitely, with agriculture and towns like Catal Huyuk blooming, and matristic societies continuing to flourish in the warm parts of the earth. If the outside influences that came to change them had not occurred (more of this in a moment), I don't believe that population growth in the matristic cultures would have been a problem. As time went on, the women managing the burgeoning matristic towns would have learned to accommodate growth based on improvements in survival rates vis-a-vis new food combinations, and year-to-year fluctuations in crop yield. In line with their history of clever cultural innovations, they certainly might have utilized various means of birth control known to non-industrial peoples (and chimpanzees) in order to ensure that group size did not get out of hand and degrade the quality of life that was everything to them.

But the women of the classical matristic era were not allowed to do this. They were not given time to demonstrate that humans can successfully manage the size of their groups, even when new types of food make it possible to feed more mouths, and even when modes of production lead to a surplus of food (long considered by orthodox anthropologists and archeologists to be the trigger which *naturally* leads to social stratification).

What prevented them from doing this was the same thing that helped them to their new prosperity – the warming of world climate. The warmer weather also made life easier on the steppes, and resulted in explosive population increases among the groups living there – not only because of their r/K domestic animals but also their women, perhaps now with additional food sources, producing a good annual 'crop' of babies, a helpful resource for building armies.

As a result, the Ice People of the steppes became expansionist and began to spread in all directions. At first, accompanied by slow-moving herds and travelling on foot, they were widely scattered, with vast distances to cover. But around 4500 BCE something truly decisive happened, a dramatic increase in their mobility – the people of the western steppes became the first to domesticate the horse as a vehicle, by inventing the bit. The rest, as they say, is 'history.'

In the West, the increased speed and range provided by the horse allowed groups of Ice People to reach the Middle East. These people are now referred to as Indo-Europeans and were very pale (they are the Aryans [Sanskrit for 'noble'] of Nazi fantasies). They found the brown people (warm-adapted 'Sun People') living in the lovely towns like Catal Huyuk, farming the fragrant, fertile valleys – and simply moved in and took over.

There was essentially no resistance. The people living there were peaceful, without fortifications (in a matristic world, what need is there for parapets and blockhouses?). It was like taking candy from a baby. Archeology shows that the takeover was actually not sudden for the most part, as with a single, 'blitzkrieg' warlike invasion. It was gradual, but no less sure. The Ice People knew well from long practice (in controlling women, children, and other animals) how to subjugate and silence, and the fact that their 'targets of opportunity' were women-centered cultures made it all the easier – the invaders brought to the task millennia of practice in shutting women down.

Incredibly, given the almost total silence on the subject in our standard history books, the story of how the Ice People took over, around the entire world, is there for all to see, in archeological records and especially in the recent genetic evidence for migrations described by Cavalli-Sforza and colleagues (see chapter bibliography). The Indo-European invaders from north of the Caspian Sea, whom Marija Gimbutas calls the 'Kurgans,' came into the Middle East in several successive waves, starting around 4500 BCE. Soon after arriving, steppes-derived societies developed the horse-drawn chariot for use in warfare, even though it was based on a very inefficient harness, the 'throat and girth,' better suited to oxen; once the breast-strap method was invented in China several thousand years later, war chariots could be even more effective. Gimbutas suggests that among the motivations drawing invaders to the Middle East was the news that various metals were available there, which they desired for making better weapons (the beginning of the use of the 'terrible metals' which have enabled so much of perimeterized cultures, occasionally for good, but mostly for great ill).

The Kurgan influence spread west and north into all of Europe, where they pushed the original inhabitants out into the far reaches of the land, where some still persist as people of Celtic heritage, many of whom retain elements of their old matristic life. Ironically enough, the Indo-Europeans who took over Old Europe were themselves later invaded by other waves of cold-adapted people from the steppes (Goths, Huns, Mongols), who were a constant nightmare to people of Europe well into the Middle Ages. Later, the murderous, expansionist activities of the Aryan-loving Nazis and the pale-skinned Soviet totalitarians were simply the 20th-century expressions of repeating 'steppes-on-steppes' invasions by cold-adapted societies spawned in the cold places of the earth.

Eventually, the influence of these people from the far north was felt even in Africa, where they descended on peaceful farming communities and birthed 'native' perimeterized expansionist cultures such as the Ashanti, Benin, and Dahomey of West Africa. These groups spread out across the continent as the 'Bantu expansion,' and later collaborated enthusiastically in the slave trade with descendants of other Indo-Europeans, from Arabia, England, and France.

Still other groups of pale-faced Indo-Europeans came down from the north into India around 1300 BCE, eventually subsuming the matristic cultures there. The invaders imposed a rigid and punitive caste system *based on skin color,* with the palest people (themselves) at the top, and others ranked from there down, with the darkest people at the bottom. This caste system is still in place today, of course, and continues to perpetuate a dramatically unequal distribution of resources in India. Yet the arrival of these people in India has been described by some historians as "a springboard to Ganges civilization."

Invaders from Mongolia moved into northern China in 2300 BCE, bringing violence and stratification to the new agricultural societies there, and reached Indochina somewhat later. Their successors founded the terrible line of the Chinese dynasties, who ruled by force and violence and, like the Indo-Europeans in Europe, continued to experience the steppes-on-steppes phenomenon for thousands of years, themselves repeatedly assaulted by still other invaders from the very steppes they had left behind.

Around 1600 BCE these Mongolian-originating people may also have given rise to the Lapita culture, euphemistically described as 'very mobile' (always a bad sign – we'll see later that biologically, *high mobility* is often linked with *maleness*) which swept rapidly out of Indonesia into Australia and also into the islands of Melanesia (just north of Australia), Micronesia (north of that), and Polynesia to the east as far as Easter Island. Again, they installed violent, perimeterized chiefdom societies everywhere they went. In a later (13th-century CE) Melanesian culture, one excavation revealed that more than 40 people had been killed on the occasion of the death of a major chief. Several individuals were buried alone, couples side by side, a young girl crosswise at the man's feet, and a child's skeleton in a box was found between the chief's legs. The most common extra items in the graves were bracelets made of pig tusks – teeth for attack.

Invaders from Southeast Asia also entered New Guinea and Samoa at about the same time (1600 BCE). Similar groups had expanded into Australia somewhat earlier, around 5000 BCE, bringing a new type of stone tool and the dingo, related to the pariah dog of India. Their arrival is clearly indicated by the sudden appearance of burials marked by obvious differences in wealth.

Intermarriage between these latecomers and the older, warm-adapted Australians may have resulted in the African/Asian mix recognized in present-day Australian indigenous peoples (the signs of the invasions are still present in some versions of their folk-tales).

In the Americas, the Clovis people originating in northern Mongolia who had entered the Northern American continent around 12000 BCE, were also weapon-loving, animal-killing, and high-mobility: they moved quickly from north to south, destroying animals, particularly large mammals, as they went. These people with their advanced weapons may have been responsible for the extinction of 35 genera of large mammals in North America alone – 73% of the mammals living there at that time – and 79% of the large mammals in South America.

When they came across peaceful and matristic cultures from the ancient migrations, they made war with them and also intermarried, transforming many of these societies from partnership societies to dominator chiefdoms. Examples of these new invaders from North America include the 'mound-builder' cultures based along the Mississippi River, whose earthen tombs (resembling the 'kurgan' mounds made by the earlier invaders of Eastern Europe, and the pyramids built by still other invader societies) show clear evidence of social stratification, including people and animals killed and buried in a chief's grave, and sculptures of warriors beheading captives taken in warfare.

The Clovis people extended their influence from north to south, all the way to the tip of South America. At times they may have lived side by side for a while with some of the older cultures, forming a potential pool for hostile take-overs if any of the older groups developed a better life, such as happened with the beginnings of agriculture in Mexico. People living in the Tehuacán valley of Mexico were clearly transformed in this way; remains around this region show the same discontinuity seen everywhere else, changing over a relatively short period of time from the beginning of settled, peaceful farming, to explosive population growth and signs of stratification, followed in rapid succession by a series of violent, warlike 'civilizations.' These repressive societies included the Olmecs, the Toltecs, and their culmination, those tremendous representatives of 'man's rise to civilization' (according to Peter Farb), the Aztecs. Of course, the Aztecs themselves eventually suffered the steppes-on-steppes fate, invaded and conquered by the Spanish, themselves the pale-faced Indo-European descendants of the Kurgans.

And then there was Peru, where peaceful farming communities along the western coast attracted the attention of the expansionist, militaristic Incas; over time, the Toltecs and Aztecs of Mexico extended a net of domination much like that of the Indo-Europeans from Rome. All of these Perimeter cultures built 'artificial-volcano' pyramids like the ones in Egypt, and the

Aztecs eventually used their pyramids as the site of ritual sacrifices where radical cardiac surgery was performed on living human bodies.

Archeological Newspeak

Books on human history and archeology often refer to all these ghastly events as the 'dawn of civilization.' Most of the standard texts depict cultural changes occurring in these crucial years as a smooth continuum rather a calamitous turnaround, a 180-degree reversal, in the personal and community life of the people being invaded.

In standard texts, such events are described as a series of three basic steps. Step 1 involves the emergence of the earliest known techniques for subsistence farming which then (they say) 'remained static (sic) for many thousands of years.' Step 2 details the developments in agriculture and the building of small towns occurring in 10 KYA to 5 KYA (Catal Huyuk, Indus Valley, Indonesia, Mexico, etc.), changes often characterized as 'laying the foundation for civilization.'

Then without missing a beat, the text will report Step 3: explosive increases in population, the rapid spreading and intensification of agricultural techniques, the construction of the first fortified towns, the rise of elaborate rituals and specialized occupations, and other signs that society was becoming increasingly centralized (*not* 'centerized,' they were already that – but 'perimeterized') and hierarchical. Soon thereafter comes the emergence of warrior elites and 'monumental architecture,' routinely and joyfully heralded in these texts as sure signs of the arrival of human civilization.

As Merlin Stone, Riane Eisler and others have noted, such descriptions (clearly biased in favor of the social style of the invaders) seem to be the norm in the standard historical treatments of this period. Little or no awareness is exhibited regarding the possibility that these years did not involve a continuous process at all, but were a point of *radical discontinuity* in human history, a rapid shift from the millennia of peaceful, matristic management, to something utterly different – a change that came about as a result of invasive, external influences, not the 'natural evolution of society.'

If invaders or other steppe-originating outsiders are mentioned in these standard texts, it is only in passing, as though the tremendous changes that transformed the agricultural matristic societies were somehow intrinsic to them, and not the devastating results of intrusive influences *from outside*. If details of the goddess cultures themselves are noted at all, it is in somewhat embarrassed and stilted language, noting that there may have been a 'fertility cult' signaled by 'representations of female genitalia' and carvings showing 'the ample figure of a mother goddess.' In other words, there seems to be no suspicion that the step from stage 2 to stage 3 was not only gigantic, it was *backward*, away from true biological adaptive living, honoring the carrying capacity of the land, and harmonious relations between humans and the world that supported them, to something very different. Step 3, in short, seems to qualify (from our standpoint) as "The Fall" far more than does the story told in Genesis (we'll talk about Genesis in a later chapter).

After The Fall, things rapidly deteriorated. Soon, complex cities began sprouting like evil mushrooms – Uruk, Babylon, Cairo, Mohenjo-Daro in India, Zhengzhou in China, Dong Son in Vietnam, etc., etc. The new metros popping up around the world contained monumental palaces with vast open plazas, luxurious great houses for the wealthy, vs. cramped crowded quarters for servants and slaves. Soon there was war of every description, expanding in every direction, some perpetrated by the invaders on the locals, others occurring in the steppes-on-steppes mode, invader vs. invader, but all made murderously efficient by technological developments in metallurgy, hailed un-ironically in many archeological texts as 'new means for man to control his environment.'

As one might expect in societies so oriented to death and destruction, tombs of rulers grew larger and larger. In Egypt, the invaders built the first pyramid around 2600 BCE, about 180 feet high; within 100 years, the Great Pyramid at Giza was almost three times higher, and involved quarrying, transporting (without wheels) and hoisting vertically 1100 2.5-ton stone blocks every day for 23 years. Who needs any other evidence of the perimeterization of these societies – such ridiculous, ludicrous waste of resources says loud and clear that the left-brain guys were firmly in control.

Such societies are called 'patriarchies,' which technically means 'rule by the fathers.' However, that term vastly inflates the dignity of the people doing such silly things, and is also ethologically inaccurate. To me, 'father' means a big, gentle, loving, middle-brain male who always defers to the guidance of the women of the house. I would substitute the word 'juvenarchy' in place of patriarchy, to emphasize that in ethological terms, the rulers of these new societies are *juvenile males*. Sometimes reading about what they've done and go on doing, I give up and call it 'idiarchy' – just plain idiotic. If they had not been so damned efficient at torture, misery, and mayhem, their pitiful pratfalls while attempting to run human society would be pure vaudeville.

Pyramids are an interesting detail, by the way. The form has been traced to the volcano-god religions of cold-adapted peoples from the Asian steppes – volcano fields, some active even today, are found all around the Caspian Sea, and a line of volcanoes extends east along the southern border of the steppes as far as the Pacific. The uses that pyramids were often put to (ritual murder, royal burial, etc.) clearly align with the associations of volcanoes with death and destruction. As mentioned before, pyramidal forms, from smaller mounds to structures hundreds of feet high were built around the world during a short period of time – used for tombs in Egypt and Mesopotamia, and sites for factory-farm-like killings of captive humans in the Americas. Of course, their phallic nature reminds us they are also a wonderful icon for the Perimeter societies which built them, combining an idiotic waste of resources with immense cost of human life, in the service of just another form of male display. (Perhaps even the two-foot-high conical hats worn by the short, stocky Kurgans to make them look taller were little volcano symbols – the platform shoes of their time.) And dominator cultures from the steppes that eventually moved into Polynesia did not need to build pyramids for ritual killings – they found real volcanos there, and so naturally, threw people in, as part of ceremonies validating their right to rule.

Unbelievably, in spite of all this, archeology texts commonly praise pyramids as signs of advanced civilization, products of 'great states.' The same texts often express the idea that the pyramid form was developed independently in different parts of the world, an expression of 'convergent evolution.' Such a theory regarding human cultural artifacts is suspect, because it seems to ignore the tremendous extent of human migration (the invasions) immediately preceding these troubled times, and also fails to credit the robustness of cultural memory, where the idea of a thing can be retained intact for many years, even if it is not expressed during every generation. Thus the Indo-Europeans who left behind the volcano fields of the Caspian Sea, eventually erected fake volcanos (pyramids) when they had the resources, both in Egypt and Mesopotamia. Similar phallic buildings (though not geometrically pyramids, per se) were built by invaders in India, Southeast Asia, and China.

As for the pyramids of Central and South America, it is not at all unreasonable to suppose that the perimeterized Clovis people, recently arrived in the Americas from the volcanic steppes, could have brought the idea of monumental 'volcano-gods' with them, and erected symbols of them once conditions allowed – that is, as soon as they could gain control over peaceful farming peoples already in place, seize their resources, and force them into the literally murderous work of building fake fire-mountains, lifting the Perimeter-male rulers and priests, like their earth-spurning gods, toward the sky.

Chapter Five Summary: What does it mean?

Pyramids are a good place to end this chapter. The Ice People and their successors still run things around the globe; they claim they are the Owners, that they can use the whole world – animal, vegetable, mineral – for their profit, that they also own us as a species. They are the boss, we are the workers; they are the team, we are the equipment.

We all know the drill. We are repeatedly taught, from elementary school through college, the gory, monotonous, embarrassing details of the 'history' of the last 10,000 years. History as presented in schools is *post-invader political history*, the fireside stories of competition between one group of Perimeter males and another. Unfortunately, most of the people who get caught in the middle, and end up miserable, enslaved, or dead, are the members of the old Center – the polytropic women, the middle-brain men, and children, children, children.

We are only taught *Perimeter history*: males displaying in various ways to other males, the pissing contests of kings and governments, armies and navies. This story conveniently ignores 99% of human life, focusing only on the few Perimeter males at the top of the heap, like paying attention to a wannabe-alpha chimp male banging two kerosene cans together and monopolizing the bananas (story told by Jane Goodall in her book of the unwittingly prescient title, *In the Shadow of Man*).

Such 'histories' rarely even mention the millennia of matristic management of human life. Thousands of generations of human societies are left a blank. Girls and women are not told about Catal Huyuk (except maybe to be embarrassed if they get a guilty glimpse of those 'fertility-cult' artifacts). Schoolchildren are not told that women invented virtually everything we depend on today (other than weapons) as the basis of 'modern human culture.' Tens of thousands of years when humans lived peacefully within the groups that these women fashioned don't make it into descriptions of what came eons before the 'glory that was Greece,' etc. The matristic era of human history, long by any measure – twenty or more times longer than the miniscule amount of the time since the Greeks and Romans – is summarily dismissed as unimportant, primitive 'pre-history.'

Nor do these histories mention the fact that the natural color of human skin is the color of living earth – brown to black. The perimeters are fond of cursing, and they've found lots of negative words to damn people whose skin actually has color (instead of the melanin-challenged state they are for some reason so proud of). Even the new politically-correct phrase they've invented, "people of color," implies that the de-pigmented skin of the invaders from the north is the norm. And vanishingly few schoolchildren, whatever their color, are told that it was when we were all brown that human society began, and flourished for millennia – matristic, peaceful, inclusive of all. *Remember: when we were all brown, we were all human, because we were all Center*.

But of course history is written by the winners, in this case the Perimeter males (who confusingly enough, can themselves come in all colors). The Big Lie of conventional history is that the de-pigmented people from the north invented 'civilization.' In fact, they did no such thing – rather, they destroyed the peaceful, matristic civilization of our forebears. The 'ancient history' they claim for themselves, the time of the first attacks on the truly ancient cultures, is like yesterday in the human span of time, not old at all.

It is not surprising, then, to find that none of the societies that have been the invaders' legacy – the Greeks, Romans, Egyptian and Chinese dynasties, Brahmins, expansionist monarchies and totalitarian and colonialist states of every kind in every country on every continent of the world, with their death cults, showy tombs, war, and their body-hating, puritanical 'sterility-cult' religions – none of these defines 'civilization' at all. They are grandiose, self-congratulatory, wet dreams. They are predatory displays of cold-adapted, reduced-brain juvenile males who would not know a civilized human society if they bumped into it in the night.

We are sometimes told these perimeterized societies are 'successful,' simply because they are 'still here' and they have grown so big. But as we've said, their reign has not been all that long, compared to the millennia of peaceful AMH life that went before. And they are not successful at all – from the first, they have embodied overgrowth, overkill, and overproduction. For the last 10,000 years we've been slowly drowning in artifacts, population, and new and horrible ways to make war. Big is not necessarily better. More and more may be worse and worse.

As all other animals on the planet have always known, as the matristic human societies through their peaceful millennia knew, 'enough' and 'sufficient' are nature's real watchwords, the criteria biology uses to decide who wins and who loses. The bad news is that the Perimeter males don't know the meaning of 'enough' (they don't seem to have any concept of negative feedback at all – later we'll discuss the biological origin of this seemingly maladaptive trait), and these last 10,000 years in which they've been able to starve the rest of us to feed their greed and personal selfishness may have already eaten up the only chance we have to survive.

The good news is, Perimeters are not the only ones here. They don't have all the votes. I sincerely believe that the only reason humanity is still around is simply this: *the vast majority of human beings are, as they always have been, the People of the Center, polytropics and middle-brains,* the women and men who are still best fitted for the life we've lived infinitely longer than this poor substitute called 'modern civilization.' What the Perimeters have created is literally a death cult (look at prisons, look at wars, look at religions), a poor trade for the life-affirming structure and values of the matristic, peaceful Center, where everyone is supported and everyone has a place at the table.

At the heart of Neural Rainbow Theory, however, is this notion: we mustn't be surprised that modern-day Perimeters are destructive and stupid. It is in the neurobiological nature of Perimeters to attack the Center – they are the human versions of the exiled, asocial juvenile-male lions killing and eating lion cubs.

But we don't have to put up with it. Like whales and rabbits and elk, humans are still made by the old rules. Biology goes on generating the full rainbow, so there's still more of us than there are of them. We can make the same decision that many matristic societies have made before us – *to simply stop creating the asocial Perimeters.* They are a waste of a pregnancy, a continuing threat to everybody, *made by biology only to be thrown away.* We can ourselves stop this kind of human waste.

If this sounds radical and even vaguely 'eugenic,' we need to remember the 'lost' acorns, that asocial brains are an epigenetic side-effect, destined for the non-reproductive Perimeter, non-contributors to the future. But if there is no place they can go, where their psychological nature does not threaten the generative power of the Center, something else must be done. If there is no 'away,' the next best thing is to gift every human child with the highest quality of life possible, and not force anyone to be Perimeters at all.

In Volumes Two and Three of this book I will examine exactly where we are today, see what we have left after the debacle of the last 10,000 years, and try more fully to assess the balance between the bad news and the good news. We've seen who we are, biologically and neurobiologically, where we came from, and what happened very recently (in archeological time) to spin things off on a tangent. How far have we gone off the main path for our species? Is it too late to get back on? Where is the Grandmother-Leader who can point the way – and will she be too pissed-off after all this time to show us how to be saved?

* * *

The last word in this chapter needs to be given to the *QRS rules* discussed earlier. QRS is the acronym that NRT uses to summarize biology's basic guidelines for reproduction *which must be followed* if any species is to survive and flourish – to reliably produce a *Quality* next generation at *Replacement* levels in a *Sustainable* way. As part of that discussion, we posed the question as to whether and how the rules apply to humans, and now that we know more about human history, the answer, as I said before, may be all too obvious.

First, as to 'whether:' *of course the rules apply to us* – just as they apply to all other organisms on Earth. But the more challenging issue here is the 'how' – and that's where our brief survey of the stages of human history can be enlightening, not only in terms of how but also why.

To understand this, we need to note that: 1) as a *global species* (that is, other than a few regional exceptions), Stage-3 humans (over the past 10,000 years and up through today) have been and are breaking not one, not two, but *all 3 QRS rules*; and 2) most of us have been persuaded this is perfectly OK, a view promulgated by the Owners who have taken us over (more about them in Volume Two), who repeatedly assure us not only that AMH is 'above the law' of biology, but also that our species is caught inescapably in an eternal crisis mode.

The Economy of Scarcity (EoS) that may have been the genuine start of The Change that put us on the Wrong Path (that is, the lack of year-round plant food in the far North where the cold worked its terrible changes on us), has been *artificially maintained* in multiple ways by the Owners (always to *their* advantage – *they* don't live in an EoS, they live in EoA, an Economy of Abundance – it is everyone else who has to suffer EoS). We are told that is 'the nature of things,' the 'human condition' – and they have even recently institutionalized the Eternal Crisis mode in things like the Eternal War on Terror, etc.

None of that is true – it is part of the Original Big Lie. The Earth is here to support us, we are among its children, and it *can* support us with an Economy of Abundance for all, as it does for all other species – *but only if we acknowledge the QRS rules and honor them*. But the Owners have also worked hard to make sure that we *cannot* do that, by striking at the very heart of any biological organism – from the beginning, *they have seized and weaponized reproduction,* and year by year, century by century, millennium by millennium, are employing all the perverted ways they have transformed it to run us into the ground (more about the 'weaponizing' techniques in later chapters).

I used to say that gender – in the largest sense, as defined and discussed in earlier chapters, ranging from brain types and social roles, to the social organization categories based on both – is the 'elephant in the room' for many professions concerned with understanding animal including human behavior. Gender in that sense is – I think, surprisingly and shockingly – often ignored, or set aside (and thus diminished and marginalized) as 'sexual behavior' or 'reproductive strategies' whenever authors turn to 'higher things,' in discussions of issues such as psychology, personality, violence, religion, philosophy, the arts, propensity for certain disorders – and certainly human history.

But since I've been thinking and writing about NRT, I've come to believe that *gender is not the elephant in the room, it **is** the room.* My essay *First Things* in the Volume Three Appendix explores that idea for all of biology – from single cells to nation-states – but for the moment, and particularly given the QRS rules and their significance for so much of human life (including the questionable possibility of a future for our species), *I also believe that biology 'agrees' that 'gender is the room.'* As will be explored in *First Things,* Persistence is one of four basic attributes of living things that distinguish them from non-living ones, and as such, anything that fosters or threatens persistence, of the individual or the species, is of critical interest to all organisms.

The chapters of the first part of this book have tried to make that case by outlining the many ways that individual differences such as brain types contribute to *species organization* as a device for establishing and maintaining persistence. Again, by interpreting 'gender' as anything and everything that contributes to persistence, we can recognize that the first thing we should seek to know about a species is its gender design and gender behavior. These are not special-case issues, peripheral matters, psychological curiosities, or social constructs, but *fundamental biological components of species infrastructure* that can make or break a species' campaign to survive.

Darwin said the greatest mystery was the origin of species (though by 'mystery' he clearly meant 'most interesting and significant thing to study'). I've suggested that an even more significant object for our curiosity and attention – the one on which our future as a species may depend – is how biology's arrangements for reproduction in the service of continuation are *designed to be accomplished for our species*. Because if we are standing in our own way about this – impeding our own persistence or even hastening our end by what we are doing – we clearly need to know more, and know it fast, before we find out we discovered the truth too late.

◈

Chapter Five Bibliography

Adams CJ (1991) The sexual politics of meat; A feminist-vegetarian critical theory. NY: The Continuum Pub Co.

Alexander, RD (1971) The search for an evolutionary philosophy of man. Royal Society of Victoria [Australia] Proceedings 84(1): 99-119.

Alexander, RD (1979) Darwinism and human affairs. Seattle: Univ. of Washington Press.

Alexander, Richard (1987) The biology of moral systems. NY: Aldine de Gruyter.

Allman WF (1995) The Stone Age present. NY: Simon & Schuster.

Ardrey R (1961) African genesis. NY: Dell.

Austen HI (1990) The heart of the goddess; Art, myth, and meditations of the world's sacred feminine. Berkeley: Wingbow Press.

Banner LW (1992) In full flower; Aging women, power, and sexuality. NY: Vintage Books.

Barash D (1979) The whisperings within; Evolution and the origin of human nature. NY: Penguin Books.

Barash D, NR Barash (2005) Madame Bovary's ovaries; A Darwinian look at literature. NY: Bantam Dell.

Baring A, J Cashford (1992) The myth of the Goddess: Evolution of an image. NY: Penguin Books.

Boulle P (1963) Planet of the apes. NY: Signet.

Boyd R, JB Silk (2006) How humans evolved; 4th edition. NY: W. W. Norton & Co.

Calvin WH (1991) The throwing Madonna; Essays on the brain, 2nd ed. NY: Bantam.

Cavalli-Sforza LL, P Menozzi, A Piazza (1996) The history and geography of human genes [Abridged paperback edition]. Princeton NJ: Princeton Univ. Press.

Cavalli-Sforza LL (2000) Genes, peoples, and languages. NY: North Point Press.

Clayton PA, MJ Price (Eds) (1988) The seven wonders of the ancient world. NY: Barnes & Noble Books.

Crosby AW (1972) The Columbian exchange; Biological and cultural consequences of 1492. Westport CT: Greenwood Press.

Diamond J (1992) The third chimpanzee; The evolution and future of the human animal. NY: HarperPerennial.

Diamond J (1997) Guns, germs, and steel; the fates of human societies. NY: WW Norton & Co.

Donahue P (1985) The human animal; Who are we? Why do we behave the way we do? Can we change? NY: Simon & Schuster.

Eisler RT (1987) The chalice and the blade; our history, our future. San Francisco: Harper & Row.

Eisler RT (1995) Sacred pleasure; Sex, myth, and the politics of the body. HarperSanFrancisco.

Erndl KM (1993) Victory to the mother; The Hindu goddess of northwest India in myth, ritual, and symbol. Oxford: Oxford Univ. Press.

Fagan BM (1987) The great journey; The peopling of ancient America. London: Thames & Hudson.

Farb P (1968) Man's rise to civilization as shown by the Indians of North America from primeval time to the coming of the industrial state. NY: EP Dutton & Co.

Finnegan R (1970) Oral literature in Africa. Oxford Univ. Press.

Freud S (orig 1930; translation by J Strachey, 1961) Civilization and its discontents. NY: WW Norton & Co.

Friedan B (1963) The feminine mystique. NY: Dell Pub. Co.

Gadon E (1989) The once and future goddess. San Francisco: HarperOne.

Garn, SM (1961) Human races. Springfield IL: Charles C. Thomas.

Gimbutas M (1989) The language of the goddess: Sacred images and symbols of Old Europe. (Intro by Joseph Campbell) San Francisco: Harper & Row.

Gimbutas M (1997) The Kurgan Culture and the Indo-Europeanization of Europe: Selected articles from 1952 to 1993 (J Indo-European Studies Monograph, MR Dexter Ed). Washington DC: Institute for the Study of Man.

Giraldeau L-A, T Caraco (2000) Social foraging theory. Princeton NJ: Princeton Univ. Press.

Gleason J (1987) Oya; In praise of the goddess. Boston: Shambhala.

Goodall J (as J Van Lawick-Goodall) (1971) In the shadow of man. Boston: Houghton-Mifflin.

Goodison L, C Morris (Eds) (1998) Ancient goddesses; The myths and the evidence. Madison WI: Univ. of Wisconsin Press.

Goodrich NL (1989) Priestesses. NY: HarperPerennial.

Gottfried RS (1983) The Black Death; Natural and human disaster in medieval Europe. NY: The Free Press.

Grun B (1991) The timetables of history; A horizontal linkage of people and events, 3rd English ed. [based on W Stein's Kulturfahrplan, orig copyright 1946] NY:

Simon & Schuster.

Hay MJ, S Stichter (Eds) (1995) African women south of the Sahara, 2nd ed. NY: John Wiley & Sons.

Hooks B (1995) Killing rage; Ending racism. NY: Henry Holt & Co.

Horan JL (1996) The porcelain god; A social history of the toilet. Secaucus NJ: Carol Publishing Group.

Huizinga J (orig 1938) Homo ludens; A study of the play-element in culture. (2014 edition) Mansfield Centre CT: Martino Fine Books.

Hyde L (1998) Trickster makes this world: Mischief, myth, and art, 1st ed. NY: Farrar, Strauss, & Giroux.

Jackson K, J Stamp (2003) Building the great pyramid. Buffalo NY: Firefly Books.

Johnson B (1988) Lady of the beasts; Ancient images of the goddess and her sacred animals. HarperSanFrancisco.

Karlen A (1984) Napoleon's glands; And other ventures in biohistory. NY: Warner Books, Inc.

Keller SR, EO Wilson (Eds) (1993) The biophilia hypothesis. Washington DC: Island Press.

Kohn GC (Ed) (1995) Encyclopedia of plague and pestilence. NY: Facts on File Inc.

Kolbert E (2015) The sixth extinction; An unnatural history. London: Picador.

Krause A, B Puppe, J Langbein (2017) Coping style modifies general and affective autonomic reactions of domestic pigs in different behavioral contexts. Frontiers in Behavioral Neuroscience 11: art. 103 (13 pp). doi:10.3389/fnbeh.2017.00103.

Lauter JL (2012) SPINE: A new sociobiology for the 21st Century based on socio-psycho-immuno-neuro-endocrinology (SPINE), I. Prenatal hormones, six genders, and brain-based social roles. Plenary Lecture to 87th Research Conference of the SouthWest and Rocky Mountain (SWARM) division of the American Association for the Advancement of Science (AAAS), Tulsa OK. [Unpublished; excerpt in Appendix]

Le Guin UK (1985) Always coming home. NY: HarperCollins.

Lefkowitz MR, MB Fant (1982) Women's life in Greece and Rome. Baltimore: The Johns Hopkins Univ. Press.

Lerner G (1986) The creation of patriarchy. NY: Oxford Univ. Press.

Lewontin R (1982) Human diversity. NY: Scientific American Books, Inc.

Massey MC (1985) Feminine soul: The fate of an ideal. Boston: Beacon Press.

MacLean PD (1973) A triune concept of the brain and behavior. Toronto: Univ. of Toronto Press.

MacLean PD (1990) The triune brain in evolution; Role in paleocerebral functions. NY: Plenum Press.

MacLean PD (1996) The limbic system and evolution of mammalian family-related behavior. AAAS Annual Meeting and Science Innovation Exposition 162: A62.

McNeill WH (1976) Plagues and peoples. Garden City NY: Anchor Books.

Mead M (1949) Male and female. NY: William Morrow & Co.

Mendor BDS (2000) Inanna; Lady of Largest Heart; Poems of the Sumerian High Priestess, Enheduanna. Austin: Univ. of Texas Press.

Miles R (1988) The women's history of the world. NY: Harper & Row.

Molnar S (1975) Human variation; Races, types, and ethnic groups. Prentice-Hall.

Montagu A (1965) The human revolution. NY: Bantam Books.

Montagu A, E Darling (1967) The prevalence of nonsense. NY: Dell Pub Co.

Morain L, M Morain (1998) Humanism as the next step. Amherst NY: The Humanist Press.

Morgan E (1982) The aquatic ape; A theory of human evolution. NY: Stein & Day.

Morris D (1967) The illustrated naked ape; A zoologist's study of the human animal. NY: Crown Pubs. Inc.

Morris D (1967) The naked ape. NY: McGraw-Hill.

Morris D (1969) The human zoo. NY: McGraw-Hill.

Morris R, D Morris (1966) Men and apes. NY: McGraw-Hill.

Mutén, B (Ed) (1994) Return of the Great Goddess [images and poems] NY: Stewart, Tabori & Chang.

Newman JL (1995) The peopling of Africa; a geographic interpretation. New Haven: Yale Univ. Press.

Oldham L, I Camerlink, G Arnott, A Doeschl-Wilson, M Farish, SP Turner (2020) Winner–loser effects overrule aggressiveness during the early stages of contests between pigs. Nature.com/scientific reports 10: 13338.

Olson C (Ed) (1990) The book of the goddess; Past and present. NY: Crossroad.

Partridge CG, MD McManes, R Knapp, BD Neff (2016) Brain transcriptional profiles of male alternative reproductive tactics and females in bluegill sunfish. PLoSONE 11(12): e0167509. (21 pp) doi: 10.1371/journal.pone.0167509.

Peters D (1991) From the beginning; The story of human evolution. NY: Morrow Junior Books.

Previté-Orton CW (1952 1st ed) The shorter Cambridge medieval history, Vol. 1, The later Roman Empire to the twelfth century, Vol. 2, The twelfth century to the Renaissance. Cambridge: Cambridge Univ. Press.

Quinn D (1994) Providence; The story of a fifty-year vision quest. NY: Bantam.

Quinn D (1995) Ishmael. NY: Bantam.

Richardson HW (1971) Nun, witch, playmate; The Americanization of sex. Lewiston NY: Edwin Mellen Press.

Rifkin RF, L Dayet, A Queffelec, B Summers, M Lategan, F d'Errico (2015) Evaluating the photoprotective effects of ochre on human skin by in vivo SPF assessment: Implications for human evolution, adaptation and dispersal. PLOS (open access) https://doi.org/10.1371/journal.pone.0136090.

Rothkrug P & RL Olson (1991) Mending the earth; A world for our grandchildren. Berkeley CA: North Atlantic Books.

Sagan C (1977) The dragons of Eden; Speculations on the origin of human intelligence. NY: Ballantine Books.

Sagan C, A Druyan (1992) Shadows of forgotten ancestors; A search for who we are. NY: Ballantine Books.

Sahlins M (1972) Stone Age economics. NY: Aldine de Gruyter.

Sahlins M (1976) The use and abuse of biology; An anthropological critique of sociobiology. Ann Arbor: Univ. of Michigan Press.

Sale K (1990) The conquest of Paradise; Christopher Columbus and the Columbian Legacy. NY: Penguin Books.

Schmookler AB (1984) The parable of the tribes; The problem of power in social evolution. Berkeley CA: Univ. of California Press.

Shepsut A (1993) Journey of the priestess; The priestess traditions of the ancient world. London: The Aquarian Press.

Sherman PW, JUM Jarvis, RD Alexander (1991) The biology of the naked mole rat. Princeton NJ: Princeton Univ. Press.

Sjoo M & B Mor (1987) The great cosmic mother; Rediscovering the religion of the earth, 2nd ed. San Francisco: HarperOne.

Stanford CB (1999) The hunting apes; Meat eating and the origins of human behavior. Princeton NJ: Princeton Univ. Press.

Stephenson J (1993) Women's roots; Status and achievements in Western Civilization, 4th ed. Ventura CA: Diemer, Smith Pub. Co.

Stolley PD, T Lasky (1995) Investigating disease patterns; the science of epidemiology. NY: Scientific American Library.

Stone M (1976) When god was a woman. San Diego: Harcourt Brace & Co.

Stone M (1990) Ancient mirrors of womanhood; A treasure of goddess and heroine lore from around the world, 2nd ed. Boston: Beacon Press.

Streep P (1994) Sanctuaries of the goddess; The sacred landscapes and objects. Boston: Little, Brown, & Co.

Stringer C, R McKie (1996) African exodus; the origins of modern humanity. NY: Henry Holt & Co.

Tannahill R (1992) Sex in history, 2nd ed. Scarborough House Pubs.

Tannahill R (1996) Flesh & blood; A history of the cannibal complex, 2nd ed. NY: Little, Brown & Co.

Tanner NM (1981) On becoming human; A model of the evolution from ape to human and the reconstruction of early human life. Cambridge: Cambridge Univ. Press.

Trager J (Ed) (1979) The people's chronology; A year-by-year record of human events from prehistory to the present. NY: Holt, Rinehart & Winston,

Tudge C (1996) The time before history; 5 million years of human impact. NY: Scribner.

Veblen T (1899 1st ed, Macmillan;1994 Dover Pubs) The theory of the leisure class.

Ward MC (1996) A world full of women. Boston: Allyn & Bacon.

Weisman A (2007) The world without us. NY: Thomas Dunne Books.

White E, D Brown (1973) The first men; The emergence of man [Time-Life Books]. Waltham MA: Little, Brown & Co.

Wilson EO (1975, 1st edition; 2000, 25th memorial edition) Sociobiology. Cambridge MA: Harvard Univ. Press.

Wilson EO (1998) Consilience; the unity of knowledge. NY: Random House.

Wilson EO (2002) The future of life. NY: Random House.

Wilson PJ (1983) Man the promising primate; The conditions of human evolution, 2nd ed. New Haven CT: Yale Univ. Press.

Wilson PJ (1988) The domestication of the human species. New Haven: Yale Univ. Press.

Wolkstein D, SN Kramer (1983) Inanna; Queen of heaven and earth – her stories and hymns from Sumer. NY: Harper & Row.

Wright R (1994) The moral animal; Why we are the way we are – The new science of evolutionary psychology. NY: Vintage Books.

Yalom M (1997) A history of the breast. NY: A.A. Knopf.

Zinsser H (1934 1st ed; 2007 9th ed) Rats, lice, and history; a history of pestilence and plagues. Boston: Little, Brown.

* * *

Chapter Five Figures & Tables

** PREVIEW **

Neural Rainbow

VOLUME TWO
The Rainbow Distorted

Chapter Six
"Why didn't we know? Newspeak & the big coverup"

(excerpt = first six pages)

⤜ Chapter Six ⤛

WHY DIDN'T WE KNOW?
NEWSPEAK & THE BIG COVERUP

(excerpt limited to the first six pages)

At the end of Chapter Five, we asked if there is a Grandmother (the experienced, polytropic, wise woman counsellor of mammalian groups) who can tell us what to think about our situation today, what we are like as a species here and now, 10,000 years after the invasions began. We want to ask her for the answer to the puzzle that has challenged and confounded so many philosophers, scientists, and everyday people – what *is* human nature after all, and how can we understand this awful thing that's been called the "human condition?"

I would like to find her (we might call her Neural Rainbow Woman) sitting under a shade tree in the afternoon, watching the moving clouds and grass, surrounded by the members of the group with whom she has spent her life, adults of different ages dozing, talking, or laughing quietly, children playing or taking naps. She might start by admitting the last 10,000 years have indeed been hard, and that over these last few millennia, human history certainly hasn't looked very mammalian. In many ways, as we indicated at the end of Chapter Five, it seems like our species as a whole has reverted from being mammals to something more like invasive small-brained reptiles or sharks in a feeding frenzy – wreaking havoc and mayhem on everything in sight, especially on ourselves and our children.

But then Neural Rainbow Woman would quickly go on to reassure us that in the only ways that count, we are as we have always been. We are still mammals, still highly social, we still have that gyroscope in our neurobiology which prepares us for life in a peaceful Center/Perimeter society, like virtually all other mammals. And remember, she would add, all the invasions – the ones that occurred around the world starting around 10,000 years ago and the many others since then – still have not achieved complete perimeterization of human society. Every human culture we know about, whether present or past, reveals to us – in the details of its political and economic structure, the nature of its artifacts, and even aspects of its daily life – the 'footprints' of its *history,* that is, how much or how little it has been shifted away from the Center values of the human mainstream by the perimeterizing influence of the invaders and their successors. In this, Neural Rainbow Woman might agree with Richard Lewontin who notes that "nothing in human evolution makes sense except in the light of history" [revising Theodosius Dobzhansky's 1973 original, "nothing in biology makes sense except in the light of evolution"] – though as we'll see, our conclusions will be different from Lewontin's.

Introduction: Three classes of human societies

Chapter Five described the stages of human evolution in terms of the same five social-organization categories (SOCs) used by all animals, and predicted not only that Anatomically Modern Humans (AMH) began, like almost all mammals, using a Center/Perimeter (C/P) lifestyle, but also that later events transformed our C/P first into peaceful 50:50 groups, and then into violent, hierarchically-organized forms of 50:50 that have been unlike C/P in almost every way.

The events leading to the last stage, referred to as Stage Three of human history in that chapter, were summarized as the 'descent of the Ice People,' consisting of a series of invasions by northern-AMH groups who had been radically changed both biologically and culturally by millennia of life in the far North, returning south and disrupting the peaceful lifestyle of warm-region AMH groups, a series of events which changed the warm-adapted groups almost beyond recognition.

Because of the deep changes in human society which resulted from these invasions, they serve as a handy landmark defining another classification of human groups, based on the *amount of change* the invasions brought about in the originally peaceful AMH 50:50 groups, as seen from society to society. All human cultures since that time, including those present today, no matter their apparent variety, can be classified into three basic classes around the 'hinge' of the invasions:

1) *Mainstream human cultures*. These are the societies which, either because they remained physically out of reach of the invasions, or if contacted, did not succumb to their influence, remained essentially the same as all warm-adapted AMH had been living for millennia, before the time when other groups moved north onto the steppes. NRT refers to these 'unchanged ones' as the "Old People," the "Sun People," who stayed in warm regions compatible with our biology, and were not substantially affected by the invasions. *Because these societies form an unbroken connection with our pre-invasion past, NRT defines them as 'mainstream cultures,' the enduring legacy of the peaceful 50:50 human life described as Stage Two in Chapter Five.* They live according to the Center values that sustained our C/P and peaceful 50:50 ancestors: female-managed, cooperation rather than competition, equable distribution of resources, and an emphasis on biologically-informed nurturing behaviors supporting individuals as

members of a community dedicated to fostering the persistence of the group.

2) *Pure-Perimeter human cultures.* These are societies which are essentially copies of the cultures of the invaders; thus they are the "New People," the "Ice People," whose brain-type distributions and culture were radically changed by millennia spent in a harsh, cold environment, which led them to adopt the Perimeter values discussed earlier: males over females, competition not cooperation, unequal distribution of resources, and violence of all kinds, targeting human women and children as well as other animals. Although these cultures may contain individuals that would *not* be relegated to the C/P perimeter (polytropics and middle-brains), they are called 'pure' because in these groups, supreme power is held by and flows from those who *are* themselves 'pure' Perimeter types – left-brain, Focal-Asocials, who rule these cultures with an iron hand, through intimidation, domination, and violence.

3) *Perimeterized human cultures.* These are hybrid blends of the first two. This class is represented by a great variety of cultures which have been 'perimeterized' to different extents as a result of these last ten millennia of continuing invasions – whether physical or cultural. Their features can be confusing to analyze because they represent a 'palimpsest,' a set of superimposed layers (like geologic strata) of influences which have waxed and waned over the years – some more Center, some more Perimeter, creating a hodge-podge mix of Center *and* Perimeter values which can be found side-by-side even in institutionalized religions (which typically do not distinguish between the two sets of values, another source of confusion for their followers). Most current human cultures are in this third category, and their many internal contradictions have given rise to the widespread personal and professional despair regarding the degraded 'human condition,' which unfortunately for many has become accepted as the hallmark of our species.

Thus this classification system is based not only on human history as described in previous chapters, but more fundamentally, as we have seen, on patterns of human neurobiology, and its sensitivity to environmental conditions experienced over tens of thousands of years. In fact, any human society (or any human group, for that matter – even 20 people at a time or fewer) can be identified as one of these three classes by using a relatively simple rubric NRT refers to as the "Center/Perimeter (C/P) touchstone."

The C/P touchstone involves evaluating the precepts and practices of a group according to how they reflect the two sets of values we've talked about before – either those of the mammalian Center (woman-based wisdom for conceiving and bringing up children, a 'partnership' model of social structure, equitable distribution of resources, fairness and support to all members, recognition of the primacy of women as sources of advice and counsel, etc.), vs. the values of the mammalian Perimeter ('lone wolf' independence, rigidly stratified hierarchies, unequal distribution of resources based on violence and competition, a 'dominator' model of social structure, glorification of violence, denigration of features associated with women and children, etc.).

Later in this book we will describe the C/P touchstone in the form of a questionnaire, a checklist for analyzing the expression of C/P values as reflected in almost every facet of everyday life. However, for the moment we will limit ourselves to a brief illustration using the C/P touchstone to classify a few sample societies.

For instance, the touchstone would classify the Pueblo peoples of the American Southwest as a 'Mainstream' human society. Groups such as the Zuni and Hopi are strongly Center-valued – they have long been recognized as egalitarian, with fair practices designed to encourage contribution from all members according to individual abilities, and also to ensure equal distribution of resources. There is a clear recognition of the primacy of women as wise counsellors, while males are provided with ways to contribute that make use of middle-brain characteristics such as physical strength, good social skills, artistic ability, and dancing.

As suggested above, there are others besides the Pueblo who were not radically changed by invaders. Such people either evaded the intruders by staying out of their way or 'under their radar,' or were internally strong enough to resist influences felt from afar. In different places around the world, these groups continue to live as they always have, in the old modified-Center way – that is, in peaceful 50:50 groups, without any of the stress indicators we've identified as danger signs for animal societies (such as violence toward group members or neighbors, immune-system problems, or overpopulation).

In all of these groups representing the human Mainstream, NRT predicts that very few if any left-brain types will be found – based on the neuro-socioethologic reasoning outlined in earlier chapters, polytropics and middle-brains should be the rule. This is the same pattern, carefully adjusted by psychological and cultural management, that, as mentioned earlier, human beings established for themselves around 100,000 years ago and have maintained through the vast majority of human history.

In marked contrast, societies of the second type, Pure-Perimeter, are founded on and devoted to Perimeter values, thus marking them as direct inheritors of the invaders. One vivid example of this type of society is one that became all too well-known during the early 21st century, the Taliban regime of Afghanistan. Afghanistan under the Taliban was an excellent expression of a pure invader society: rigidly hierarchical and stratified, with left-brain males on top, rigidly controlling middle-brain males and polytropic females even to the most private aspects of their lives by means of extreme violence. Interestingly enough, Afghanistan provided such a regime with a congenial and historically appropriate home – a steppes-like environment that was, in fact, one of the areas from which the original invaders attacked the Mediterranean Goddess cultures in the 5th millennium BCE (Before Common Era).

In such Pure-Perimeter types of society, NRT predicts that all three brain-types are present (though perhaps not in equal numbers), and this observation leads us to emphasize again a very important point – that even in "pure Perimeter" invader cultures, *not all individuals are left-brain types*. As we've said, the root problem in these societies, the thing that generates extreme violence and the resulting chronic misery of most of their citizens, is not that *everyone* is a left-brain (and perhaps hurt during childhood), but rather that any left-brains are made at all. And in these repressive cultures, the left-brains may make up more than 1/3 of the population. Given the neurobiological nature of left-brains, originally destined for the socially-primitive life of the mammalian Perimeter, such a substantial ratio of the population may function as a critical mass, leading naturally to stratified hierarchies dominated by a few 'top dogs' who rule through psychological, economic, and physical forms of terror.

Obviously, most human societies today fall into the third or hybrid category – 'Perimeterized.' These take a great variety of forms, ranging from small groups in the jungles of New Guinea (such as the Sepik River cultures studied by Margaret Mead and others) to the giant, anthill-like accumulations of people in industrialized countries such as the United States. But just as is true for individual differences, the variety of these hybrid societies becomes comprehensible if they are seen as different mixes of a few basic elements, in this case, the mix of Center vs. Perimeter values. The degree of mixture might even be quantified – 90% Center/10% Perimeter, 30% Center/70% Perimeter, etc. This approach might be helpful to anthropologists for identifying strands of similarities underlying the surface differences between groups. [The checklist we'll review later could be used to make such a classification, and it could obviously be expanded and eventually calibrated against emerging information about human migrations and mutual influences, as reflected in things such as linguistic history and genetic analysis, as mentioned in Chapter Five.]

* * *

Neural Rainbow Woman would probably point out that we are not to blame for somehow 'forgetting' about the invasions, and the terrible changes they brought to human life. She would tell us that *the truth of our human history has been obscured purposefully through an active process of cover-up*, the Big Lie about human nature and human history. It was begun by the invaders almost immediately after they arrived, and goes on being promulgated even (and perhaps especially) today.

In this chapter and the next one, we'll review how that Lie was framed from the beginning, how it was engineered, and why it has made almost all humans, scientists as well as lay people, 'forget' who we really are, forget that human life was ever different than it is now, forget that there was ever any other definition of human life than the Perimeter. Building on Lewontin's comment, we might say that certainly "nothing in human evolution *can* make sense except in the light of history" – but one has to know the *whole* story, and as we'll see, the Perimeters have put impressive amounts of effort into 'painting-over' the view of *all* AMH history (most of it happening long before they took over), and replacing it with their own version – so we see the past only 'through a glass darkly' instead of in the full-spectrum sunlight of the truth.

(to continue reading, please see Volume Two)

APPENDIX

1. Volume One master list of figures & tables, by chapter

2. Expanded Table of Contents for all three volumes

3. Earlier treatments of Neural Rainbow Theory
(citations, with titles and abstracts/excerpts)

VOLUME ONE – Master list of figures & tables

Volume One
CONTENTS
(repeated from front of book)

The Origins of the Rainbow

❧

Earlier Treatments of Neural Rainbow Theory
(citations, with abstracts/excerpts)

Lauter JL (1996) The Brain of Isis. Presented to Southwest Women's Conference, University of Oklahoma, Norman OK.

Abstract & introduction
In Egyptian mythology, Isis was a figure representing the divinity and multipotentiality of women. She was credited with powers in art, science, writing, mathematics, childbearing and child rearing, and the wisdom to govern and judge. In sculptures and paintings, she was occasionally accompanied by Osiris, who was identified as her brother/lover/husband/son and often portrayed as about 1/4 her size, even as an adult man. In one version of their story, Osiris is captured by a demon, cut into pieces, and imprisoned in the trunk of a tree. Isis finds him, frees his fragmented body from the rigid trunk and reassembles the pieces, and brings him back to life.

As I sit down at my computer to write this, I am 50 years old. As a neuroscientist, I have studied the human brain and behavior for the last two decades of those 50 years. I've read literature and written poetry for more than 30 years, and I've been a student of human nature all my life. My everyday experiences observing people, and the lessons I've learned from art and science, lead me to believe that this old story of Isis bears an uncanny resemblance to the most modern conceptions of the biological bases of gender. I believe that a closer examination of this story in terms of a modern "translation" may give us some clues as to how the most fundamental aspects of human biology related to gender differences and the nervous system can account for the sometimes puzzling varieties of human behavior.

Thus I would like to tell the story of Isis in a new way, using vocabulary and concepts borrowed from several sciences, including ethology, embryology, psychology, and developmental neuroscience. As is true in most of modern science, these disciplines are typically pursued independently of each other, separated and isolated from each other much like the fragments of Osiris' body. I believe that if we bring them together, and draw on all their insights in a gestalt and synthesizing way, we will see that the story they tell can be comprehended as a coherent and re-integrated whole. The story that I will recount here may seem at first to represent a point of view on human behavior that is very new, but it is in fact – as the Isis story makes clear – very old, familiar and taken for granted by millions of human beings for tens of thousands of years.

So I am really offering old wine in new bottles, just as Dr. Benjamin Spock did in his first book on childrearing. He began that book by acknowledging that although what he was going to describe would seem revolutionary compared to the recommendations of contemporary pediatricians, in reality all he was going to recount for his readers was what women already knew, and had known since there were any women to know it: "You already know more than you think you do."

The story I am going to tell is exactly the same. We as humans *already know* the essence of it in our hearts and bodies and brains. I find that when I share this story with others, whether they are women or men, seniors or adolescents, high-schoolers

283

or PhDs, they all always smile – with recognition, self-knowledge, and, I think, relief, that what they have always known, even without knowing that they know, is in fact the truth, and can be backed up by the latest scientific facts. They tell me it is a relief to have it said, out in the open, finally brought back to light and life– like poor dismembered Osiris.

The scientific terms that give the story so much credibility for me as a scientist, and make me believe even more that it is true – are in actuality only a "local habitation and a name" as Shakespeare would say. The knowledge and the facts of the case connect our modern present with the distant past, reaching far beyond even the time when there were any creatures living on this planet recognizable as members of our own species.

* * *

Lauter JL (1999) The Center, the Perimeter, and the Neural Rainbow; The human brain and ways of being human – A neuroscientist suggests some new approaches to understanding individual differences, human types, social evolution, and the nature of good and evil. [Unpublished MS; limited circulation]

Excerpt
Part One
NEUROTYPOLOGY – THE "NEURAL RAINBOW"

Long before a human baby is born, its future self is being shaped by powerful forces working inside the womb. As with all mammals, the mother's body provides a safe haven, the original Garden of Eden, for the developing child, surrounding it with warmth and all the nutrients it needs to grow and become strong -- and many aspects of prenatal life involve the brain.

Right Brain & Left Brain. Researchers have long known that the brain does much more than think. It also controls the heart, shapes gender behavior, and governs the immune system. Thus learning more about the brain may help us understand why certain people are prone to heart attacks or breast cancer, and why children with reading problems are often left-handed.

Virtually all the patterns which create individual differences are laid down before birth, and the old idea that the baby is born as a "tabula rasa" (blank slate) is rapidly fading. The updated view is that an individual's biological outline is so complete before birth, that experience acts more like a proofreader than a writer, and the events of a life are the unfolding of a plot line pretty much established in the womb.

A person's brain "story" may depend on the right and left sides of the brain, and the way they grow before birth. Originally scientists described the left brain as "dominant" because it regulated thinking and speech. The right side was dismissed as primitive and limited, good only for controlling the muscles on the left side of the body. Later, researchers found that the right brain has its own areas of "dominance," such as perception of emotions and orientation in space. Thus the two sides came to be seen as having equal-and-opposite functions.

However, the latest evidence suggests that the two sides of the brain are related in a very different way, with the right side functioning as the greater set, the "mother" of the brain and body, overseeing everything from general health, to the coordination

284

of complex abilities related to right- vs. left-side skills. The right brain maintains connections not only between the two sides of the brain, but also between the brain and the rest of the body. It manages our sleep cycles, tells us what tastes good, supports the heart through the calming, "parasympathetic" part of the autonomic nervous system (the part that guarantees good digestion, a calm heart, and healthy sexual function), and keeps the immune system active and strong. The right brain also has many functions related to the larger world, and the "macro" functioning of the body and brain. For instance, it manages balance, provides the "big picture" of gestalt awareness, helps us tell whether people around us are happy or sad, gives us three-dimensional spatial awareness, and the ability to identify things seen or heard at a distance.

* * *

Lauter JL (2008) How is your brain like a zebra? A new human neurotypology. Bloomington IN: Xlibris. [Excerpt is from an addendum section titled "Bigger Pictures" based on a Q&A format, which was omitted from the 2008 edition, and is here published for the first time]

Excerpt
1. Do animals other than humans have brain types, too?
Short Answer: My best guess is yes, the three brain types are probably found in one form or another in all mammals, and maybe even in birds and fish. My own research has focused on humans, but work on other animals suggests that similar patterns exist in them. Studying brain types by looking exclusively at humans can only tell us so much – in fact, in order to figure out *why* humans have brain types at all, we have to look at other animals.

Gaining a larger perspective by looking at brain patterns in more than one species may reveal why there are three major categories, and why each should be represented in about one-third of the population, etc. Finally, the reason brain types exist at all becomes pretty obvious, once you start looking at other animals.

Long Answer: Social Organization in Mammals, Two Kinds of Males, Mammalian Social Roles
1) Social Organization in Mammals. Let's start with mammals. Remember the last nature film you saw on any kind of mammal – elephants, elk, wild horses. The most common social organization among mammals, *found in virtually all mammalian species,* involves two major social subdivisions. I call these the "center" and the "perimeter." In mammals that live this way (center/perimeter, or C/P), the *center* consists of the groups formed by the women and children of the species. Female membership in these multigenerational groups is very stable over time – ethologists report the groups consist of two or more "matrilines" of grandmothers, mothers, and daughters, who spend all their lives in the same community, composed of the same set of families in which their ancestors lived all their lives. These groups can justifiably be considered the "center" of the species, for it is here where the children – the guarantors of the species' future – are conceived, born, and raised.

In many ways, the center groups depend on the wisdom of their older members, the grandmothers. The grandmothers lead the group, model group behavior, and provide the group's memory, reminding them where the best food is and where water can be found, even in the driest years. Bonding in center groups is complex and strong, so that for mammals, a center group is almost a "colonial organism," like the microscopic creatures known as Volvox, where each unit functions less like an individual than a supporting and supported part of the whole.

The second social subdivision is the "perimeter." This is where most of the males live – on the non-reproductive margin of the species. It is critical to understand that with non-human mammals, the perimeter is literally just that – *a geographical area outside the center*. It occupies the space in between center groups, a kind of no-man's land – though actually it is a no-woman's land, since only males live there. When boys in the center groups reach puberty, the perimeter is where they go, and the perimeter is where they then spend most if not all their lives – in a perpetual exile, away from the centers, wandering in small, unstable bands or living as solitaries. Ethologists refer to most of these males as "juvenile males" no matter their age, because for most of them, their social identity is fixed at puberty. Relationships in the perimeter are fleeting and short-lived; life there is more about competition, risk-taking, and violence than cooperation and mutual, lifelong support.

* * *

Lauter JL (2011a) A new natural-selection approach to social organization in humans and other animals, based on the neurological effects of sex hormones. Part I: Propositions One and Two, linking economics, social-organization categories (SOCs), and social roles. Prepared for 86th Research Conference of the SouthWest and Rocky Mountain (SWARM) regional division of the American Association for the Advancement of Science (AAAS), Wichita KS. [Unpublished]

Abstract

This and the companion paper overview three propositions of a new natural-selection approach to the connection between social organization and neurological function, which in general posits that *the organizational effects of sex hormones serve as a major biological technology for shaping individuals to function in the social organization of their species*. Proposition One begins with the concept, generally accepted among ethologists, that **the economics of a species (food sources, need for shelter, predator presence, etc.) represent a niche for which social organization is an adaptation.** One example of this is the distribution of adults. For instance, if each adult requires a fairly large territory to survive, members of a species live as solitaries; a slightly more congenial habitat allows adults to live in pairs; and more abundant resources are associated with a variety of "center-perimeter" (for term cf. Lauter, 2005, 2008) arrangements. Proposition One of the new approach additionally suggests that the apparent heterogeneity of styles of social organization observed in different types of animals can all be interpreted as variations on a few basic themes, or social-organization categories (SOCs). Proposition Two posits that, just as the economics of a species is a niche for which SOCs are an adaptation, **SOCs in turn are a niche for** which social roles are an adaptation. Specifically, each SOC is seen as depending on a *combination of one or more social roles,* selected from a relatively small set of roles defined in terms of *behavioral feature sets* (not just a bimodal distinction based on gender) that together provide the necessary support for that SOC.

* * *

Lauter JL (2011b) A new natural-selection approach to social organization in humans and other animals, based on the neurological effects of sex hormones. Part II: Proposition Three, connecting social roles to hormone-mediated brain types. Prepared for 86th Research Conference of the SouthWest and Rocky Mountain (SWARM) regional division of the American Association for the Advancement of Science (AAAS), Wichita KS. [Unpublished]

Abstract
Following up on the previous paper's review of Propositions One and Two, this presentation outlines <u>Proposition Three</u> of this new approach, which hypothesizes that just as SOCs are a niche for which social roles are an adaptation (Prop. 2), **social roles in turn are a niche for which brain types are an adaptation.** More specifically, the idea is that a continuum of *brain-shaping by sex hormones* is employed by biology, in humans and other animals, to fit each individual to fulfill one of the social roles on which the social organization of its species depends. This component of the new theory draws on the Trimodal Model of Brain Organization (Lauter 1998, 1999, 2001. 2003, 2004, 2007, 2008), which describes a neurotypology of individuals produced via a continuum of prenatal, perinatal, and postnatal exposure to sex hormones. Under the Trimodal Model, the result is *three principal brain types,* each of which is characterized by a *coordinated profile of features* (e.g., sidedness, sensorimotor skills, personality – including different degrees of social capability such as "emotional intelligence," and general mental and physical health). Previous discussions of the Trimodal Model have focused on implications for human individual differences in academic skills, athleticism, and propensity for disorders ranging from autism and hyperactivity to chronic pain and Alzheimer's Disease. Proposition Three goes well beyond educational and clinical implications in humans to invoke a larger biological importance for the three brain types – specifically, that each coordinated profile of features associated with each of the three principal brain types is predicted to match one of the social roles identified in Proposition Two. Thus SOCs can be distinguished not only by particular sets of social roles, but also by *different distributions of brain types.*

* * *

Lauter JL (2012) SPINE: A new sociobiology for the 21st Century based on socio-psycho-immuno-neuro-endocrinology (SPINE). Prenatal hormones, three brain types/six genders, brain-based social roles, and social organization categories. Plenary Lecture to 87th Research Conference of the SouthWest and Rocky

Mountain (SWARM) division of the American Association for the Advancement of Science (AAAS), Tulsa OK. [Unpublished]

Abstract
The Trimodal Model of Brain Organization is a meta-theory describing a new neurotypology of *systematic phenotypic variation*, based on the epigenetic effects of hormones working during brain development (Lauter 1997, 1998, 2001, 2004, 2008). To date, discussions of the Trimodal Model have focused on the psychological, medical, and educational impacts of these developmental processes in humans (e.g., ZebraBrain.net). However, the model also suggests that the same brain-shaping mechanisms provide a neurobiological basis for more general relations linking *individual neuropsychology* with the details of *social organization*, for all animal species that employ sexual reproduction, including humans. Under the rubric of SPINE (emphasizing its origins in Socio-Psycho-Immuno-Neuro-Endocrinology), this approach offers a new perspective that goes well beyond the limited concepts of 'selfish genes' and personal 'agendas' that characterize many studies in sociobiology, evolutionary psychology, etc. Specifically, the model posits a 'waterfall' series of niches and adaptations related to social life. That is, just as the economics of a species can be considered as a niche for which social organization is an adaptation, in turn social organization can be seen as a niche for which a certain set of social roles is an adaptation, and the social roles themselves can in turn be characterized as niches for which the 'brain types' described by the Trimodal Model are an adaptation. Such a neuroethological approach provides both: a) a new means of formulating the neurological basis of animal (including human) social interactions, considered at the 'whole-organism' level; and b) a set of universal patterns linking individual neurology with group function that may be *applicable across all animal species*. Perhaps of equal importance, the Trimodal Model's approach to social organization also highlights the difficulties that arise if individuals are not allowed to fulfill their 'wired-in' social roles, or are forced into roles for which they are not fitted. Either of these situations may prove extremely maladaptive not only for individual psychological and physical health, but also for the very existence of a species. Applications of these issues to human societies will be briefly discussed.

About the Author

Beginnings

Judith Lauter was born in Austin, Texas. When she was nine, her family moved to Michigan where she later met her husband, the poet Ken Lauter, in a poetry-writing seminar at the University of Michigan taught by Donald Hall (US Poet Laureate, 2006-7). The couple has subsequently lived in Arizona, Colorado, Missouri, Oklahoma, and now make their home in Nacogdoches TX.

Although Judith's early education reflected a mix of interest in science and humanities, especially literature, she focused on humanities due largely to a lack of encouragement from friends and family regarding a scientific career (uncommon for a female during the early post-WWII years). She enjoyed poetry and fiction, learning languages (three years of Spanish, one of Russian in high school), and began writing poetry (in both English and Spanish), published a few poems, and won a series of regional prizes for her poetry and short stories.

Her focus on the humanities persisted during her English-literature undergraduate work at the Univ. of Michigan Honors College, where she continued publishing, and won two Hopwood Writing Awards for poetry. At UM she also took two more years of Spanish, two years of Classical Greek, a series of Art History courses concentrating on Eastern Art (enough hours to earn an informal minor), and several courses in the natural sciences, including a year in geology which tempted her to switch majors (but again she was dissuaded by the gender gap – virtually all geology students and faculty were male).

In fall 1965, Judith and Ken (also an English major) met in Donald Hall's writing class, and the following spring they graduated together – he with an MA in English, she with a BA. He took a teaching job at the Univ. of Arizona, and in fall 1966 they moved to Tucson, married, and Judith enrolled in the UA Creative-Writing MA program (later to become an MFA). She went on writing and publishing poems, and began giving poetry readings, usually in tandem with Ken.

However, toward the end of the master's work, a series of five events occurred that opened new outlets for her long-repressed fascination with science: 1) in a graduate course in the History of English she was introduced to linguistics as the *science of language;* 2) she read a recently-published book (Licklider 1965) on the revolutionary promise of computers for automated information storage and retrieval that also mentioned the importance of new developments in *language sciences*; 3) she found an even newer book (Brown 1970) on the *psychology of language*, including language development in children; 4) she took a part-time job as secretary to the UA department chair of Speech and Hearing Sciences, where she began learning about the variety of sciences practiced in a field she had never heard of (she would spend her entire subsequent career teaching and doing research in such departments); and finally, 5) a third new book (Koestler 1968) on the evolution of the nervous system made her realize that *the brain* was a blank space on her intellectual map, with virtually untapped potential for explaining the vast variety of human behavior she had read about for years in literature.

After finishing the Creative Writing MA (her thesis a poetry collection entitled *Epithalamion*), she again encountered gender-based discouragement – this time about pursuing a PhD in English – and guided by those five recent events, she began looking for something different. Continuing her job in the S&H department, she enrolled in new kinds of courses – computer sciences, psychology, library science, and neuroanatomy and neurophysiology (taught by an MD/PhD researcher who studied the neural bases of motor control) in the new UA Medical School.

More details about all these developments are included in her autobiographical volumes (titles below). Everything that happened in Judith's intellectual future from then on came directly from the radical departures in educational focus she made during those years.

Later education and work history

Two years later, her computer and library-science classes at UA (emphasizing computer applications) led Judith to the Library & Information Science MA program at the University of Denver, which she completed in the summer of 1971 (a 2nd MA degree), graduating as a professional librarian with an emphasis on special (e.g., medical) libraries. Her thesis described a novel linguistic strategy for improving the accuracy of computer-based literature searches.

Ken was working on a PhD in English at DU, but with Judy's new MA, they decided to move to St. Louis where she had landed a job as a medical librarian at the Washington University School of Medicine Library (WUSML), which was doing its own pioneering work in computer applications. Ken got a scholarship for the Wash U English PhD program, along with a Schubert Playwriting Fellowship.

In addition to her full-time job at WUSML (now the Bernard Becker Library), Judith enrolled in the interdisciplinary Wash U Linguistics MA program, which developed into essentially a degree in speech and hearing sciences, since she took most of her courses at the prestigious Central Institute for the Deaf Research Center located on the Wash U Medical School campus. As she grew familiar with the cutting-edge clinical and research facilities at CID, she discovered with relief that there were no 'discouraging words' about her joining this new academic community – at CID, women formed the majority of students at all levels – and senior faculty soon recruited her into their PhD program. She completed her Linguistics MA thesis in 1974, a chronological linguistic analysis of improvements in speech-sound production by a young woman who had suffered a traumatic brain injury, followed over the first six months of recovery.

For the next five years Judith worked on a PhD in 'Communication Sciences,' a new name for the degree, created by CID to fit her basic-science interests (as compared to the standard clinical designations of Speech Pathology or Audiology). Her doctoral coursework included classes in psychology, psychophysics (including psychoacoustics), neurophysiology, embryology, clinical neurology, and communication sciences and disorders; and she worked in classrooms, clinics, and laboratories learning from teachers such as James D. Miller (speech perception – CID), Charles Watson (auditory psychophysics – CID), Randy Monsen (speech acoustics and intelligibility – CID), Rao Vemula (computer-based waveform analysis – WUSM Biomedical Computer Laboratory), Hallowell Davis (inner-ear anatomy, computer-based evoked potentials – CID and WUSM Otolaryngology), Stanley Finger (neural bases of animal behavior – WU Psychology), James Simmons (neurophysiology of animal communication – WU Psychology), Nobuo Suga (cortical neurology of echolocation – WU Biology), Thomas Woolsey (somatosensory neurophysiology – WUSM Anatomy and Neurobiology), W. Maxwell Cowan (developmental neurobiology – Chair of WUSM Anatomy and Neurobiology, later Chief Scientific Officer of the Howard Hughes Medical Institute), and Ira Hirsh (psychoacoustics – CID Director of Research, WU Psychology).

Judith's doctoral dissertation, directed by Ira Hirsh, took a novel psychoacoustic approach to dichotic listening, and described auditory asymmetries in terms of interactions between individual differences and physical dimensions of speech and nonspeech stimuli. Postdoctoral work at CID included research projects on the physiological correlates of individual differences in brain asymmetries studied at several levels of the nervous system, conducted in collaboration with other groups at WUSM, including measurements of evoked potentials with faculty in Otolaryngology, and research on regional cerebral blood flow conducted in the PETT-VI laboratory at the Mallinckrodt Institute of Radiology.

In 1985 she took a research appointment in affiliation with the Department of Speech and Hearing Sciences at the University of Arizona, where she supported her work through a six-year series of grants from the Air Force Office of Scientific Research. One grant involved collecting speech samples from English, Japanese, Spanish, Chinese, and Diné (Navajo) speakers.

During this time she gained additional hands-on experience with a variety of noninvasive methods for studying the human brain, ranging from more work with evoked potentials and PET, to research using quantitative electroencephalography (qEEG), magnetic resonance imaging (MRI), and magnetoencephalography (MEG), pursued in collaboration with researchers in the UA departments of Psychology, Education, and Speech and Hearing Sciences, the University of Arizona School of Medicine (Neurology), University of Wisconsin/Madison (Communication Sciences and Disorders), University of Tennessee Medical Center in Knoxville (Speech-Language Pathology, and the Brain & Spine Institute), and the Los Alamos National Laboratory (MEG laboratory).

In 1991 Judith joined the faculty of the University of Oklahoma Health Sciences Center (OUHSC). There she founded and served as Director of the Center for Communication Neuroscience (CCNS). Her work emphasized collaborative projects with a number of departments on both the medical and main campuses of OU, including Neurology, Psychiatry, Dentistry, Public Health, Pediatrics, Otolaryngology, and Psychology; the Oklahoma City Public Schools; the Veterans Administration OKC Health Care Center; and private clinical programs including NeuroNet and Lindamood-Bell Learning Processes. While at OUHSC, she served as Public Liaison for the Oklahoma Center for Neuroscience, for which she created and coordinated NeuroNights, a monthly series of community-outreach programs offering the public the opportunity to interact with neuroscientists and clinicians on a variety of topics regarding the human brain and its disorders (this series is still active after more than 20 years).

In 2001, she accepted an appointment to the faculty of the Department of Human Services at Stephen F. Austin State University in Nacogdoches Texas. There she established and served as Director for the Human Neuroscience Laboratory (HNL), for which she designed and equipped a 1200 sq-ft laboratory space in a new building. She collaborated with SFA programs in Communication Sciences and Disorders, Counseling, Visual Impairment, the School Psychology Doctoral Program, and the SFA School of Music. HNL research programs included: 1) developing new ways to use inexpensive noninvasive technologies to study human brain and behavior; 2) specifying individual differences in terms of 'neurological fingerprints' making it possible to compare and contrast individuals in new ways; 3) exploring the neural bases of many types of human characteristics, ranging from gender behavior and personality, to propensity for disorders such as autism, chronic pain, nicotine addiction, hyperactivity, dyslexia, and Alzheimer's Disease; and 4) further work on designing multi-assessment, multidimensional testing techniques for coordinated use of a variety of noninvasive tools for linking behavior, peripheral physiology, and central function, based on measurement methods such as speech and voice acoustics, dichotic listening, electromyography (EMG), electrocardiography (ECG), eye-movement tracking, otoacoustic emissions (OAEs), Repeated Evoked Potentials (REPs), magnetic resonance imaging (MRI), quantitative electroencephalography (qEEG), and positron emission tomography (PET).

Outcomes include a suite of new theoretical and methodological approaches for the study of functional brain organization in humans, including: the EPIC Model of Functional Asymmetries, the Handshaking Model of Brain Function, the Trimodal Model of Brain Organization, and the Auditory Cross-Section (AXS) Test Battery.

* * *

Dr. Lauter has produced more than 50 scientific publications (articles, chapters, books, educational videos) and presented more than 160 scholarly lectures to research conferences in the U.S. and internationally, describing her basic, applied, and theoretical research. Her popular-neuroscience book, *How is Your Brain Like a Zebra? A New Human Neurotypology* (2008, Xlibris; ZebraBrain.net) explores the epigenetic neuro-organizational effects of sex hormones, and their implications for a variety of issues in psychology, sociology, education, and clinical practice.

Her work has been published in journals representing communication sciences and disorders, education, psychology, learning disorders, and brain imaging, including: *Perceptual and Motor Skills, Brain and Cognition, Biological Psychiatry, Speech Communication, Ear and Hearing, Hearing Research, British Journal of Audiology, Current Opinion in Otorhinolaryngology and Head & Neck Surgery, Folia Phoniatrica et Logopedica, Scandinavian Audiology, Journal of the Acoustical Society of America, Journal of Developmental and Learning Disorders, Neuroimage, Behavioral Research Methods Instrumentation and Computers, Human Brain Mapping, Frontiers in Bioscience,* and *Annals of the New York Academy of Sciences.* An abbreviated *curriculum vitae* with details on work-history, scientific publications and presentations, and funded projects, is available on the Author Page at ZebraBrain.net. See also JudithLauter.com.

Current activities

Since retiring from her faculty position in 2012, Judith has published 11 books of poetry-and-images, many of them with samples of her digital art and nature photography, plus three volumes of a planned eight-volume autobiographical series. She has also shown and sold digital-art pieces and photographs at a number of regional art centers (reproductions are available at FineArtAmerica.com).

Ten of the poetry-and-images books were published by Xlibris: *Year of Haiku* (2013); *Light from the Left – Poems on paintings by Rembrandt* (2013); *Sonora Spring Haiku* (2013); *Pineywoods Summer Haiku* (2014); *Rockies Autumn Haiku* (2014); *Coastal Bend Winter Haiku* (2014); *LaNana Creek Haiku* (2014); *Lady Slipper Trail Haiku* (2016); *Konza Tallgrass Prairie Haiku* (2017); *The Long Hot Summer 2022* (2022). *The Poet in the Park – Wallace Stevens and Elizabeth Park*, another book of poetry and images, with a set of informative endnotes, was published by the SFASU Press in 2017.

Her autobiographical books (all with Xlibris) include: *Green is Certain – An autobiography with selected poems, Vol. I, 1944-1962*; *Green is Certain – An autobiography with selected poems, Vol. II, 1962-1966*; *Perturbations – An autobiography with selected poems, Tucson & Denver 1966-1971*. The first volume of the next title *Becquerel's Plate – An autobiography with selected poems and scientific works, Vol. I, St. Louis 1971-1985*, is currently in progress.

Born of water

caught in light and air, rainbows
remind us who we
are – and bring us back to Earth.

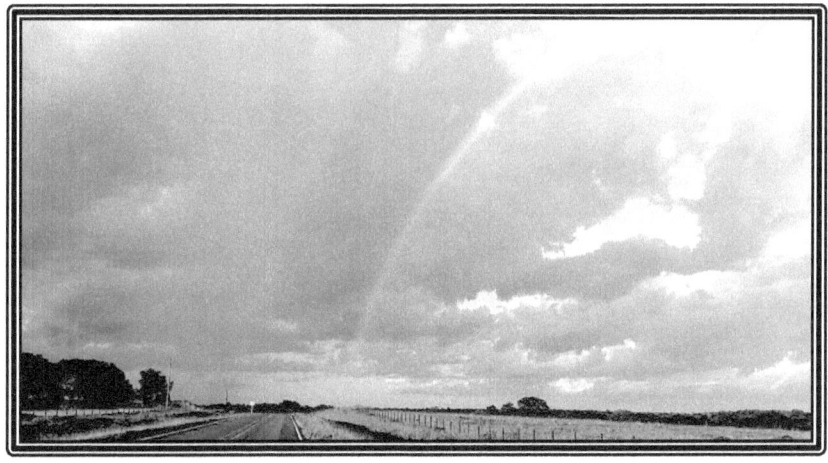

293

www.ingramcontent.com/pod-product-compliance
Lightning Source LLC
Chambersburg PA
CBHW021351210526
45463CB00001B/66